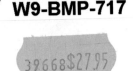

Fifth Edition

Appleton & Lange's Review of
PHARMACY

Fifth Edition

Appleton & Lange's Review of
PHARMACY

Gary D. Hall, MS
Professor of Pharmaceutics

Barry S. Reiss, PhD
Professor of Pharmaceutics

Albany College of Pharmacy
Union University
Albany, New York

APPLETON & LANGE
Norwalk, Connecticut

0-8385-0162-1

Notice: The author(s) and the publisher of this volume have taken care to make certain that the doses of drugs and schedules of treatment are correct and compatible with the standards generally accepted at the time of publication. Nevertheless, as new information becomes available, changes in treatment and in the use of drugs become necessary. The reader is advised to carefully consult the instruction and information material included in the package insert of each drug or therapeutic agent before administration. This advice is especially important when using new or infrequently used drugs. The publisher disclaims any liability, loss, injury, or damage incurred as a consequence, directly or indirectly, of the use and application of any of the contents of this volume.

Prentice Hall International (UK) Limited, *London*
Prentice Hall of Australia Pty. Limited, *Sydney*
Prentice Hall Canada, Inc., *Toronto*
Prentice Hall Hispanoamericana, S.A., *Mexico*
Prentice Hall of India Private Limited, *New Delhi*
Prentice Hall of Japan, Inc., *Tokyo*
Simon & Schuster Asia Pte. Ltd., *Singapore*
Editora Prentice Hall do Brasil Ltda., *Rio de Janeiro*
Prentice Hall, *Englewood Cliffs, New Jersey*

Library of Congress Cataloging-in-Publication Data

Hall, Gary D.
    Appleton & Lange's pharmacy review.—5th ed. / Gary D. Hall,
Barry S. Reiss.
        p. cm.
    Includes bibliographical references.
    ISBN 0–8385–0162–1
    1. Pharmacy—Examinations, questions, etc. I. Reiss, Barry S.,
1944–   . II. Title. III. Title: Appleton & Lange's pharmacy
review. IV. Title: Pharmacy review.
    [DNLM: 1. Pharmacy—examination questions. QV 18 H176a 1993]
RS97.H35 1993
615'.1'076—dc20
DNLM/DLC
for Library of Congress   92–48535
                                                         CIP

Acquisitions Editor: Jamie L. Mount
Production Editor: Sondra Greenfield
Designer: Penny Kindzierski

PRINTED IN THE UNITED STATES OF AMERICA

CONTENTS

Preface

Pharmacy licensing examinations are designed to determine whether a candidate has the requisite ability to carry out the responsibilities of the profession. A candidate preparing for the licensing examination must be prepared to demonstrate competence in many areas, any one of which may be the subject for in-depth questioning.

This book is designed as a self-testing tool for the pharmacy student to identify individual areas of strength and weakness, to suggest areas for further review, and to impart new concepts and other information useful to both the student and the practicing pharmacist. The book consists of three major sections: *Chapters 1* through *6* concentrate upon specific disciplines in order to improve the student's competence in each. Within each chapter, some questions dealing with related subject matter have been grouped together, while others have intentionally not been categorized, necessitating a return to certain areas of study in later questions to reinforce prior learning. In each chapter, questions are followed by an *Answers and Explanations* section, which we feel is the keystone of our book. Some comments are quite extensive and represent miniature reviews while others are limited to brief specifics. In every instance, the cited references offer a way for more extensive review.

Chapter 7 consists of patient profiles, each accommpanied by a series of related questions. Information obtained from the questions and commentaries in *Chapters 1* through *6* will probably aid in answering questions in *Chapter 7*.

The final section, *Chapter 8*, is a practice examination to test the reader who has faithfully completed all of the previous material.

There are also two appendices: The first lists over 200 drugs by generic names that the authors considered most likely to be dispensed by pharmacists. Included in the table are trade or brand names, manufacturing companies, a brief description of therapeutic uses, and common dosage forms and strengths. While it is not necessary to memorize the name of the company manufacturing a certain product, many individuals find it easier to relate a trade name to a company. To complete the cycle, the second appendix serves as a cross-reference of trade names with generic names.

We trust that this book will not be viewed as simply a means to review material for the licensing examination. Passing this examination does not guarantee continued competence throughout a long professional career. Practicing pharmacists must not only retain their previously acquired knowledge and skill, but must remain up to date on contemporary modes of practice. We hope that this book will serve as both a means for self-assessment of competence to practice, as well as a valuable guided review. A statement listing professional competency in pharmacy originally prepared by the California State Board of Pharmacy appears on the next page. Many of the test items in this book relate to these competencies.

Professional Competence in Pharmacy

A competent pharmacist is one who is able to confer with a physician about the care and treatment of his or her patient. The pharmacist should appreciate the essentials of the clinical diagnosis and understand the medical management of the patient. He or she should also be informed about the drugs that may be used in the treatment of the patient,—their mechanism of action; their combinations and dosage forms; the fate and disposition of the drugs (if known); the factors that may influence the physiological availability and biological activity of the drugs from their dosage forms; how age, sex, or secondary disease states might influence the course of treatment; and how other drugs, foods, and diagnostic procedures may interact to modify the activity of the drug.

A competent pharmacist is one whose overall function is to ensure optimum drug therapy. He or she should know the appropriate indications and dosage regimen for the drug therapy being undertaken as well as the contraindications and potential untoward reactions that may result during therapy. He or she should also be informed as to the proprietary products that might interact adversely with or be useful adjuncts to drug therapy, facilitating administration or improving overall patient care.

A competent pharmacist must be aware of the proposed therapeutic actions of proprietary medications, their composition, and any unique applications or potential limitations of their dosage forms. He or she should be able to objectively appraise advertising claims. At the patient's request, he or she should be able to ascertain the probable therapeutic usefulness of a certain drug in resolving the patient's complaints.

A competent pharmacist should be able to review a scientific publication and summarize the practical implications of the findings as they may relate to the clinical use of drugs. He or she should be able to analyze a published report of a clinical trial in terms of the appropriateness of the study design and the validity of the statistical analysis, and should be able to prepare an objective summary of the significance of the data and the authors' conclusions.

A competent pharmacist is a specialist as to the stability characteristics and storage requirements of drugs and drug products, the factors that influence the release of drugs from dosage forms, and the effect of the site of administration or its environment within the body on the absorption of a drug from the administered dosage form. Most importantly, the pharmacist understands the effect of the interaction of all these factors on the onset, intensity, or duration of therapeutic action.

A competent pharmacist should be precisely informed as to the legal limitations on procurement, storage, distribution, and sale of drugs; the approved use of a drug as specified by federal authorities and acceptable medical practice; and his or her legal responsibilities to the patient when drugs are used in experimental therapeutic procedures.

A competent pharmacist should be able to recommend the drug and dosage form that are are most likely to fulfill a particular therapeutic need, supporting his or her choice objectively with appropriate source material. In addition, he or she should be capable of identifying a drug, within a reasonable period of time, on the basis of its color, shape, and proposed use, as described in reference books or other sources.

On the basis of symptoms described in an interview with the patient, a competent pharmacist should know what additional information he or she must obtain from the patient. Based on this information, he or she should be able to refer the patient to the proper medical practitioner, specialist, or agency that would be of most help.

A competent pharmacist should be aware of drug toxicities, as well as the most effective means of treatment for them.

A competent pharmacist should be able to instruct patients on the proper administration of prescription and proprietary drugs. He or she should know which restrictions should be placed on food intake, other medication, and physical activity.

A competent phamacist should be able to communicate with other healthcare professionals or laymen on appropriate subjects, ensuring that the recipient understands the contents of the message being communicated.

A competent pharmacist should be capable of compounding appropriate drugs or drug combinations in acceptable dosage forms.

Finally, a competent pharmacist is a person who takes appropriate measures to maintain his level of competency in each of the areas described above.

Helpful Hints

There are several ways to maximize learning from this review book. For example, the reader could answer a short series of questions before looking for the answers at the end of each chapter. Keeping score will make these chapters function as miniature tests. Unfortunately, when challenged by multiple-choice questions, even in the nonthreatening environment of a self-learning program, our behavioral response is often predictable. When more than 75% of the questions are answered correctly, satisfaction and confidence dominate. As the percentage of missed questions increases, frustration and even panic develop. Such reactions lead to a self-limiting response: namely, the quick memorization of answers. Keep in mind, however, that while you may have increased your knowledge by one fact, you may not have maximized your learning experience. Do you really expect to see the same question on another examination? Do you realize why the other answer choices are not correct? Have you read the explanations of all the questions even those you answered correctly? Hopefully, these explanations will contain additional tidbits of information that will increase your knowledge base. If the question mentions a drug with which you are not familiar, be sure to look up the drug in one of the reference sources at your disposal. The next time you see that drug may be when it is the subject of a question. Some questions may concern topics with which you are not familiar. This is a perfect opportunity for learning!

Rather than blindly guessing at the answers, seek information in the cited reference or other sources, then attempt to answer the question. If your answer does not agree with the one given in this book, check further in another source. Keep digging—learning cannot be passive. Recognize that a question stating "which of these does NOT" or "all of these EXCEPT" gives you four positive facts or statements. These, in themselves, have expanded your knowledge base.

References

The references listed below represent a valuable collection of source material that can be used to review and expand one's knowledge of pharmacy. To maintain an up-to-date personal library, the reader should obtain at least a general pharmaceutical science book (eg, references 1, 20, and 29), a pharmacology book (reference 6), a book with a clinical pharmacy orientation (reference 11 or 19), and a publication discussing the use of drug therapy in managing certain disease states (reference 16). Although it is not necessary to purchase the latest editions of all reference books, sources describing drugs, drug products, and therapy that are periodically updated are of significant value. Examples include annuals (references 9 and 25) and the monthly version of reference 3.

The last line of each explanation in this review book includes a number identifying the reference source for each question and answer. The first number in the cited reference indicates the "e" source, while the second provides the page number. For example, (1:117; 20:218) refers to page 117 in the first source (*Remington's Pharmaceutical Sciences*) and page 218 in the twentieth source (*Dispensing of Medication*). The USP/DI has been cited as three sources (18a, b, and c), reflecting the three volumes. Citations referring to Koda-Kimble's *Applied Therapeutics* include the case study number followed by the page on which the case appears.

Because of frequent updates, the authors have chosen to cite the bound editions of reference 3 (*Facts and Comparisons*). Those using the loose-leaf edition with monthly updates can readily locate the cited drug in the index. The annuals 9 and 25 (*A.S.H.P. Drug Information and Physicians' Desk Reference*) are cited by section only rather than by page.

1. Osol A. *Remington's Pharmaceutical Sciences*. 18th ed. Easton, Pa: Mack Publishing Co; 1990.
2. American Pharmaceutical Association. *Handbook of Nonprescription Drugs*. 9th ed. Washington, DC: American Pharmaceutical Association; 1990.
3. Kastrup EK, Olin BR. *Facts and Comparisons* Philadelphia, Pa: Facts and Comparisons Division, JB Lippincott Co; 1992.
4. AMA Division of Drugs. *Drug Evaluations Annual*. Chicago, Ill: American Medical Association; 1992.
5. Evans WE, Schentag JJ, Jusko WI. *Applied Pharmacokinetics*. 2nd ed. San Francisco, Calif: Applied Therapeutics; 1986.
6. Gilman AG, Rall TW, Nies AS, et al. *Goodman and Gilman's Pharmacological Basis of Therapeutics*. 8th ed. New York, NY: Pergamon Press; 1990.
7. Avery GS. *Drug Treatment*. 3rd ed. New York, NY: Publishing Sciences Group Inc; 1987.
8. Hansten PD, Horn JR. *Drug Interactions and Updates*. 5th ed. Vancouver, Wash: Applied Therapeutics; 1990.

9. AHFS Drug Information 92. Bethesda, Md: American Society of Hospital Pharmacists; 1992.

10. Product Literature: drug package inserts current in 1992.

11. Herfindal ET, Gourley DR, Hart LL. *Clinical Pharmacy and Therapeutics*. 5th ed. Baltimore, Md: Williams & Wilkins Co; 1992.

12. Martin AN, Swarbrick J, Cammarata A. *Physical Pharmacy*. 3rd ed. Philadelphia, Pa: Lea & Febiger; 1983.

13. Turco S, King RE. *Sterile Dosage Forms*. 3rd ed. Philadelphia, Pa: Lea & Febiger; 1987.

14. Tatro DS. *Drug Interaction Facts*. St. Louis, Mo: J B Lippincott Co; 1992.

15. Sacher RA. *Widmann's Clinical Interpretation of Laboratory Tests*. 10th ed. Philadelphia, Pa: FA Davis Co; 1991.

16. Wilson JD, Braunwald E, Isselbacher KJ, et al. *Harrison's Principles of Internal Medicine*. 12th ed. New York, NY: McGraw-Hill Co; 1991.

17. Winter ME. *Basic Clinical Pharmacokinetics*. 2nd ed. San Francisco, Calif: Applied Therapeutics; 1988.

18a. USP Convention Inc. USP DI Volume I—Drug Information for the Health Care Professional. 12th ed. Rockville, Md: USPC Inc; 1992.

18b. USP Convention Inc. USP DI Volume II—Advice for the Patient. 12th ed Rockville, Md: USPC Inc; 1992.

18c. USP Convention Inc. USP DI Volume III—Approved Drug Products and Legal Requirements. 12th ed. Rockville, Md: USPC Inc; 1992.

19. Koda-Kimble MA, Young LY. *Applied Therapeutics*. 5th ed. Vancouver, Wash: Applied Therapeutics; 1992.

20. King RE. *Dispensing of Medication*. 9th ed. Easton, Pa: Mack Publishing Co; 1984.

21. Trissel LA. *Handbook on Injectable Drugs*. 7th ed. Bethesda, Md: American Society of Hospital Pharmacists; 1992.

22. Catania PN, Rosner MM. *Home Health Care Practice*. Palo Alto, Calif: Health Markets Research; 1986.

23. Stoklosa MJ, Ansel HC. *Pharmaceutical Calculations*. 9th ed. Philadelphia, Pa: Lea & Febiger; 1991.

24. Ansel HC, Popovich NG. *Introduction to Pharmaceutical Dosage Forms*. 5th ed. Philadelphia, Pa: Lea & Febiger; 1990.

25. *Physician's Desk Reference*. 46th ed. Oradell, NJ: Medical Economics Co; 1992.

26. Morris W. *The American Heritage Dictionary of the English Language*. New York, NY: American Heritage Publishing Co; 1982.

27. Gibaldi M. *Biopharmaceutics and Clinical Pharmacokinetics*. 4th ed. Philadelphia, Pa: Lea & Febiger; 1991.

28. *Stedman's Medical Dictionary*. 25th ed. Baltimore, Md: Williams & Wilkins; 1990.

29. Banker GS, Rhodes CT. *Modern Pharmaceutics*. 2nd ed. New York, NY: Marcel Dekker; 1989.

30. Notari RE. *Biopharmaceutics and Pharmacokinetics*. 4th ed. New York, NY: Marcel Dekker; 1987.

31. Traub S. *Interpreting Laboratory Data*. Bethesda, Md: American Society of Hospital Pharmacists; 1992.

CHAPTER 1

Pharmacology

Since 1940, the book cited in our bibliography as reference 6 has been known to successive classes of pharmacy students as simply "Goodman and Gilman." On page 1 of the current edition, the following statement can be found: "In its entirety, pharmacology embraces the knowledge of the history, source, physical and chemical properties, compounding, biochemical and physiological effects, mechanisms of action, absorption, distribution, biotransformation and excretion, and therapeutic and other uses of drugs. Since a drug is broadly defined as any chemical agent that affects processes of living, the subject of pharmacology is obviously quite extensive."

The test items in this chapter deal with some of these areas of pharmacology. Related questions may be found in chapters on biopharmaceutics and pharmacokinetics and clinical pharmacy.

Questions

DIRECTIONS (Questions 1 through 165): Each of the numbered items or incomplete statements in this section is followed by answers or by completions of the statement. Select the ONE lettered answer or completion that is BEST in each case.

1. An adverse effect commonly associated with the use of theophylline products is

    (A) hypertensive crisis *hypotension*
    (B) skin rash
    (C) insomnia
    (D) tardive dyskinesia
    (E) corneal lesions

2. Which of the following is NOT true of epinephrine?

    (A) It is therapeutically effective after oral or parenteral administration.
    (B) It will tend to elevate arterial blood pressure.
    (C) It is a bronchodilator.
    (D) It may be administered by inhalation.
    (E) It will cause vasoconstriction in mucous membranes.

3. Which of the following is true of epinephrine?

    (A) Its aqueous solutions are stable indefinitely.
    (B) It is a specific beta₂ agonist.
    (C) It is a specific beta₁ agonist.
    (D) It is an alpha-adrenergic agonist.
    (E) It is an ingredient in many OTC remedies.

4. Dipivefrin can best be described as a(n)   *Dipivefrin → epi*

    (A) active metabolite
    (B) preservative
    (C) buffer
    (D) chelating agent
    (E) prodrug

5. Heparin does NOT

    (A) inhibit blood clotting
    (B) inhibit thrombosis
    (C) inhibit activation of the fibrin-stabilizing factor (Factor VIII)

    (D) lyse existing clots
    (E) prolong clotting time

6. Diltiazem is used primarily for its ability to produce

    (A) cough suppression
    (B) analgesia
    (C) skeletal muscle relaxation
    (D) calcium channel blockade
    (E) emesis

7. Streptokinase is indicated for the treatment of

    (A) impaired fat absorption
    (B) pulmonary emboli
    (C) tuberculosis
    (D) neoplastic disorders
    (E) psoriasis

8. Which of the following metals has been found useful in the treatment of rheumatoid arthritis?

    (A) platinum
    (B) gold
    (C) copper
    (D) silver
    (E) mercury

9. As an antiarrhythmic drug, procainamide is most similar in action to which of the following agents?

    (A) lidocaine   *Class IA*
    (B) phenytoin   *Quinidine*
    (C) flecainide   *procainamide*
    (D) quinidine   *disopyramide*
    (E) amiodarone

10. The antiarrhythmic action of tocainide (Tonocard) and mexiletine (Mexitil) most closely resembles that of   *Class IB*

    (A) lidocaine
    (B) verapamil
    (C) quinidine
    (D) acebutolol
    (E) disopyramide

11. Acetylcysteine is an agent used clinically as a

(A) laxative
(B) cough suppressant
(C) hemostatic
(D) mucolytic
(E) diagnostic agent

12. Which of the following agents may be added to local injections of lidocaine HCl in order to prolong its effect?

local vasocons.

(A) epinephrine
(B) sodium carboxymethylcellulose
(C) atropine sulfate
(D) norepinephrine
(E) succinylcholine chloride

13. Cholestyramine resin is most commonly used to treat

(A) hyperkalemia
(B) hyperglycemia
(C) hypernatremia
(D) hyperlipidemia
(E) hyperchlorhydria

14. The agent most similar in action to cholestyramine is

(A) chlorpheniramine
(B) colestipol
(C) cholecalciferol
(D) choline salicylate
(E) clomiphene

15. Which of the following drugs does NOT lower plasma lipoprotein concentrations?

(A) nicotinamide
(B) clofibrate
(C) probucol
(D) cholestyramine
(E) lovastatin

16. A drug that has been shown to have a high level of antagonism for both histamine and 5-hydroxy-tryptamine (5-HT) is

(A) chlorpheniramine (Chlor-Trimeton)
(B) tripelennamine (PBZ)
(C) promethazine (Phenergan)
(D) diphenhydramine (Benadryl)
(E) cyproheptadine (Periactin)

17. Idoxuridine (Herplex) is an effective treatment for dendritic keratitis, which is caused by

(A) *E. coli*
(B) Herpes simplex
(C) *Staphylococcus aureus*
(D) *Clostridium difficile*
(E) *Pseudomonas aeruginosa*

18. Which of the following agents is NOT an antifungal agent?

(A) natamycin
(B) trifluridine
(C) undecylenic acid
(D) clioquinol
(E) ciclopirox olamine

19. Tretinoin is used therapeutically

(A) as a urinary acidifier
(B) as an antifungal agent
(C) in the topical treatment of acne
(D) in the treatment of tuberculosis
(E) as an ophthalmic irrigant

20. An agent that would be most likely to cause drug-induced bronchospasm is

(A) nadolol
(B) hydrochlorothiazide
(C) isoproterenol
(D) reserpine
(E) aminophylline

21. Dopamine (Intropin) is

(A) an alpha and beta agonist
(B) primarily a beta agonist
(C) primarily an alpha agonist
(D) a beta-adrenergic blocker
(E) an alpha-adrenergic blocker

22. Which of the following has NOT been used extensively for the treatment of parkinsonism?

(A) Tofranil
(B) Cogentin
(C) Artane
(D) Kemadrin
(E) Symmetrel

23. Albuterol (Proventil, Ventolin) is a(n)

(A) beta-receptor agonist
(B) alpha-receptor agonist
(C) beta-receptor antagonist
(D) alpha-receptor antagonist
(E) alpha- and beta-receptor agonist

24. Which of the following is a pharmacologic action of histamine?

(A) capillary constriction
(B) stimulation of gastric secretion
(C) elevation of blood pressure
(D) skeletal muscle paralysis
(E) anti-inflammatory activity

25. Which of the following agents is NOT an H₁-receptor antagonist?

    (A) astemizole (Hismanal)
    (B) azatadine (Optimine)
    (C) triprolidine (Actidil)
    (D) promethazine (Phenergan)
    (E) nizatidine (Axid)

26. Which of the following would NOT be an expected effect of inhaling the smoke of cannabis (marijuana)?

    (A) anorexia
    (B) increase in pulse rate
    (C) perceptual changes
    (D) vascular congestion of the eyes
    (E) hypertrichosis

27. Of the following glucocorticoids, which one has the greatest anti-inflammatory potency when administered systemically?

    (A) hydrocortisone (Cortef)
    (B) prednisone (Meticorten)
    (C) triamcinolone (Aristocort)
    (D) dexamethasone (Decadron)
    (E) cortisone (Cortone)

28. Benzoyl peroxide is commonly employed in the treatment of

    (A) psoriasis
    (B) pinworms
    (C) lice
    (D) viral infections
    (E) acne

29. Augmentin is a product that contains amoxicillin and potassium clavulanate. Potassium clavulanate

    (A) is an antifungal agent
    (B) prevents the urinary excretion of amoxicillin
    (C) prevents first-pass metabolism of amoxicillin
    (D) is a buffer
    (E) inhibits beta-lactamase enzymes

30. Which of the following hormones is released from the posterior pituitary gland?

    (A) adrenocorticotropic hormone (ACTH)
    (B) oxytocin
    (C) thyroid-stimulating hormone (TSH)
    (D) follicle-stimulating hormone (FSH)
    (E) growth hormone

31. During ovulation, peak plasma concentrations of which of the following hormones will be reached?

    (A) follicle-stimulating hormone (FSH)
    (B) luteinizing hormone (LH)
    (C) both FSH and LH
    (D) progesterone
    (E) both progesterone and LH

32. Liotrix is a thyroid preparation that contains
    I. dessicated thyroid
    II. levothyroxine sodium
    III. liothyronine sodium

    (A) I only
    (B) III only
    (C) I & II only
    (D) II & III only
    (E) I, II, & III

33. Methimazole (Tapazole) is used for the same therapeutic indication as

    (A) thyroglobulin
    (B) papaverine
    (C) lisinopril
    (D) dextranomer
    (E) propylthiouracil

34. A phenothiazine derivative commonly used for its antihistaminic effect is

    (A) chlorpromazine
    (B) promazine
    (C) promethazine
    (D) prochlorperazine
    (E) thioridazine

35. Carbamazepine (Tegretol) is indicated for the treatment of

    (A) enuresis
    (B) trigeminal neuralgia
    (C) endometriosis
    (D) psoriasis
    (E) attention deficit disorder

36. Of the following anxiolytic agents, the one that possesses the least sedating action is

    (A) diazepam (Valium)
    (B) buspirone (BuSpar)
    (C) meprobamate (Miltown, Equanil)
    (D) chlordiazepoxide (Librium)
    (E) oxazepam (Serax)

37. Which of the following is NOT true of theophylline?

    (A) relaxes the smooth muscle of the respiratory tract
    (B) is chemically related to caffeine
    (C) increases the contractile force of the heart
    (D) causes central nervous system depression
    (E) stimulates the production of gastric secretions

38. Penicillins are believed to exert their antibacterial effect by which of the following mechanisms?

    (A) detergent effect on the bacterial cell membrane
    (B) inhibition of bacterial cell wall synthesis
    (C) destruction of the bacterial cell nucleus
    (D) inhibition of protein synthesis
    (E) steric hindrance of membrane amino acids

39. The antibacterial mechanism of the penicillins is most similar to that of

(A) clindamycin (Cleocin) *rib 50S sub*
(B) tetracycline HCl (Achromycin) *rib 50S sub*
(C) ciprofloxacin (Cipro) *DNA gyrase inhib*
(D) cefaclor (Ceclor) *cell wall synth*
(E) gentamicin (Garamycin) *30s rib subunit*

40. Which of the following agents can be administered with ampicillin and other penicillins to achieve higher blood levels of the penicillin?

(A) aspirin
(B) penicillamine (Cuprimine) *↑ amp levels*
(C) probenecid (Benemid)
(D) nitrofurantoin (Furadantin)
(E) epinephrine

41. One milligram of pure potassium penicillin G is equivalent to approximately how many penicillin units of activity?

1 mg = 1600 units
250 = 400,000 units

(A) 37
(B) 600
(C) 1600
(D) 250,000
(E) 600,000

42. Which of the following agents is most similar in action to ampicillin?

(A) amoxicillin (Amoxil)
(B) oxacillin (Prostaphlin)
(C) penicillin V potassium (Pen Vee K)
(D) dicloxacillin (Pathocil)
(E) benzyl penicillin

43. Chlorhexidine gluconate is most similar in action to

(A) hexachlorophene *Phisohex*
(B) chlorpheniramine *H₁ blocker*
(C) calcium gluconate *Ca supplement*
(D) quinidine gluconate *anti arrhythmic*
(E) chloroquine phosphate *aralen (antimalarial)*

rheumatoid arthritis or chelator

44. Penicillamine is a drug used therapeutically

(A) in the treatment of gram-positive infections
(B) as a diagnostic agent for penicillin allergy
(C) as a chelator of various metals
(D) in the treatment of gram-negative infections
(E) as an antifungal agent

45. Polymyxin B is pharmacologically and microbiologically similar to

(A) ampicillin (Polycillin)
(B) colistin (Coly-Mycin S)
(C) kanamycin (Kantrex) *— aminoglycoside*
(D) penicillin G
(E) tetracycline (Achromycin)

— gram neg — nephrotox

46. Potentially fatal aplastic anemia is a toxic effect associated with

(A) demeclocycline (Declomycin)
(B) chloramphenicol (Chloromycetin) *meningitis*
(C) nitrofurantoin (Furadantin)
(D) clindamycin (Cleocin)
(E) cefadroxil (Duricef)

47. Which of the following agents is effective against penicillinase-producing staphylococci?

(A) dicloxacillin (Pathocil)
(B) penicillin V potassium (V-Cillin K)
(C) ticarcillin (Ticar)
(D) piperacillin (Pipracil)
(E) amoxicillin (Amoxil)

① cloxacilli
② dicloxac
③ oxacillin
④ nafcillin
⑤ methacill

48. Which of the following antagonizes the action of sulfonamides?

(A) streptomycin
(B) penicillin G
(C) morphine
(D) para-aminobenzoic acid (PABA)
(E) tetracycline

49. Sulfones such as dapsone are employed commonly in the treatment of

inhib folic acid
antimalarial
anti leprosy

(A) urinary tract infections
(B) thrush
(C) systemic fungal infections
(D) leprosy
(E) pseudomembranous enterocolitis

50. Which of these tetracyclines has the longest duration of action?

(A) tetracycline (Achromycin) *t½ 6 –12 H*
(B) doxycycline (Vibramycin) *t½ 22 – 24 H*
(C) demeclocycline (Declomycin) *t½ 10 –17 H*
(D) minocycline (Minocin) *t½ 11 –26 H*
(E) oxytetracycline (Terramycin) *t½ 6 –10 H*

51. Tricyclic antidepressants are believed to exert their antidepressant action by

(A) potentiating GABA activity
(B) blocking beta-adrenergic receptors
(C) blocking alpha-adrenergic receptors
(D) increasing the metabolic breakdown of biogenic amines
(E) inhibiting biogenic amine reuptake into adrenergic nerve terminals

52. Which of the following agents is NOT indicated for the treatment of depression?

(A) haloperidol (Haldol)
(B) phenelzine (Nardil)
(C) fluoxetine (Prozac)
(D) trazodone (Desyrel)
(E) doxepin (Sinequan)

53. A common adverse effect related to the chronic use of aluminum antacids is

(A) nausea and vomiting
(B) constipation
(C) flatulence
(D) diarrhea
(E) gastrointestinal bleeding

54. Which of the following is NOT a fat soluble vitamin?

(A) cholecalciferol
(B) vitamin A
(C) tocopherol
(D) phytonadione
(E) pyridoxine

55. Carbidopa can best be classified as a drug that

(A) reverses symptoms of Parkinson's disease
(B) exerts an anticholinergic action
(C) is a skeletal muscle relaxant
(D) is a neuromuscular blocking agent
(E) is a dopa-decarboxylase inhibitor

56. Methylxanthines such as caffeine and theophylline exert all of the following pharmacologic effects EXCEPT

(A) cardiac stimulation
(B) diuresis
(C) relaxation of smooth muscle
(D) peripheral vasoconstriction
(E) central nervous system stimulation

57. Which of the following anorectic drugs is more likely to cause CNS depression than stimulation?

(A) diethylpropion HCl (Tenuate)
(B) fenfluramine HCl (Pondimin)
(C) phentermine HCl (Ionamin)
(D) phendimetrazine tartrate (Plegine)
(E) mazindol (Sanorex)

58. Lactase enzyme is available for the treatment of

(A) lactose intolerance
(B) galactokinase deficiency
(C) Hansen's disease
(D) phenylketonuria
(E) hypochlorhydria

59. Isotretinoin (Accutane) is a drug employed in the treatment of severe recalcitrant cystic acne. Which of the following is NOT an adverse effect associated with its use?

(A) hyperglycemia
(B) hypertriglyceridemia
(C) pseudotumor cerebri
(D) conjunctivitis
(E) fetal abnormalities

60. Which of the following is true of isotretinoin (Accutane)?

(A) It may be safely used in pregnant patients after the first trimester.
(B) It is a derivative of vitamin D.
(C) It is applied topically to severe acne lesions.
(D) Its use is contraindicated in patients with diabetes.
(E) It commonly causes cheilitis.

61. Endorphins are

(A) a new class of topical anti-inflammatory agents
(B) endogenous opioid peptides
(C) neuromuscular blocking agents
(D) biogenic amines believed to cause schizophrenia
(E) endogenous chelating agents

62. Which of the following is true of "crack"?

  I. It is a free-base form of cocaine.
 II. It is generally smoked.
III. Its use results in CNS stimulation.

(A) I only
(B) III only
(C) I & II only
(D) II & III only
(E) I, II, & III

63. A uricosuric drug is one that

(A) decreases flow of urine
(B) increases flow of urine
(C) blocks excretion of uric acid in the urine
(D) promotes excretion of uric acid in the urine
(E) aids in the reabsorption of uric acid

64. Alteplase (Activase) is employed clinically as a(n)

(A) xanthine oxidase inhibitor
(B) ulcer adherent complex
(C) plasma expander
(D) tissue plasminogen activator
(E) keratolytic

65. A disadvantage in the use of cimetidine (Tagamet) is its ability to cause

(A) hair loss
(B) decreased prolactin secretion
(C) gastric hyperparesis
(D) inhibition of hepatic enzyme activity
(E) esophageal reflux

66. A drug that decreases the production of uric acid is

(A) allopurinol
(B) chloroquine
(C) probenecid
(D) phenylbutazone
(E) propoxyphene

67. Hypoparathyroidism is a disorder that would most logically be treated with

(A) d-alpha tocopherol acetate
(B) nicotinamide
(C) calcium pantothenate
(D) phytonadione
(E) dihydrotachysterol

68. A drug found to be useful in reducing elevated serum cholesterol is

(A) calcitriol (Rocaltrol)
(B) encainide (Enkaid)
(C) lovastatin (Mevacor)
(D) butorphanol (Stadol)
(E) selegiline (Eldepryl)

69. Which of the following is NOT an anabolic steroid?

(A) stanozolol
(B) nandrolone
(C) norethindrone   progestin
(D) oxymetholone
(E) oxandrolone

70. Nerves in the human body that transmit their impulses by releasing acetylcholine are known as _____ nerves.

(A) adrenergic
(B) choleretic   Cholinergic
(C) axillary
(D) cholinergic
(E) neurogenic

71. Pentoxifylline (Trental) can best be classified pharmacologically as a(n)

(A) hemorheologic agent
(B) skeletal muscle relaxant
(C) CNS depressant
(D) bronchodilator
(E) antipsychotic

72. Which of the following is NOT true of methadone?

(A) is available commercially under the name Dolophine
(B) can be given orally or parenterally
(C) is a narcotic antagonist
(D) is an addicting drug
(E) has significant analgesic activity

73. An example of a pure narcotic antagonist is

(A) naloxone HCl (Narcan)
(B) buprenorphine (Buprenex)
(C) nalbuphine HCl (Nubain)
(D) butorphanol (Stadol)
(E) sufentanil (Sufenta)

74. The ergot alkaloids have been found to be useful in the treatment of migraine headaches and are also used extensively as

(A) nasal decongestants
(B) uterine stimulants
(C) skeletal muscle relaxants
(D) local anesthetics
(E) antineoplastic agents

75. Which of the following is NOT a pharmacologic effect of morphine?

(A) constriction of the pupils
(B) CNS depression
(C) diarrhea
(D) respiratory depression
(E) nausea and vomiting

76. An active metabolite of the anticonvulsant drug primidone (Mysoline) is

(A) phenobarbital
(B) dopamine
(C) phenytoin
(D) methsuximide
(E) trimethadione

77. Etidronate disodium (Didronel) is an agent primarily indicated for the treatment of

(A) Paget's disease
(B) Ménière's syndrome
(C) Crohn's disease
(D) Hansen's disease
(E) Parkinson's disease

78. An agent used for the same indication as etidronate disodium (Didronel) is

(A) dantrolene (Dantrium)
(B) salmon calcitonin (Calcimar)
(C) carmustine (BiCNU)
(D) chenodiol (Chenix)
(E) bretylium tosylate (Bretylol)

79. Prednisone is an agent that exhibits several pharmacologic functions. These include
    I.   glucocorticoid activity
    II. mineralocorticoid activity
    III. diuretic activity

    (A) I only
    (B) III only
    (C) I & II only
    (D) II & III only
    (E) I, II, & III

80. Which of the following agents is indicated for use as an antiemetic agent?

    (A) colestipol (Colestid)
    (B) guanfacine (Tenex)
    (C) difenoxin (Motofen)
    (D) methoxsalen (Oxsoralen)
    (E) ondansetron (Zofran)

81. Amrinone (Inocor) is most similar in action to

    (A) propranolol (Inderal)
    (B) lidocaine (Xylocaine)
    (C) hydralazine (Apresoline)
    (D) disopyramide (Norpace)
    (E) digoxin (Lanoxin)

82. Which of the following is a vasodilating drug with marked platelet-suppressing activity.

    (A) nitroglycerin
    (B) nylidrin (Arlidin)
    (C) pentaerythritol tetranitrate (Peritrate)
    (D) dipyridamole (Persantine)
    (E) hydralazine (Apresoline)

83. Lactulose (Cephulac, Chronulac)

    (A) is an antidiarrheal agent
    (B) reduces blood ammonia levels
    (C) is a potent antiemetic agent
    (D) causes systemic acidosis
    (E) releases ammonia in the GI tract

84. The active laxative principle formed by hydrolysis of castor oil in the GI tract is

    (A) pyruvic acid
    (B) vitamin A
    (C) ricinoleic acid
    (D) benzaldehyde
    (E) carvone

85. The dose of liothyronine sodium that is approximately equivalent to 60 mg of Thyroid USP in its ability to produce a clinical response is

    (A) 120 µg
    (B) 0.4 µg
    (C) 250 µg

    (D) 25 µg
    (E) 100 µg

86. Acid rebound is most likely to occur with the use of large doses of which of the following antacids?

    (A) aluminum phosphate
    (B) aluminum hydroxide
    (C) magnesium trisilicate
    (D) calcium carbonate
    (E) magnesium hydroxide

87. Chronic use of aluminum hydroxide gel may deplete a patient of

    (A) sodium
    (B) chloride
    (C) calcium
    (D) phosphate
    (E) thiamine

88. Patients who are sensitive to aspirin should avoid the use of

    (A) nystatin (Mycostatin)
    (B) piroxicam (Feldene)
    (C) enalapril (Vasotec)
    (D) haloperidol (Haldol)
    (E) minoxidil (Loniten)

89. Aspirin is believed to inhibit clotting by its action on which of the following endogenous substances?

    (A) prostacyclin
    (B) thromboxane
    (C) fibrinogen
    (D) vitamin K
    (E) albumin

90. The primary site of action of triamterene (Dyrenium) and spironolactone (Aldactone) is the

    (A) proximal tubule
    (B) descending loop of Henle
    (C) ascending loop of Henle
    (D) distal tubule
    (E) glomerulus

91. Which of the following beta-adrenergic blocking agents also exhibit alpha₁-adrenergic blocking action?
    I.   nadolol (Corgard)
    II. pindolol (Visken)
    III. labetelol (Normodyne, Trandate)

    (A) I only
    (B) III only
    (C) I & II only
    (D) II & III only
    (E) I, II, & III

92. Which of the following drugs is most useful in the relief of acute attacks of gout?

    (A) probenecid
    (B) aspirin
    (C) sulfinpyrazone (Anturane)
    (D) colchicine
    (E) allopurinol (Zyloprim)

93. Prolonged activity (8–10 hours) is an advantage in the use of which of the following topical decongestants?
    I. phenylephrine
    II. oxymetazoline
    III. xylometazoline

    (A) I only
    (B) III only
    (C) I & II only
    (D) II & III only
    (E) I, II, & III

94. Use of auranofin (Ridaura) may result in the development of

    (A) damage to the auditory nerve
    (B) blood dyscrasias
    (C) damage to the optic nerve
    (D) precipitation of an acute attack of gout
    (E) electrolyte depletion

95. The major effects of Opium Tincture USP are related to its content of

    (A) morphine
    (B) papaverine
    (C) codeine
    (D) dihydrocodeinone
    (E) alfentanil

96. After oral administration, the greatest amount of iron absorption occurs in the

    (A) duodenum
    (B) stomach
    (C) sigmoid portion of the large intestine
    (D) transverse portion of the large intestine
    (E) ascending portion of the large intestine

97. Iron is required by the body to maintain normal

    (A) digestion
    (B) immunological function
    (C) bone growth
    (D) oxygen transport
    (E) vitamin absorption

98. Regular use of sublingual doses of organic nitrates (eg, nitroglycerin) is likely to result in the development of

    (A) hepatotoxicity
    (B) nephrotoxicity
    (C) peptic ulcer disease
    (D) tolerance
    (E) respiratory impairment

99. Which of the following is NOT true of regular insulin?

    (A) It is a clear product.
    (B) It may be administered SC or IV.
    (C) It is shorter acting than other insulins.
    (D) All regular insulin products currently marketed in the United States are prepared at neutral pH.
    (E) When mixing regular insulin with another insulin in the same syringe, always draw the regular insulin into the syringe last.

100. Lovastatin (Mevacor) is contraindicated for use in patients who

    (A) are hypersensitive to aspirin
    (B) are pregnant
    (C) have bronchial asthma
    (D) are more than 25% over ideal body weight
    (E) are diabetics

101. Which of the following drugs is available in a transdermal dosage form for use in the prevention of nausea and vomiting associated with motion sickness in adults?

    (A) metoclopramide
    (B) fluoxetine
    (C) atropine
    (D) clonidine
    (E) scopolamine

102. Which of the following drugs is indicated for the treatment of primary nocturnal enuresis?

    (A) ritodrine (Yutopar)
    (B) desmopressin acetate (DDAVP)
    (C) metolazone (Zaroxolyn)
    (D) amiloride (Midamor)
    (E) mannitol (Osmitrol)

103. An example of a benzodiazepine that is not metabolized to active metabolites in the body is

    (A) diazepam
    (B) chlordiazepoxide
    (C) lorazepam
    (D) triazolam
    (E) halazepam

104. Which of the following antimicrobial agents would be MOST useful in the treatment of an infection caused by beta-lactamase–producing staphylococci?

    (A) dicloxacillin
    (B) cefazolin
    (C) cephalexin
    (D) amoxicillin
    (E) bacampicillin

105. Gastric intrinsic factor is a glycoprotein that is required for the gastrointestinal absorption of

   (A) cyanocobalamin   V B12
   (B) folic acid
   (C) iron
   (D) thiamine
   (E) calcium

106. Gingival hyperplasia, hirsutism, and ataxia are adverse effects associated with the use of

   (A) minoxidil (Loniten)
   (B) chlorpromazine (Thorazine)
   (C) phenytoin (Dilantin)
   (D) enalapril (Vasotec)
   (E) ciprofloxacin (Cipro)

107. Timolol maleate is a drug used in the treatment of glaucoma. Which of the following best describes the action it exerts on the eye?

   (A) miotic
   (B) mydriatic
   (C) interferes with the enzyme carbonic anhydrase
   (D) acts as an osmotic diuretic
   (E) decreases the production of aqueous humor

108. The ophthalmic beta-adrenergic blocking agent with the LEAST likelihood of producing respiratory impairment is

   (A) carteolol (Ocupress) nonselective w/ISA
   (B) metipranolol hydrochloride (OptiPranolol) B2
   (C) levobunolol hydrochloride (Betagan) nonselective
   (D) timolol (Timoptic) non selct
   (E) betaxolol (Betoptic) B1 selective

109. Pilocarpine is employed in the treatment of glaucoma. It is believed to act as a(n)

   (A) mydriatic
   (B) cycloplegic
   (C) carbonic anhydrase inhibitor
   (D) miotic
   (E) anticholinergic

110. Which of the following is NOT an effect of atropine on the human body? anticholinergic

   (A) cardiac stimulation
   (B) diminished sweating
   (C) stimulation of gastric secretion
   (D) reduction of gastrointestinal tone
   (E) mydriasis

111. Which of the following statements best describes the mechanism of action of antihistaminic drugs?

   (A) They interfere with the synthesis of histamine in the body.
   (B) They form inactive complexes with histamine.

   (C) They block the receptor sites on which histamine acts.
   (D) They stimulate the metabolism of endogenous histamine.
   (E) They are alpha-adrenergic blockers.

112. Haloperidol (Haldol) differs from chlorpromazine (Thorazine) in that haloperidol

   (A) is not a phenothiazine
   (B) does not produce extrapyramidal effects
   (C) is not an antipsychotic agent
   (D) does not cause sedation
   (E) cannot be administered parenterally

113. Tamoxifen (Nolvadex) is an agent that can best be described as a(n)

   (A) gonadotropin-releasing hormone analog
   (B) androgen
   (C) estrogen
   (D) progestin
   (E) antiestrogen

114. Which of the following is NOT true of auranofin (Ridaura)?

   (A) It is an orally administered form of gold.
   (B) It may cause thrombocytopenia in some patients.
   (C) It is currently the only drug that is curative for arthritis.
   (D) Therapeutic effects do not appear until at least 3 months of therapy have elapsed.
   (E) Its use may result in renal impairment.

115. Advantages of acetaminophen over aspirin include all of the following EXCEPT

   (A) no alteration of bleeding time
   (B) greater anti-inflammatory action   none
   (C) no occult blood loss
   (D) no appreciable effect on uric acid excretion
   (E) less gastric irritation

116. The use of clozapine (Clozaril) has been associated with the development of

   (A) meningitis
   (B) hypercalcemia
   (C) hyperuricemia
   (D) thrombocytopenia
   (E) agranulocytosis

117. Which of the following is true of propoxyphene HCl (Darvon)?

   (A) It has about the same analgesic activity as an equivalent dose of codeine.
   (B) It has significant analgesic and antipyretic properties.
   (C) It has analgesic and anti-inflammatory properties but has no antipyretic properties.

(D) The analgesic property of this drug resides only in the dextrorotatory isomer (1-propoxyphene).

(E) It is administered with meperidine to reduce meperidine's adverse effects.

118. Although classified as antibiotics, dactinomycin (Cosmegen) and plicamycin (Mithracin) are used in cancer chemotherapy because they have a(n)

(A) immunosuppressant effect
(B) antiviral effect
(C) cytotoxic effect
(D) anabolic effect
(E) ability to "sterilize" the blood

119. The anti-inflammatory effect of aspirin is due to

(A) an anticoagulant effect
(B) an antigen–antibody reaction
(C) inhibition of the synthesis of prostaglandins
(D) increased membrane permeability of inflamed tissue
(E) stimulation of endogenous hydrocortisone production

120. The "first-dose" effect is characterized by marked hypotension and syncope upon taking the first few doses of medication. This effect is seen with the use of

I. doxazosin (Cardura)   *Least doxazosin*
II. prazosin (Minipress)
III. terazosin (Hytrin)

(A) I only
(B) III only
(C) I & II only
(D) II & III only
(E) I, II, & III only

121. Carbon monoxide exerts its toxic effects primarily by

(A) reacting with body enzymes to produce acidic substances
(B) paralyzing the muscles of the diaphragm
(C) reacting with amino acids in the body to form ammonia
(D) inhibiting the gag reflex
(E) decreasing the oxygen-carrying capacity of the blood

122. The most serious potential consequence of ingestion of a liquid hydrocarbon such as kerosene or gasoline is

(A) dissolution of the mucoid coat of the esophagus
(B) the corrosive action of the poison on the stomach lining
(C) the paralysis of peristaltic motion of the GI tract
(D) the aspiration of the poison into the respiratory tract
(E) the destruction of body enzymes by the poison

123. A specific antidote for the treatment of poisoning due to the oral ingestion of excessive iron would be the administration of

(A) potassium permanganate solution
(B) deferoxamine mesylate
(C) acetic acid solution
(D) normal saline
(E) sodium bicarbonate

124. Which of the following agents is classified pharmacologically as a carbonic anhydrase inhibitor?

(A) acetazolamide (Diamox)
(B) spironolactone (Aldactone)   *K sparing*
(C) chlorthalidone (Hygroton)
(D) bumetanide (Bumex)   *loop*
(E) amiloride (Midamor)   *Ca channel*

125. The thiazide diuretics decrease the excretion of

(A) sodium   *↑ excretion K, Na, Cl*
(B) urea   *↓ " uric acid, calcium*
(C) uric acid
(D) bicarbonate
(E) creatinine

126. The renal excretion of amphetamines can be diminished by alkalinization of the urine. Which of the following would tend to diminish the excretion rate of amphetamine sulfate?

(A) methenamine mandelate
(B) acetazolamide
(C) tetracycline HCl
(D) ammonium chloride
(E) niacin

127. An agent employed in relieving signs and symptoms of spasticity resulting from multiple sclerosis is

(A) baclofen (Lioresal)
(B) buspirone (Buspar)
(C) ursodiol (Actigall)
(D) mexiletine (Mexitil)
(E) amiodarone (Cordarone)

128. Which of the following drugs inhibits the metabolism of ethanol?

(A) phenylbutazone   *NSAID*
(B) disulfiram
(C) chlorpheniramine   *H1*
(D) meprobamate
(E) carbamazepine   *inducer*

129. Which of the following is NOT an MAO inhibitor?

(A) pargyline
(B) isocarboxazid
(C) cyclobenzaprine   *Flexeril*
(D) tranylcypromine   *Parnate*
(E) phenelzine   *Nardil*

130. A drug that is indicated for the treatment of both diarrhea and constipation is

(A) bisacodyl (Dulcolax)
(B) lactulose (Cephulac)
(C) magnesium sulfate
(D) polycarbophil (Mitrolan)
(E) senna (Senokot)

131. Which of the following is a microsomal enzyme inducer?

(A) indomethacin
(B) clofibrate
(C) tolbutamide
(D) phenobarbital
(E) ibuprofen

132. The thiazide derivative diazoxide (Hyperstat)

vasodilator

(A) is a stronger diuretic than hydrochlorothiazide
(B) is a pressor agent
(C) produces about the same diuretic response as an equal dose of hydrochlorothiazide
(D) produces diuresis in normotensive subjects only
(E) is not a diuretic

133. Which of the following are broad spectrum antifungal agents?

I. nystatin — *yeast*
II. griseofulvin — *tinnea*
III. miconazole — *yeast & tinnea*

(A) I only
(B) III only
(C) I & II only
(D) II & III only
(E) I, II, & III

134. Which of the following barbiturates is used as an intravenous anesthetic?

(A) phenobarbital
(B) amobarbital
(C) thiopental sodium
(D) pentobarbital sodium
(E) talbutal

135. The most useful drug in the treatment of diabetes insipidus is

(A) chlorpropamide (Diabinese)
(B) glucagon
(C) insulin
(D) lypressin (Diapid)
(E) glyburide (Micronase)

136. A pharmacist receives a prescription order for indomethacin (Indocin) capsules. He should consult with the physician if the medication record indicates that the patient

(A) has gout
(B) has arthritis
(C) is hypertensive
(D) has insomnia
(E) has a peptic ulcer

137. The sulfonylureas (eg, Orinase, Glucotrol) are believed to exert their hypoglycemic effect by

(A) stimulating the release of insulin from the pancreas
(B) inhibiting the breakdown of endogenous insulin
(C) enhancing the effectiveness of the small amounts of insulin that the diabetic can produce
(D) increasing the peripheral utilization of glucose
(E) decreasing the desire for sugar consumption

138. Which of the following oral hypoglycemic drugs has the longest serum half-life?

(A) acetohexamide (Dymelor) *6hr*
(B) chlorpropamide (Diabinese) *36 hr t/2 10*
(C) glyburide (Diabeta, Micronase)
(D) tolbutamide (Orinase) *4-5hr.*
(E) all of the above have about the same serum half-life

139. Vidarabine (Vira-A) is an antiviral agent indicated for the treatment of

(A) rubella
(B) herpes simplex encephalitis
(C) influenza
(D) rubeola
(E) smallpox

140. Which of the following statements regarding methenamine mandelate is NOT true?

(A) After oral ingestion formaldehyde is formed in acid urine.
(B) It is maximally effective at a pH below 5.5.
(C) It should be given with sulfonamides to enhance effectiveness of therapy.
(D) It is contraindicated in renal insufficiency.
(E) Ammonia is produced in acid urine after its oral ingestion.

Sulfonamides + methenamine cause ppt in acidic urine

141. Zidovudine (Retrovir) is indicated for the treatment of patients with
    I.   AIDS
    II. herpes simplex infections
    III. influenza A virus infection
    (A) I only
    (B) III only
    (C) I & II only
    (D) II & III only
    (E) I, II, & III

142. Which of the following is true of alteplase (Activase)?
    (A) It is derived from bovine tissue.
    (B) It is an anticoagulant.
    (C) It is derived from porcine tissue.
    (D) It is a thrombolytic agent.
    (E) It is administered intramuscularly.

143. Which of the following agents is NOT employed in the treatment of bronchial asthma?
    (A) ipratropium bromide (Atrovent)
    (B) dyphylline (Lufyllin)
    (C) beclomethasone dipropionate (Vanceril)
    (D) flunisolide (AeroBid)
    (E) beractant (Survanta)

144. Diclofenac sodium (Voltaren) is most similar in action to
    (A) buspirone (Buspar)
    (B) dicyclomine (Bentyl)
    (C) chlorzoxazone (Paraflex)
    (D) ketoprofen (Orudis)
    (E) mecamylamine (Inversine)

145. Cromolyn sodium (Intal, Nasalcrom, Opticrom) is a drug that is
    (A) effective in acute asthmatic attacks
    (B) a synthetic corticosteroid
    (C) a histamine antagonist
    (D) a stabilizer of sensitized mast cells
    (E) a theophylline derivative

146. A calcium channel blocker that is employed parenterally in the treatment of cardiac arrhythmias is
    (A) isradipine (DynaCirc)
    (B) verapamil (Calan)
    (C) nifedipine (Procardia)
    (D) diltiazem HCl (Cardizem)
    (E) felodipine (Plendil)

147. Which of the following antibiotics is a third-generation cephalosporin?
    (A) cefoxitin (Mefoxin)
    (B) cefaclor (Ceclor)
    (C) cephalexin (Keflex)
    (D) cefonicid (Monocid)
    (E) ceftriaxone (Rocephin)

148. Reflex sympathetic stimulation is an adverse effect most likely to be associated with the use of which of the following drugs?
    (A) reserpine (Serpasil)
    (B) minoxidil (Loniten)
    (C) hydrochlorothiazide (HydroDIURIL)
    (D) nadolol (Corgard)
    (E) clonidine (Catapres)

149. Which of the following is TRUE of buprenorphine (Buprenex)?
    I.   It is available only for parenteral use.
    II. It is an opioid.
    III. It is indicated for the treatment of inflammatory bowel disease.
    (A) I only
    (B) III only
    (C) I & II only
    (D) II & III only
    (E) I, II, & III

150. Which of the following is NOT progestin?
    (A) mestranol
    (B) norethindrone
    (C) ethynodiol diacetate
    (D) levonorgestrel
    (E) norethynodrel

151. Which of the following beta-adrenergic blocking agents has intrinsic sympathomimetic activity?
    (A) esmolol (Brevibloc)
    (B) atenolol (Tenormin)
    (C) metoprolol (Lopressor)
    (D) pindolol (Visken)
    (E) propranolol HCl (Inderal)

152. Danazol (Danocrine) can best be classified as a(n)
    (A) alkylating agent
    (B) progestin
    (C) androgen
    (D) corticosteroid
    (E) estrogen

153. Metolazone (Diulo, Zaroxolyn) is most similar in action to
    (A) spironolactone (Aldactone)
    (B) furosemide (Lasix)
    (C) triamterene (Dyrenium)
    (D) chlorthalidone (Hygroton)
    (E) acetazolamide (Diamox)

154. Potassium supplementation is LEAST likely to be required in a patient using

   (A) ethacrynic acid (Edecrin)
   (B) chlorthalidone (Hygroton)
   (C) amiloride (Midamor)
   (D) acetazolamide (Diamox)
   (E) furosemide (Lasix)

155. Acyclovir (Zovirax) is indicated for the treatment of

   (A) influenza caused by influenza A virus strains
   (B) pseudomembranous enterocolitis
   (C) mumps
   (D) measles
   (E) shingles

156. A drug that is effective in the treatment of alcohol withdrawal syndromes and in the prevention of delirium tremens is

   (A) disulfiram (Antabuse)
   (B) methadone (Dolophine)
   (C) phenytoin (Dilantin)
   (D) haloperidol (Haldol)
   (E) chlordiazepoxide (Librium)

157. Which of the following is TRUE of bacitracin?

   (A) It is too sensitizing to use topically.
   (B) Nephrotoxicity limits its parenteral use.
   (C) It is an aminoglycoside antibiotic.
   (D) It is most effective in treating *Pseudomonas* infections
   (E) Its exhibits cross-resistance with the penicillins.

158. Which of the following agents would be effective when administered orally to relieve symptoms of Parkinson's disease?

   (A) reserpine (Serpasil)
   (B) dopamine (Intropin)
   (C) haloperidol (Haldol)
   (D) chlorpromazine (Thorazine)
   (E) selegiline (Eldepryl)

159. Sucralfate (Carafate) is employed in the treatment of

   (A) diabetes insipidus
   (B) duodenal ulcers
   (C) dysmenorrhea
   (D) urinary tract infections
   (E) diabetes mellitus

160. An advantage of albuterol (Proventil) over isoproterenol (Isuprel) in the treatment of bronchial asthma is that albuterol

   (A) has more beta agonist activity than isoproterenol
   (B) has no effect on the heart
   (C) has alpha-adrenergic activity
   (D) is more selective for beta$_2$-adrenergic receptors
   (E) has a more rapid onset of action

161. Fosinopril (Monopril) can best be classified as a(n)

   (A) beta-adrenergic blocking agent
   (B) vasodilator
   (C) potassium-sparing diuretic
   (D) angiotensin-converting enzyme inhibitor
   (E) alpha-adrenergic blocking agent

162. Which of the following is TRUE of beclomethasone dipropionate (Beclovent, Vanceril) aerosol?

   (A) It should only be used in the treatment of an acute asthmatic attack.
   (B) It should not be used in a patient who is currently using a theophylline product.
   (C) If used in conjunction with a bronchodilator administered by inhalation, the bronchodilator should be used first.
   (D) The aerosol form is also useful in the treatment of status asthmaticus.
   (E) Beclomethasone is not systemically absorbed by this route.

163. Agents useful in the treatment of bronchial asthma usually

   (A) block both alpha- and beta-adrenergic receptors
   (B) stimulate alpha receptors but block beta receptors
   (C) stimulate beta receptors but block alpha receptors
   (D) stimulate alpha and/or beta receptors
   (E) inhibit acetylcholinesterase activity

164. Which of the following cancer chemotherapeutic agents is classified as an antimetabolite?

   (A) fluorouracil (Adrucil)
   (B) cyclophosphamide (Cytoxan)
   (C) mechlorethamine (Mustargen)
   (D) chlorambucil (Leukeran)
   (E) cisplatin (Platinol)

165. Which of the following antihistamines would be LEAST likely to cause sedation?

(A) diphenhydramine (Benadryl)
(B) terfenadine (Seldane)
(C) promethazine (Phenergan)
(D) dimenhydrinate (Dramamine)
(E) tripelennamine (PBZ)

DIRECTIONS (Questions 166 through 250): Each group of items in this section consists of lettered headings followed by a set of numbered words or phrases. For each numbered word or phrase, select the ONE lettered heading that is most closely associated with it. Each lettered heading may be selected once, more than once, or not at all.

Questions 166 through 170

MATCH the numbered drug with the lettered antihypertensive mechanism most closely associated with it.

(A) vasodilator
(B) centrally acting adrenoreceptor agonist
(C) diuretic
(D) beta blocker
(E) angiotensin-converting enzyme inhibitor

166. atenolol (Tenormin) D

167. hydralazine (Apresoline) A

168. ramipril (Altace) E

169. amiloride HCl (Midamor) C

170. guanabenz acetate (Wytensin) B

Questions 171 through 182

MATCH the lettered side effect, adverse effect, or hypersensitivity reaction with the associated numbered drug.

(A) positive Coombs' test
(B) Stevens–Johnson syndrome
(C) gynecomastia
(D) peripheral neuritis
(E) bronchospasm

171. spironolactone (Aldactone) C

172. metoprolol (Lopressor) E

173. methyldopa (Aldomet) A

174. sulfasalazine (Azulfidine) B

(A) nephrotoxicity, ototoxicity
(B) discoloration of urine and sweat
(C) tardive dyskinesia
(D) gingival hyperplasia
(E) alopecia

175. rifampin (Rifadin) B

176. phenytoin D

177. netilmicin (Netromycin) A

178. thioridazine (Mellaril) C

(A) photosensitization
(B) hemorrhagic cystitis
(C) cholestatic jaundice
(D) dysgeusia
(E) agranulocytosis

179. clozapine (Clozaril) E

180. erythromycin estolate (Ilosone) C

181. cyclophosphamide (Cytoxan) B

182. captopril (Capoten) D

Questions 183 through 198

MATCH the lettered pharmacologic category with the associated numbered drug.

(A) anticonvulsant
(B) antianxiety agent
(C) antidepressant
(D) antiemetic
(E) antipsychotic

183. haloperidol (Haldol) E

184. bupropion (Wellbutrin) C

185. ondansetron (Zofran) D

186. alprazolam (Xanax) B

(A) gastrointestinal stimulant
(B) antipsychotic agent
(C) skeletal muscle relaxant
(D) antihistamine
(E) monoamine oxidase inhibitor

187. metoclopramide (Reglan) A

188. phenelzine (Nardil) E

189. dantrolene (Dantrium) *C*

190. terfenadine (Seldane) *D*

    (A) calcium channel antagonist
    (B) anti-inflammatory
    (C) antineoplastic
    (D) anticholinergic
    (E) hypoglycemic

191. piroxicam (Feldene) *D*

192. trihexyphenidyl (Artane) *D*

193. bepridil (Vascor) *A*

194. tamoxifen (Nolvadex) *C*

    (A) xanthine oxidase inhibitor
    (B) hypnotic
    (C) diuretic
    (D) antifungal
    (E) hypoglycemic

195. allopurinol (Zyloprim) *A*

196. clotrimazole (Lotrimin) *D*

197. estazolam (ProSom) *B*

198. glyburide (Micronase) *E*

Questions 199 through 213

MATCH the lettered therapeutic indication most closely corresponding to the numbered brand name.

    (A) systemic candidiasis
    (B) absence seizures
    (C) peptic ulcer
    (D) bronchial asthma
    (E) hypertension

199. Nizoral *A*

200. Axid *C*

201. Depakote *B*

202. Prinivil *E*

203. Intal *D*

    (A) bronchial asthma
    (B) muscle spasm
    (C) hypertension
    (D) glaucoma
    (E) gout

204. Benemid *E*

205. Sectral *B* *Acebutolol*

206. Tornalate *A*

207. Betagan *D*

208. Lioresal *B*

    (A) pain
    (B) urinary tract infection
    (C) manic–depressive illness
    (D) vulvovaginal candidiasis
    (E) angina pectoris

209. Maxaquin *B* *fluuroquinolone*

210. Buprenex *A*

211. Eskalith *C*

212. Minitran *E*

213. Mycostatin *D*

Questions 214 through 218

MATCH the lettered antihypertensive agent with the numbered adverse effect with which it is most closely associated.

    (A) diazoxide (Hyperstat)
    (B) doxazosin (Cardura)
    (C) procainamide (Procan SR)
    (D) guanethidine (Ismelin)
    (E) reserpine (Serpasil)

214. syncope after first dose *B*

215. drug-induced SLE *C*

216. mental depression *E*

217. drug-induced inhibition of ejaculation *D*

218. sodium retention *A*

Questions 219 through 223

Deficiencies of certain substances may result in disease. MATCH the lettered substance believed to be deficient in the body with the numbered resulting disease.

    (A) ascorbic acid
    (B) cyanocobalamin
    (C) niacin
    (D) vitamin A
    (E) thiamine

219. pellagra C

220. pernicious anemia B

221. beriberi E

222. scurvy A

223. nyctalopia D

Questions 224 through 228

MATCH the lettered antimicrobial agent with the numbered disease for which it would be a drug of choice.

    (A) netilmicin
    (B) griseofulvin
    (C) ethambutol
    (D) pentamidine isethionate
    (E) vancomycin

224. *Pneumocystis carinii* D

225. *Pseudomonas aeruginosa* A

226. pseudomembranous colitis E

227. tinea capitis B

228. tuberculosis C

Questions 229 through 234

The numbered group of laxatives below is preceded by a lettered list of mechanisms by which laxatives act. MATCH the mechanism with the laxative. Letters may be used more than once.

    (A) draws water into intestinal tract by osmosis
    (B) forms bulk by absorbing water
    (C) softens stools by lubrication
    (D) softens stools by lowering surface tension
    (E) stimulates intestinal wall

229. phenolphthalein E

230. polycarbophil B

231. mineral oil C

232. docusate calcium D

233. psyllium B

234. sodium biphosphate A

Questions 235 through 239

MATCH the lettered antineoplastic drug with the most appropriate numbered category.

    (A) carboplatin (Paraplatin)
    (B) fluorouracil (Adrucil)
    (C) doxorubicin HCl (Rubex)
    (D) flutamide (Eulexin)
    (E) vinblastine sulfate (Velban)

235. antimetabolite B

236. alkylating agent A

237. hormone D

238. mitotic inhibitor E

239. antibiotic C

Questions 240 through 244

MATCH the lettered adverse drug reaction most closely associated with the use of the numbered drug.

    (A) ototoxicity
    (B) conjunctivitis
    (C) flushing
    (D) drowsiness
    (E) pneumonitis

240. Isordil C

241. Blenoxane E

242. Nebcin A

243. Paxipam D

244. Accutane B

    (A) hypokalemia
    (B) tardive dyskinesia
    (C) hyperkalemia
    (D) fluid retention
    (E) nephrotoxicity
    (F) aplastic anemia

245. Bumex A

246. Premarin D

247. Garamycin E

248. Chloromycetin F

249. Midamor C

250. Trilafon B

Answers and Explanations

1. (C) Theophylline products tend to cause insomnia, palpitations, nausea, vomiting, and many other adverse effects. *(3:861)*

2. (A) Epinephrine is a sympathomimetic agent that produces alpha$_1$- as well as beta$_1$- and beta$_2$-adrenergic agonist activity. It can, therefore, be expected to produce bronchodilation, cardiac stimulation, and vasoconstriction. Because it is rapidly destroyed in the GI tract, it is generally administered by IM or SC injection or by inhalation. *(3:844)*

3. (D) Epinephrine is a nonspecific alpha$_1$- as well as a beta$_1$- and beta$_2$-agonist. Its rapid destruction in the GI tract limits its use in oral OTC or Rx products. Aqueous solutions of epinephrine undergo oxidation upon standing. *(3:856)*

4. (E) Dipivefrin (Prefrin) is a prodrug that is much more rapidly (17X) absorbed into the anterior chamber than epinephrine. Once absorbed, the drug is converted to epinephrine by enzymatic hydrolysis. It produces the same therapeutic effects as epinephrine with fewer adverse effects. *(3:2045)*

5. (D) Heparin is an anticoagulant that affects many steps in the coagulation pathway, thereby preventing thrombosis formation and prolonging clotting time (when administered in therapeutic doses). Heparin will not dissolve existing clots but will prevent their extension. *(3:253)*

6. (D) Diltiazem (Cardizem) is a calcium channel blocking agent employed in the treatment of angina pectoris. Sustained release forms of the drug are also employed in the treatment of hypertension. *(3:660)*

7. (B) Streptokinase (Kabikinase, Streptase) is a thrombolytic enzyme that acts with plasminogen to produce a complex that converts plasminogen to the proteolytic enzyme plasmin, which degrades fibrin clots. Streptokinase is usually administered intravenously. *(3:275,280)*

8. (B) Gold compounds such as auranofin (Ridaura), gold sodium thiomalate (Myochrysine), and aurothioglucose (Solganal) are used to suppress or prevent, but not cure, arthritis and synovitis. Auranofin is administered orally, while the other compounds are administered by the IM route. All gold compounds may cause serious adverse effects, including dermatitis, renal damage, and blood dyscrasias. *(3:1141–45)*

9. (D) Procainamide and quinidine are both classified as Group 1A antiarrhythmic drugs. These are local anesthetics or membrane stabilizers that depress phase 0 and prolong the duration of the action potential. *(3:586–88)*

10. (A) Tocainide (Tonocard), mexiletine (Mexitil), and lidocaine (Xylocaine) are classified as Group 1B antiarrhythmic agents. They slightly depress phase 0 and may shorten the action potential. *(3:586–88)*

11. (D) Acetylcysteine (Mucomyst) is primarily employed as a mucolytic in the treatment of respiratory diseases in which mucus is produced. It is also used as an antidote in the treatment of acetaminophen poisoning. *(3:877–9)*

12. (A) Epinephrine is available in combination with lidocaine in a number of different products. It is used to cause local vasoconstriction, thereby reducing the rate of lidocaine removal from the local injection site. *(3:2495)*

13. (D) Cholestyramine (Questran) is an anion exchange resin that binds bile acids in the intestine, causing them to be removed in the feces. This causes further breakdown of cholesterol to bile acids, as well as a decrease in low-density lipoproteins (LDL) and serum cholesterol levels. *(3:821)*

14. (B) Colestipol (Colestid) is an anion exchange resin similar in action to cholestyramine that reduces low-density lipoprotein and serum cholesterol levels. *(3:821)*

15. (A) Nicotinamide, unlike nicotinic acid (niacin), does not lower plasma lipoprotein concentrations or cause vasodilation. It does, however, produce the same vitamin actions as nicotinic acid. *(3:21)*

16. (E) Cyproheptadine (Periactin), an antihistamine,

is an H_1-receptor antagonist. Unlike other antihistamines, however, cyproheptadine also antagonizes the action of 5-hydroxytryptamine (5-HT, serotonin), which makes it particularly useful as an antipruritic agent. *(3:925)*

17. (B) Dendritic keratitis is an ophthalmic viral infection caused by the action of herpes simplex virus. Idoxuridine (Herplex) blocks herpes simplex virus reproduction and thereby helps to control this condition. *(3:2099)*

18. (B) Trifluridine (Viroptic) is an antiviral product employed in the treatment of herpes simplex infections. The other compounds are all antifungal agents. *(3:2099)*

19. (C) Tretinoin (Retin-A) is vitamin A acid. It appears to be useful in the topical treatment of acne because of its ability to stimulate mitotic activity and increase the turnover of follicular epithelial cells. It does not have antimicrobial activity. *(3:2164)*

20. (A) Nadolol (Corgard) is a beta-adrenergic blocking agent. Such drugs should be avoided in patients with bronchospastic disorders because they may cause bronchoconstriction. *(3:708)*

21. (A) Dopamine (Intropin, Dopastat) is an endogenous catecholamine that is a precursor for epinephrine. It acts directly and indirectly on alpha- and beta$_1$-adrenergic receptors to produce an inotropic effect, increased cardiac output, and increased systolic pressure. It is commonly employed in the treatment of shock syndrome. *(3:679)*

22. (A) Tofranil is a tricyclic antidepressant, while Cogentin, Artane, and Kemadrin are anticholinergic drugs used in treating Parkinson's disease. Symmetrel appears to cause dopamine release, thereby improving Parkinson's disease symptoms. *(3:1472)*

23. (A) Albuterol is an agonist acting on beta$_1$- and beta$_2$-adrenergic receptors to produce bronchodilation and potential cardiac stimulation. Albuterol is considered to be beta$_2$-specific, making it less likely than many other sympathomimetic agents to cause cardiac stimulation. *(3:844)*

24. (B) Histamine is an endogenous substance that can cause capillary dilation as well as stimulate gastric acid secretion. *(6:578–9)*

25. (E) Nizatidine (Axid) is an H_2-receptor antagonist used in inhibiting gastric acid secretion. The other agents are H_1-histamine receptor antagonists used in treating allergic symptoms. *(3:1520)*

26. (E) Hypertrichosis is an excessive growth of body hair. It is not associated with cannabis use. The other effects are common cannabis effects.
(6:550–2)

27. (D) Dexamethasone is about 25 times as potent as hydrocortisone, five to six times as potent as pred-

nisone, four to six times as potent as triamcinolone, and 20 to 25 times as potent as cortisone. *(3:438)*

28. (E) Benzoyl peroxide is an oxidizing agent found in many OTC products that are used in the treatment of acne. It is believed to exert an antibacterial effect, thereby reducing the level of *Propionibacterium acnes* on the skin surface. *(3:2170)*

29. (E) Potassium clavulanate is an agent capable of inactivating beta-lactamase enzymes that are often found in microorganisms resistant to penicillin. The addition of potassium clavulanate to ampicillin extends the spectrum of antimicrobial coverage of ampicillin to include beta-lactamase–producing organisms. *(3:1639)*

30. (B) Oxytocin is an endogenous hormone produced by the posterior pituitary gland. It is a uterine stimulant that promotes uterine contractions, particularly during labor. The other hormones are released by the anterior pituitary gland. *(3:415)*

31. (C) During the menstrual cycle, levels of follicle-stimulating hormone (FSH) and luteinizing hormone (LH) vary widely. At the time of ovulation the concentration of each of these hormones reaches a peak, coinciding with the release of the ovum and the complete development of a mature endometrial wall. *(6:1348)*

32. (D) Liotrix consists of a uniform mixture of synthetic levothyroxine sodium (T_4) and liothyronine sodium (T_3) in a ratio of 4:1 by weight. It is used in products such as Euthroid and Thyrolar as a thyroid hormone supplement. *(3:501)*

33. (E) Methimazole (Tapazole) and propylthiouracil are antithyroid agents that inhibit synthesis of thyroid hormone and thus are useful in the treatment of hyperthyroidism. *(3:504)*

34. (C) Promethazine (Phenergan) is a phenothiazine derivative with antihistaminic as well as antiemetic and sedative properties. The other agents listed are also phenothiazines but do not exert any significant antihistaminic action. *(3:923)*

35. (B) Carbamazepine (Tegretol) is an anticonvulsant drug indicated for the treatment of trigeminal neuralgia as well as a variety of seizure disorders. Patients using this drug must be carefully monitored for the development of aplastic anemia and agranulocytosis. *(3:1392)*

36. (B) Buspirone (BuSpar) is a relatively new anxiolytic agent which, unlike the benzodiazepines, barbiturates and carbamates, does not produce significant sedative, muscle relaxant, or anticonvulsant effects. *(3:1208)*

37. (D) Theophylline use is associated with bronchodilation, central nervous system and cardiac stimulation, and stimulation of gastric acid secretion. Because theophylline and caffeine are both methylxanthines, they share many common pharmacologic effects. *(3:858)*

38. (B) Penicillins and other beta-lactam antimicrobial agents act by being incorporated into an actively growing bacterial cell wall. This causes defects in the cell wall, causing disintegration and destruction of the bacterial cell. Since human cells do not have cell walls, they are not adversely affected by such antimicrobial agents. *(6:1066–7)*

39. (D) The mechanism of action of the penicillins is most similar to cephalosporins such as cefaclor (Ceclor); both have a beta lactam ring incorporated into their structure and exhibit a similar mechanism of action. *(6:1066–7)*

40. (C) Probenecid is a uricosuric and renal tubular blocking agent. It is capable of inhibiting the tubular secretion of penicillins and cephalosporins, thereby increasing the plasma levels of these drugs and prolonging their action in the body. *(3:1148)*

41. (C) Penicillin G potassium strength is usually measured in milligrams or units. Each milligram of the pure drug is equivalent to 1600 units of activity. Thus, 250 mg of penicillin G is approximately equivalent to 400,000 units of activity. *(3:1613)*

42. (A) Ampicillin and amoxicillin are both aminopenicillins that are virtually identical in their antimicrobial spectrum. Amoxicillin has more complete absorption than ampicillin, a three-times-daily dosing regimen, and fewer GI adverse effects than ampicillin. Amoxicillin also reaches higher blood levels than an equal dose of ampicillin. *(3:1637)*

43. (A) Chlorhexidine (Hibiclens) and hexachlorophene (pHisoHex) are antiseptic agents used in surgical scrub and bacteriostatic skin cleanser products. Both provide a residual bacteriostatic effect on the cleansed surface, which helps sustain a lowered bacterial count. Chlorhexidine is also used in antiseptic mouthwash products such as Peridex. *(3:2305–5)*

44. (C) Penicillamine (Cuprimine, Depen) is a chelating agent used in treating Wilson's disease, a disorder characterized by an excessive level of copper in the body. It is also capable of binding with iron, mercury, lead, and arsenic. Penicillamine has also been used in the treatment of rheumatoid arthritis. *(3:2532)*

45. (B) Polymyxin B and colistin (Coly-Mycin S) are closely related chemical compounds that are cationic detergents and act as antimicrobial agents. They have the strongest antimicrobial action against gram-negative organisms. Because of their potential for producing severe nephrotoxicity, they are rarely used systemically. *(6:1138)*

46. (B) Chloramphenicol (Chloromycetin) is a broad-spectrum antimicrobial agent. Its use has been asso-ciated with the development of serious and sometimes fatal blood dyscrasias, including aplastic anemia. As a result, chloramphenicol is only indicated for the treatment of serious infections that are not responsive to less dangerous drugs. *(3:1711)*

47. (A) Dicloxacillin (Dynapen, Pathocil) is one of several antimicrobial drugs resistant to beta-lactamase (penicillinase) enzymes produced by some microorganisms. Other drugs resistant to such enzymes include methicillin, oxacillin, nafcillin, and cloxacillin. *(3:1624–9)*

48. (D) Sulfonamides exert their bacteriostatic action by competitively antagonizing para-aminobenzoic acid (PABA). Sulfonamide resistance may occur if an organism produces excessive amounts of PABA or if PABA-containing products are used concurrently with a sulfonamide drug. *(3:1804)*

49. (D) Dapsone is a sulfone that is bactericidal and bacteriostatic against *Mycobacterium leprae*, the organism believed to be the cause of leprosy (Hansen's disease). *(3:1895)*

50. (B) Doxycycline is the longest acting of the tetracyclines, having a normal serum half-life of 15 to 25 hours. Half-lives for other tetracyclines are tetracycline (6 to 12 hours), demeclocycline (12 to 16 hours), minocycline (11 to 18 hours), and oxytetracycline (6 to 12 hours). *(3:1723)*

51. (E) Tricyclic antidepressants such as amitriptyline exert three major pharmacologic actions: They inhibit the reuptake of biogenic amines into adrenergic nerve terminals, induce sedation, and produce peripheral and central anticholinergic actions. *(3:1220)*

52. (A) Haloperidol (Haldol) is an antipsychotic agent; the other agents have antidepressant activity. *(3:1279)*

53. (B) Aluminum-containing antacids (eg, aluminum hydroxide) tend to cause constipation because of their astringent effect on the GI tract. They may also bind phosphate, thus potentially lowering serum phosphate levels. *(6:906)*

54. (E) Pyridoxine, or vitamin B_6, is water soluble. Cholecalciferol is a form of vitamin D, tocopherol is a form of vitamin E, and phytonadione is a form of vitamin K. The latter three vitamins, as well as vitamin A, are fat soluble. *(3:22)*

55. (E) Carbidopa is a dopa-decarboxylase inhibitor that prevents peripheral decarboxylation of levodopa in the body. This reduces the adverse effects associated with peripheral dopa decarboxylation and reduces the dose of levodopa required to control a patient with Parkinson's disease. Carbidopa is available alone (Lodosyn) or in combination with levodopa (Sinemet). *(3:1468–71)*

56. (D) Theophylline and caffeine are methylxanthines. They may act in the body to produce diuresis and bronchodilation, as well as cardiac and central nervous system stimulation.   *(6:620–3)*

57. (B) Fenfluramine HCl (Pondimin) is an anorexiant which, unlike other anorexiants, depresses rather than stimulates the CNS. The other agents listed are anorexiant drugs that tend to stimulate the CNS.   *(3:1027)*

58. (A) Lactase enzyme is effective in treating symptoms of lactose intolerance. These symptoms are most evident shortly after consuming a lactose-containing food and may include bloating and diarrhea. Lactase enzyme is available as a liquid (Lactaid), caplets (Lactaid), capsules (Lactrase), or as chewable tablets (Dairy Ease). It is also added to some commercial dairy products.   *(3:196)*

59. (A) Hyperglycemia is not a problem commonly associated with the use of isotretinoin (Accutane). Cheilitis (cracked margins of the lips), conjunctivitis, and dry mouth occur in a large proportion of patients receiving this drug.   *(3:2168)*

60. (E) The use of isotretinoin (Accutane), a vitamin A derivative, is associated with an incidence of cheilitis greater than 90%. The drug is administered orally and must not be used in pregnant women because it carries a high risk of causing fetal deformities.   *(3:2166–8)*

61. (B) Endorphins are endogenous (naturally found in the body) opioid peptides that are released in response to stress.   *(6:486–7)*

62. (E) Crack is a free-base form of cocaine. It is generally smoked and rapidly absorbed through the respiratory membranes. Within seconds, it reaches the brain and produces central nervous system stimulation and euphoria. Dependence may occur with only a single dose of the drug.   *(6:541)*

63. (D) A uricosuric drug is one that promotes the excretion of uric acid in the urine. Uricosuric agents such as probenecid (Benemid) and sulfinpyrazone (Anturane) inhibit tubular reabsorption of urate and promote urate excretion. They are used to treat hyperuricemia associated with gout or gouty arthritis.   *(3:1148–51)*

64. (D) Alteplase (Activase) is a tissue plasminogen activator produced by recombinant DNA technology. It is used in the management of acute myocardial infarction. Once injected into the circulation, alteplase binds to fibrin in a thrombus and converts the entrapped plasminogen to plasmin. This produces local fibrinolysis and assists in reopening a blocked coronary blood vessel.   *(3:267)*

65. (D) Cimetidine (Tagamet) is an H_2-histamine receptor antagonist used to decrease gastric acid secretion in patients with peptic ulcer disease. It has been shown to inhibit the hepatic metabolism of drugs metabolized via the cytochrome P-450 pathway, thereby delaying metabolism and increasing serum levels. Cimetidine may affect the metabolism of drugs such as theophylline, some benzodiazepines, phenytoin, and warfarin.   *(3:1525)*

66. (A) Allopurinol (Zyloprim) is a xanthine oxidase inhibitor that does not exert a uricosuric effect but does prevent the conversion of hypoxanthine to uric acid. It is employed in the treatment of gout as well as in the management of patients receiving therapy for leukemia and other malignancies that raise uric acid levels.   *(3:1152)*

67. (E) Dihydrotachysterol is a synthetic product of tachysterol, a substance similar to vitamin D. It is used in combination with calcium and parathyroid hormone in the treatment of hypoparathyroidism.   *(3:11)*

68. (C) Lovastatin (Mevacor) is a cholesterol-lowering agent used to reduce elevated total and LDL cholesterol levels in patients with primary hypercholesterolemia when response to diet and other nondrug approaches have not been successful. Its use is associated with hepatic dysfunction and danger to the developing fetus.   *(3:825–7)*

69. (C) Norethindrone is a progestin. All of the other products are anabolic steroids.   *(3:379–80)*

70. (D) The autonomic nervous system consists of two major branches, the sympathetic (adrenergic) branch and the parasympathetic (cholinergic) branch. Each branch utilizes different neurotransmitters. For example, the sympathetic branch utilizes norepinephrine while the parasympathetic branch utilizes acetylcholine.   *(6:122)*

71. (A) Pentoxifylline (Trental), a methylxanthine derivative, is a hemorheologic agent that enhances blood flow by decreasing blood viscosity and improving erythrocyte flexibility. This is useful in patients with chronic peripheral arterial disease.   *(3:281)*

72. (C) Methadone (Dolophine) is a narcotic agonist analgesic with actions similar to those of morphine. It is twice as potent when used parenterally than when used orally. It is employed in the treatment of severe pain and in maintenance treatment of narcotic addiction.   *(3:1046)*

73. (A) A pure narcotic antagonist is one that reverses the effects of opioids without producing agonist action of its own. Naloxone (Narcan) is an example of a pure narcotic antagonist. Other drugs listed have agonist and some antagonist activity.   *(3:2508)*

74. (B) Ergot alkaloids such as ergonovine maleate (Ergotrate) and methylergonovine maleate (Methergine) are used as uterine stimulants to facilitate delivery and to manage postpartum atony and bleeding.   *(3:41̇*

75. (C) Diarrhea is not commonly associated with morphine use. Constipation is a more likely effect since morphine decreases peristaltic activity in the GI tract. Constriction of the pupils, CNS and respiratory depression, and nausea and vomiting are all effects associated with morphine use. *(3:1036)*

76. (A) Primidone (Mysoline) is an anticonvulsant drug used in a variety of convulsive disorders. Primidone and its two active metabolites, phenobarbital and phenylethylmalonamide (PEMA) have anticonvulsant activity. *(3:1386)*

77. (A) Etidronate (Didronel) is an agent used in treating Paget's disease of the bone, a condition characterized by abnormal bone resorption and the development of fractures. The use of the drug seems to decrease the dissolution of hydroxyapatite crystals, the building blocks of bone tissue. *(3:511)*

78. (B) Salmon calcitonin (Calcimar, Miacalcin) is a polypeptide hormone derived from salmon. It is similar in action to mammalian calcitonin produced in the thyroid gland. This agent inhibits bone resorption much like etidronate (Didronel) does. *(3:508)*

79. (C) The naturally occurring adrenal cortical steroids exert both salt-retaining (mineralocorticoid) and anti-inflammatory (glucocorticoid) activity. The synthetic steroids prednisone and prednisolone exert similar actions on the body. The use of these agents is often associated with fluid and sodium retention. *(3:438–44)*

80. (E) Ondansetron (Zofran) is a selective serotonin receptor antagonist used for the prevention of nausea and vomiting associated with cancer chemotherapy. It is administered by IV infusion over 15 minutes beginning 30 minutes before the start of emetogenic chemotherapy. *(3:1185–8)*

81. (E) Amrinone (Inocor), like digoxin, is a drug that produces a positive inotropic effect. In addition, amrinone also produces vasodilation. The drug is used for the short-term management of congestive heart failure in patients who have not responded adequately to digoxin, diuretics, or vasodilators. Use of the drug has been associated with the development of thrombocytopenia, arrhythmias, and GI upset. It is administered by IV bolus or infusion. *(3:569–71)*

82. (D) Dipyridamole (Persantine) inhibits platelet adhesion. It is used as an adjunct to coumarin anticoagulants in the prevention of thromboembolic complications of cardiac valve replacement. It is also used either alone or in combination with aspirin for the prevention of myocardial reinfarction and reduction of mortality after myocardial infarction. (This use is unapproved by the FDA.) *(3:250)*

83. (B) Lactulose (Cephulac, Chronulac), a synthetic disaccharide, is an analog of lactose. Unlike lactose, which is hydrolyzed enzymatically to its monosaccharide components, oral doses of lactulose pass to the colon virtually unchanged. In the colon, bacteria chemically convert the lactulose to low molecular weight acids and carbon dioxide. The acids produce an osmotic effect that draws water into the colon and makes the stools more watery. They also permit ammonia in the body to be converted to ammonium ion in the acidic colon and allow it to be eliminated in the stool. *(3:1579)*

84. (C) Ricinoleic acid, the active agent in castor oil, is formed in the small intestine. It facilitates formation and passage of a fluid stool. *(3:1562)*

85. (D) Liothyronine sodium (Cytomel) is a synthetic form of the natural thyroid hormone T_3. Approximately 25 μg of liothyronine sodium is equivalent to 60 mg (1 grain) of dessicated thyroid (Thyroid, USP). Liothyronine is useful in patients who are allergic to dessicated thyroid and require thyroid supplementation. *(3:500)*

86. (D) Calcium carbonate and sodium bicarbonate may cause rebound hyperacidity and milk-alkali syndrome, a condition that may appear in an acute or chronic form. These antacids are associated with rebound hyperacidity since they may raise the pH of the stomach to a level high enough (alkaline) to permit release of gastrin, a stimulator of hydrochloric acid release.

87. (D) Aluminum hydroxide gel may irreversibly bind phosphate in the gut, causing it to be eliminated from the body. This may be used to treat patients with hyperphosphatemia or to prevent the formation of phosphate urinary stones. *(3:1484)*

88. (B) Piroxicam (Feldene) is a nonsteroidal anti-inflammatory agent (NSAID) and should be avoided in patients who are sensitive to aspirin because of possible cross-sensitivity reactions. *(3:1111)*

89. (B) Single aspirin doses are known to prolong bleeding time, which is believed to occur by the acetylation of platelet cyclooxygenase by aspirin. This in turn prevents the synthesis of thromboxane, a prostaglandin that is a potent vasoconstrictor and inducer of platelet aggregation. *(3:1090)*

90. (D) Both triamterene (Dyrenium) and spironolactone (Aldactone) inhibit sodium reabsorption in the distal tubule. Spironolactone is an aldosterone antagonist that prevents the formation of a protein important for sodium transport in the distal tubule. Triamterene inhibits sodium reabsorption induced by aldosterone and inhibits basal sodium reabsorption. Triamterene is not an aldosterone antagonist. *(3:542)*

91. (B) Labetalol (Normodyne, Trandate) is a nonselective beta-adrenergic blocking agent primarily used for the management of hypertension. In addition to its beta-blocking action, labetalol is also able to block alpha$_1$-adrenergic receptors. This lowers standing blood pressure and may result in hypotension and syncope. *(3:722)*

92. (D) Colchicine is a substance that may be employed orally or parenterally to relieve the pain of acute gout. It appears to act by reducing the inflammatory response to deposited urate crystals and by diminishing phagocytosis. Although it relieves pain in cases of acute gout, colchicine is not an analgesic or a uricosuric agent. Vomiting, diarrhea, abdominal pain, and nausea have all been reported with the use of colchicine. Bone marrow suppression and thrombocytopenia have also been associated with colchicine use. *(3:1158)*

93. (D) Oxymetazoline (Afrin, Duration) and xylometazoline (Otrivin), when used as topical nasal decongestants, produce an effect that may persist for 8 to 12 hours. This is in sharp contrast to other topical nasal decongestant drugs such as phenylephrine, naphazoline, and tetrahydrozoline, which require dosing at 3- to 4-hour intervals. *(3:888)*

94. (B) The use of gold compounds such as auranofin (Ridaura), gold sodium thiomalate (Myochrysine), and aurothioglucose (Solganal) has been associated with a wide variety of adverse effects, including blood dyscrasias, dermatitis, and renal disorders. Patients using such compounds must be constantly monitored for adverse effects. *(3:1144)*

95. (A) Morphine is the major ingredient in Opium Tincture USP and Camporated Opium Tincture (Paregoric). It is employed in these products because of its antiperistaltic activity, particularly in the treatment of diarrhea. *(3:1042)*

96. (A) Iron is primarily absorbed in the duodenum and the jejunum by an active transport mechanism. The ferrous salt form is absorbed approximately three times more readily than the ferric form. The presence of food, particularly dairy products, eggs, coffee, and tea, in the GI tract may decrease the absorption of iron significantly while the concurrent administration of vitamin C maintains iron in the ferrous state, thereby enhancing its absorption from the GI tract. *(3:200)*

97. (D) Iron is an essential component of hemoglobin, myoglobin, and several enzymes. Approximately two thirds of total body iron is in the circulating red blood cells as part of hemoglobin, the most important carrier of oxygen in the body. *(3:200)*

98. (D) The development of tolerance to the action of nitroglycerine may occur with repeated use. Sensitivity to the action of nitroglycerin is generally restored after several hours of withdrawal from the drug. *(3:575)*

99. (E) When mixing regular insulin with other insulin products, the regular insulin should be drawn into the syringe first. This will prevent contamination of the regular insulin with the suspension products (lente, NPH). *(3:470)*

100. (B) Lovastatin (Mevacor) is a cholesterol-lowering agent contraindicated for use during pregnancy because of its great potential for causing fetal harm. The drug is in FDA pregnancy category X. *(3:826)*

101. (E) Scopolamine is available in a transdermal patch dosage form (Transderm Scōp) for prevention of nausea and vomiting associated with motion sickness in adults. It is applied to the skin behind the ear at least 4 hours before the antiemetic effect is required. The drug is then released from the transdermal product for 3 days. *(3:1178)*

102. (B) Desmopressin acetate (DDAVP) is the synthetic analog of naturally occurring human antidiuretic hormone (ADH) produced by the posterior pituitary gland. It is administered intranasally for the treatment of primary nocturnal enuresis. A single dose of the drug will produce an antidiuretic effect lasting from 8 to 20 hours. *(3:412)*

103. (D) Triazolam (Halcion) is a benzodiazepine hypnotic agent that is not metabolized to form active metabolites. Since it has the shortest half-life (1.5 to 5.5 hours) of any of the hypnotics, it is often used in elderly patients. The development of anterograde amnesia has been reported in some patients receiving therapeutic doses of triazolam. *(3:1324)*

104. (A) Dicloxacillin (Dynapen, Pathocil) is a beta-lactamase–resistant penicillin and would be suitable for treating an infection caused by beta-lactamase–producing staphylococci. Other penicillins that would also be suitable include oxacillin (Prostaphlin, Bactocill), cloxacillin (Cloxapen, Tegopen), nafcillin (Nafcil, Unipen), and methicillin (Staphcillin). All of these products are available for oral use with the exception of methicillin, which is administered either IM or IV. *(3:1624–9)*

105. (A) Cyanocobalamin, or vitamin B_{12}, is essential for proper growth, cell reproduction, formation of blood components, and many other functions. In order for cyanocobalamin to be properly absorbed from the GI tract it must combine with a glycoprotein called intrinsic factor. In the absence of proper levels of intrinsic factor, cyanocobalamin is administered parenterally. *(6:1297)*

106. (C) Phenytoin (Dilantin) is an anticonvulsant used in controlling grand mal and psychomotor seizures as well as other convulsive disorders. Adverse effects commonly associated with phenytoin use include nystagmus, gingival hyperplasia, ataxia, and many other neurological, dermatological, and hematological disorders. Because of the high frequency of adverse effects associated with the use of this drug, patients must be monitored closely during therapy. *(3:1374)*

107. (E) Timolol maleate (Timoptic) is a noncardioselective beta-adrenergic blocking agent used ophthalmically to reduce intraocular pressure in patients with chronic open-angle glaucoma and other disorders. While the exact mechanism of action of this and similar ophthalmic beta blockers has not been completely established, it appears to be due to the ability of the drug to reduce the production of aqueous humor. *(3:2047)*

108. (E) Betaxolol (Betoptic) is a beta-adrenergic blocking agent used ophthalmically to reduce intraocular pressure, particularly in patients with chronic open-angle glaucoma. Unlike other ophthalmic beta blockers, the action of betaxolol is more specific for beta$_1$-adrenergic receptors than for beta$_2$-receptors, making it less likely to affect respiratory function. *(3:2047)*

109. (D) Pilocarpine (Isopto Carpine, Pilostat) is a direct-acting miotic agent used to decrease elevated intraocular pressure. By causing miosis (constriction of the pupil), greater outflow of aqueous humor is promoted and intraocular pressure falls. Carbachol (Isopto Carbachol) is another direct-acting miotic used in situations when pilocarpine is ineffective or causes adverse effects. *(3:2052)*

110. (C) Atropine is a belladonna alkaloid capable of causing a wide range of effects in the human body. Cardiac stimulation, diminished sweating, reduction of gastric secretion and tone, and mydriasis (dilation of the pupil of the eye) are commonly associated with its administration. *(6:152–7)*

111. (C) Antihistamines are agents that competitively antagonize histamine at the H$_1$-receptor site but do not bind with histamine to inactivate it. Antihistamines do not block histamine release, antibody production, or antigen-antibody reactions. Many of these agents also produce sedation, anticholinergic, and antipruritic actions. Antihistamines are most commonly used to provide symptomatic relief of symptoms associated with perennial and seasonal allergic rhinitis and the common cold. *(3:912)*

112. (A) Haloperidol (Haldol) is an antipsychotic agent available in oral and parenteral forms. It has pharmacologic actions similar to the phenothiazines (sedation, extrapyramidal effects, etc). Chemically, haloperidol is a butyrophenone. *(3:1279)*

113. (E) Tamoxifen (Nolvadex) is an agent that has potent antiestrogenic effects because of its ability to compete with estrogen for binding sites in target tissues such as the breast. It is used in the treatment of metastatic breast cancer in women. Patients with tumors that are estrogen–receptor–positive appear to respond most favorably to tamoxifen. *(3:2400)*

114. (C) Auranofin (Ridaura) is an oral gold product used in the treatment of rheumatoid arthritis. Other gold products, such as gold sodium thiomalate (Myochrysine) and aurothioglucose (Solganal), are administered only by intramuscular injection. Use of gold products has been associated with a wide variety of adverse effects including thrombocytopenia and renal impairment. They do not cure arthritis. *(3:1141–5)*

115. (B) Acetaminophen (Tylenol, APAP) is an agent with analgesic and antipyretic actions similar to aspirin. Unlike aspirin, acetaminophen does not significantly inhibit peripheral prostaglandin synthesis, which may account for its relative lack of anti-inflammatory activity. Acetaminophen does not inhibit platelet function, affect prothrombin time, or produce GI distress. *(3:1084)*

116. (E) Clozapine (Clozaril) is an antipsychotic agent indicated for use in patients who do not respond to standard antipsychotic therapy (phenothiazines, etc). Use of clozapine has been associated with the development of agranulocytosis, a potentially life-threatening blood disorder. Patients being treated with clozapine must have a baseline white blood cell (WBC) and differential count performed before initiation of treatment, as well as a WBC count every week during treatment and for 4 weeks after discontinuing clozapine therapy. *(3:1285)*

117. (D) Propoxyphene (Darvon, Dolene) is a centrally acting narcotic analgesic with a chemical structure similar to methadone. Its analgesic activity is about one half to two thirds that of codeine. The analgesic activity of the drug is only apparent with the use of the dextrorotatory isomer. *(3:1050)*

118. (C) Dactinomycin (Cosmegen) and plicamycin (Mithracin) are antineoplastic agents classified as antibiotics because they are derived from a microbial source. These agents appear to act in a cytotoxic fashion by interfering with DNA and/or RNA synthesis. Their use is associated with the development of nausea and vomiting as well as bone marrow depression. *(3:2428–32)*

119. (C) The anti-inflammatory and analgesic action of aspirin is believed to result from its inhibition of prostaglandin synthesis. Its antipyretic action probably results from its direct action on the hypothalamus and the production of peripheral vasodilation and sweating. *(3:1090)*

120. (E) All of these agents are alpha$_1$-adrenergic blocking agents used in the treatment of hypertension. By causing dilation of arterioles and veins, both supine and standing blood pressure are lowered. The "first-dose" effect is the development of marked hypotension and syncope (fainting) upon administration of the first few doses of the drug. It can be minimized by administering low initial doses of the drug at bedtime. Dosage can be increased gradually until the drug is better tolerated. *(3:755)*

121. (E) Carbon monoxide is a colorless and odorless product of the incomplete combustion of hydrocarbons. When it is inhaled and carried to the blood, it reacts with hemoglobin to form carboxyhemoglobin. This reaction dramatically reduces the oxygen-carrying capacity of the blood and, unless corrected quickly, results in the death of the individual. *(6:1618)*

122. (D) Aspiration of a liquid hydrocarbon such as gasoline or kerosene may result in severe inflammation of pulmonary tissues, interference with gas exchange, pneumonitis, and possible death. Emesis or gastric lavage is avoided in such patients to avoid aspiration. Catharsis using magnesium or sodium sulfate may be attempted. Supportive therapy is recommended for such patients unless antimicrobial agents are required to treat respiratory infection. *(6:1622)*

123. (B) Deferoxamine mesylate (Desferal) is a chelating agent that has a high affinity for ferric iron and a relatively low affinity for calcium. It is usually administered intramuscularly in the treatment of acute iron poisoning. *(6:1611–2)*

124. (A) Acetazolamide (Diamox) is a carbonic anhydrase inhibitor used clinically in the treatment of chronic open-angle glaucoma as well as secondary glaucoma. It is also used for treatment of edema caused by congestive heart failure or drug use, or associated with certain forms of epilepsy. Since acetazolamide increases the excretion of sodium, potassium, bicarbonate, and water, many patients develop an alkaline urine. *(3:522)*

125. (C) Thiazide diuretics such as hydrochlorothiazide (Esidrix, HydroDIURIL) increase the renal excretion of sodium, chloride, and potassium while decreasing the excretion of calcium and uric acid. *(3:525)*

126. (B) Acetazolamide is a carbonic anhydrase inhibitor that increases the excretion of sodium, potassium, bicarbonate, and water, thereby alkalinizing the urine. *(3:522)*

127. (A) Baclofen (Lioresal) is a centrally acting skeletal muscle relaxant that can inhibit both monosynaptic and polysynaptic reflexes at the spinal level. It is indicated for the management of spasticity resulting from multiple sclerosis and in some patients with spinal cord injuries. Baclofen commonly causes central nervous system depression (eg, drowsiness, dizziness, and weakness). *(3:1449–50)*

128. (B) Disulfiram (Antabuse) is an aldehyde dehydrogenase inhibitor. It causes an intolerance to alcohol so that consumption of even a small amount will produce a broad array of unpleasant effects. These include flushing, throbbing headaches, nausea, sweating, and palpitations. The drug is used in the management of selected chronic alcoholics. The drug should only be used with the full knowledge and understanding of the patient. *(3:2581)*

129. (C) Cyclobenzaprine (Flexeril) is a centrally acting skeletal muscle relaxant structurally related to the tricyclic antidepressants, and not related to the MAO inhibitors. It is used as an adjunct to rest and physical therapy for relief of painful muscle spasms. *(3:1439)*

130. (D) Polycarbophil (Mitrolan) is a synthetic hydrophilic compound that is capable of absorbing large amounts of water. It is indicated for use as a bulk laxative in the treatment of constipation. It is also employed in the treatment of diarrhea, where it absorbs excess free fecal water and helps create formed stools. *(3:1569)*

131. (D) Phenobarbital and other barbiturates are capable of inducing hepatic microsomal enzymes. This results in increased metabolism and diminished pharmacologic action of drugs metabolized by these enzymes, such as warfarin, corticosteroids, and oral contraceptives. Patients using these drugs must be monitored carefully for reduced pharmacologic effects and may require dosage adjustment.

132. (E) Diazoxide (Hyperstat) is a nondiuretic antihypertensive agent structurally related to the thiazides. It is used in the emergency reduction of elevated blood pressure. Because diazoxide is rapidly and extensively bound to serum protein, it must be administered by rapid IV injection (bolus). Repeated administration of the drug may cause sodium and water retention and the need for adjuvant diuretic therapy. An oral form of diazoxide (Proglycem) is used in the management of hypoglycemia. *(3:795–7)*

133. (B) Miconazole (Micatin, Monistat) is a broad-spectrum antifungal agent effective against yeast infections (*Candida albicans*) as well as dermatophyte infections (tinea cruris, tinea corporis). Nystatin (Mycostatin, Nilstat) is employed primarily in the treatment of yeast infections, while griseofulvin is used to treat tinea infections. *(3:2219)*

134. (C) Thiopental sodium (Pentothal) is an ultrashort-acting barbiturate generally administered intravenously and used as a supplement to other anesthetic agents in the induction of anesthesia. Because of its high lipid solubility, thiopental has a very rapid onset of action (30 to 40 seconds) and a brief duration of action (20 to 30 minutes), making it a useful agent in brief surgical procedures. *(3:1346)*

135. (D) Lypressin (Diapid) is a synthetic vasopressin analog possessing antidiuretic activity without producing a pressor or oxytocic effect. It is used clinically in the management of symptoms of diabetes insipidus. Lypressin is administered as a nasal spray. *(3:411)*

136. (E) Indomethacin (Indocin) is a nonsteroidal anti-inflammatory drug (NSAID) used in the treatment of rheumatoid arthritis, ankylosing spondylitis, and other inflammatory conditions such as bursitis. The use of indomethacin and other NSAIDs is associated with serious GI bleeding, ulceration, and gastric distress. Their use should be avoided in patients with a history of peptic ulcer disease. *(3:1111)*

137. (A) The sulfonylurea hypoglycemic agents appear to reduce blood glucose levels by stimulating the release of insulin from the beta cells of the pancreas. They are only effective in patients who have some capacity for endogenously producing insulin. *(3:474)*

138. (B) Chlorpropamide (Diabinese) has a serum half-life of about 36 hours. The other sulfonylurea hypoglycemic agents have a serum half-life ranging from 2 to 10 hours. *(3:475)*

139. (B) Vidarabine (Vira-A) is an antiviral agent that possesses activity against herpes simplex virus. It is administered by slow IV infusion for the treatment of herpes simplex encephalitis and is used ophthalmically for the treatment of herpes simplex infections of the eye. *(3:1865,2101)*

140. (C) Methenamine mandelate (Mandelamine) and methenamine hippurate (Hiprex, Urex) are urinary anti-infectives that are activated in acid urine to produce formaldehyde, which is bactericidal. These agents should not be administered with sulfonamides because of the possible precipitation of the sulfonamide. *(3:1919–20)*

141. (A) Zidovudine (Retrovir) inhibits replication of some retroviruses, including HIV. It is used orally in managing patients with HIV infection who have evidence of impaired immunity. The intravenous form is used for some adult patients with symptomatic HIV infection who have a confirmed presence of *Pneumocystis carinii* pneumonia (PCP). *(3:1856)*

142. (D) Alteplase (Activase) is a tissue plasminogen activator produced by recombinant DNA technology. It is used intravenously in the management of acute myocardial infarction (AMI) patients in order to lyse thrombi obstructing coronary arteries. It is administered as soon as possible after the onset of AMI. *(3:270)*

143. (E) Beractant (Survanta) is a natural lung surfactant intended for intratracheal use for the prevention and treatment of hyaline membrane disease in premature infants. *(3:907–8)*

144. (D) Ketoprofen (Orudis) and diclofenac sodium (Voltaren) are both nonsteroidal anti-inflammatory drugs (NSAIDs). *(3:1110)*

145. (D) Cromolyn sodium (Intal, Nasalcrom, Opticrom) is a drug with antiasthmatic, antiallergy, and mast cell stabilizing activity. It has no bronchodilator or anti-inflammatory activity. Cromolyn appears to inhibit degranulation of sensitized and nonsensitized mast cells that may occur after exposure to certain antigens. Cromolyn products are prophylactically used to treat bronchial asthma, allergic rhinitis, and mastocytosis. Cromolyn should not be used in treating acute asthmatic attacks. *(3:884)*

146. (B) Verapamil (Calan, Isoptin) is a calcium channel blocking agent used orally and parenterally in the treatment of cardiac arrhythmias. Other calcium channel blocking agents are used in the treatment of angina pectoris and/or essential hypertension. Oral verapamil is also used for these indications. *(3:648)*

147. (E) Ceftriaxone (Rocephin) is a third-generation cephalosporin. Third-generation cephalosporins generally have greater gram-negative activity, less gram-positive activity, greater efficacy against resistant organisms, and higher cost than cephalosporins in first- or second-generation groups. *(3:1651)*

148. (B) Reflex tachycardia is commonly seen with the use of peripheral vasodilators such as minoxidil (Loniten) and hydralazine (Apresoline). The drop in blood pressure produced by the use of these agents causes increased renin secretion, heart rate, and output as well as sodium and water retention. This may worsen both angina and congestive heart failure. These adverse effects observed with the use of peripheral vasodilators may be managed by the concurrent administration of a beta-adrenergic blocking agent and/or a diuretic. *(3:766)*

149. (C) Buprenorphine (Buprenex) is an opioid analgesic about 30 times as potent as morphine. It is administered intramuscularly or intravenously for the relief of moderate to severe pain. *(3:1080)*

150. (A) Mestranol is an estrogen commonly employed in several oral contraceptive products (eg, Norinyl, Ortho-Novum). *(3:358)*

151. (D) Pindolol (Visken) is a nonspecific beta-adrenergic blocking agent that exhibits a high degree of intrinsic sympathomimetic activity (ISA). Drugs with this characteristic tend to reduce resting cardiac output and resting heart rate to a lesser extent than drugs lacking ISA. Other beta-adrenergic blocking agents with this effect are acebutolol (Sectral), carteolol (Cartrol), and penbutolol (Levatol). *(3:703)*

152. (C) Danazol (Danocrine) is a synthetic androgen that suppresses the pituitary–ovarian axis by inhibiting the production of pituitary gonadotropins. It is clinically used in the treatment of endometriosis, where it causes the normal and ectopic endometrial tissue to become inactive and atrophic. Danazol is also employed in the prevention of attacks related to hereditary angioedema. *(3:398)*

153. (D) Metolazone (Diulo, Zaroxolyn) and chlorthalidone (Hygroton) are thiazide-like diuretics that increase the renal excretion of sodium and chloride as well as potassium. They differ from the thiazides in that they have a different chemical structure and side effects. Metolazone has been reported to be relatively more likely to produce dizziness, headache, and fatigue than other thiazide or thiazide-like drugs. *(3:528)*

154. (C) Amiloride (Midamor) is one of three potassium-sparing diuretics currently on the market. The others include spironolactone (Aldactone) and triamterene (Dyrenium). These drugs are primarily used to enhance the action and counteract the potassium-depleting effect of thiazides and loop diuretics.

(3:542)

155. (E) Acyclovir (Zovirax) is an antiviral agent used in the treatment of infections caused by herpes simplex virus types 1 and 2 (HSV-1 and HSV-2) and varicella-zoster virus. Shingles is a painful and potentially debilitating disorder caused by varicella-zoster virus. *(3:1868)*

156. (E) Chlordiazepoxide (Librium) is a benzodiazepine used in the management of anxiety. It is also indicated in the treatment of symptoms of acute alcohol withdrawal and in the prevention of delirium tremens, a condition developed in chronic alcoholic patients experiencing withdrawal symptoms. *(3:1201)*

157. (B) Bacitracin is an antibacterial agent active against a variety of gram-positive and some gram-negative organisms. It is commonly employed in topical antimicrobial products, but is rarely used parenterally because of its ability to cause renal failure due to tubular and glomerular necrosis. When it is used parenterally, renal function of the patient should be assessed both prior to therapy and daily during therapy. If toxicity is evident, the drug should be discontinued. *(3:1779)*

158. (E) Selegiline (Eldepryl) is an antiparkinsonian drug that appears to inhibit monoamine oxidase (MAO) type B activity. By inhibiting MAO, selegiline decreases the breakdown of catecholamines, such as dopamine, norepinephrine, epinephrine, and serotonin, and permits them to accumulate to higher levels in the body. Selegiline is generally used as an adjunct to levodopa/carbidopa therapy in situations where response is deteriorating. *(3:1474)*

159. (B) Sucralfate (Carafate) is a basic aluminum salt of sulfated sucrose. In the acid environment of the stomach, the aluminum ion splits off, leaving a polar anion that is not absorbable and can only exert a local action. The anion may combine with protein-rich exudate to form an ulcer-adherent complex that covers the ulcer site and prevents the penetration of acid, pepsin, and bile salts. The drug has minimal acid neutralizing activity. Sucralfate is indicated for the treatment of duodenal ulcers. *(3:1500)*

160. (D) Albuterol (Proventil) and isoproterenol (Isuprel) are sympathomimetic bronchodilators that predominantly affect beta$_2$-adrenergic receptors. Albuterol is believed, however, to have less beta$_1$-activity than isoproterenol. This would make it less likely to stimulate the heart. *(3:844)*

161. (D) Fosinopril sodium (Monopril) is an angiotensin-converting enzyme inhibitor indicated for the treatment of hypertension. When administered orally, antihypertensive action occurs within 1 hour. Peak antihypertensive action is reached within 2 to 6 hours after dosing and persists for 24 hours. This permits single daily dosing. *(3:780)*

162. (C) Beclomethasone dipropionate (Beclovent, Vanceril) is a synthetic corticosteroid used by inhalation to control bronchial asthma. It is generally reserved for patients in whom bronchodilators and other nonsteroidal medications have not been totally successful in controlling asthmatic attacks. When used with a bronchodilator administered by inhalation, the beclomethasone dipropionate should be administered several minutes after the bronchodilator in order to enhance the penetration of the bronchodilator into the bronchial tree. *(3:874-5)*

163. (D) Sympathomimetic bronchodilators such as albuterol, terbutaline, and isoproterenol are agents that primarily stimulate beta-adrenergic receptors. Some sympathomimetic drugs (eg, ephedrine, epinephrine) also stimulate alpha-adrenergic receptors. Methylated xanthine bronchodilators such as theophylline act by inhibiting the phosphodiesterase enzyme. *(3:844,858)*

164. (A) Fluorouracil (Adrucil) is an antimetabolite drug that blocks the conversion of deoxyuridylic acid to thymidylic acid. This, in turn, interferes with the synthesis of DNA and the formation of RNA. The other agents listed are all alkylating agents. *(3:2372)*

165. (B) Terfenadine (Seldane) and astemizole (Hismanal) are antihistamines that produce a low degree of sedation. The other agents are much more likely to produce sedation as an adverse effect. *(3:912)*

166. (D) (10)

167. (A) (10)

168. (E) (10)

169. (C) (10)

170. (B) (10)

171. (C) (10)

172. (E) (10)

173. (A) (10)

174. (B) (10)

175. (B) (10)

176. (D) (10)

177. (A) (10)

178. (C) (10)

179. (E) (10)

180. (C) (10)	**216. (E)** (10)
181. (B) (10)	**217. (D)** (10)
182. (D) (10)	**218. (A)** (10)
183. (E) (10)	**219. (C)** (10)
184. (C) (10)	**220. (B)** (10)
185. (D) (10)	**221. (E)** (10)
186. (B) (10)	**222. (A)** (10)
187. (A) (10)	**223. (D)** (10)
188. (E) (10)	**224. (D)** (10)
189. (C) (10)	**225. (A)** (10)
190. (D) (10)	**226. (E)** (10)
191. (B) (10)	**227. (B)** (10)
192. (D) (10)	**228. (C)** (10)
193. (A) (10)	**229. (E)** (10)
194. (C) (10)	**230. (B)** (10)
195. (A) (10)	**231. (C)** (10)
196. (D) (10)	**232. (D)** (10)
197. (B) (10)	**233. (B)** (10)
198. (E) (10)	**234. (A)** (10)
199. (A) (10)	**235. (B)** (10)
200. (C) (10)	**236. (A)** (10)
201. (B) (10)	**237. (D)** (10)
202. (E) (10)	**238. (E)** (10)
203. (D) (10)	**239. (C)** (10)
204. (E) (10)	**240. (C)** (10)
205. (C) (10)	**241. (E)** (10)
206. (A) (10)	**242. (A)** (10)
207. (D) (10)	**243. (D)** (10)
208. (B) (10)	**244. (B)** (10)
209. (B) (10)	**245. (A)** (10)
210. (A) (10)	**246. (D)** (10)
211. (C) (10)	**247. (E)** (10)
212. (E) (10)	**248. (F)** (10)
213. (D) (10)	**249. (C)** (10)
214. (B) (10)	**250. (B)** (10)
215. (C) (10)	

Pharmaceutical Calculations

As the fraction of prescriptions requiring compounding diminishes, it seems that the importance of pharmaceutical calculations will also decline. However, the continued necessity to compound some prescriptions as well as the increased role of the pharmacist in preparing parenteral admixtures require pharmacists to maintain their calculation skills. In addition, competence in mathematics is essential in order to comprehend the scientific literature.

Most textbooks dealing with pharmaceutical calculations present the reader with many problems to solve. We have attempted to present this topic with a sampling of pharmaceutical calculations that are relevant to current pharmacy practice.

Questions

DIRECTIONS (Questions 1 through 52): Each of the numbered items or incomplete statements in this section is followed by answers or by completions of the statement. Select the ONE lettered answer or completion that is BEST in each case.

1. Which of the following units of weight measurement are identical in both the apothecary and avoirdupois systems?

    (A) drams
    (B) grains
    (C) ounces
    (D) pounds
    (E) grains and pounds

2. One thousand (1000) nanograms equals one

    (A) centigram
    (B) gram
    (C) kilogram
    (D) microgram
    (E) milligram

3. According to USP specifications, which one of the following equivalents should be used to convert a grain measurement to milligrams when compounding prescriptions?

    (A) 60 mg
    (B) 62.5 mg
    (C) 64.8 mg
    (D) 65 mg
    (E) 15.4 mg

    1 gr = 65mg

4. The minimum quantity that can be weighed on a balance with a sensitivity requirement of 6 mg if an error of 5% is permissible would be

    (A) 6 mg
    (B) 24 mg
    (C) 60 mg
    (D) 120 mg
    (E) 180 mg

SR = min amt (x)(%error)

5. How many mg of codeine phosphate are being consumed daily by a patient taking the following prescription as directed?

Rx		
Codeine Phosphate		200 mg
Robitussin-PE	q.s.	120 mL

Sig: ʒ i t.i.d. p.c. & h.s.

tsp tid after meals & QHS
20 ml / day

    (A) 6.25
    (B) 8.25
    (C) 19
    (D) 25
    (E) 33

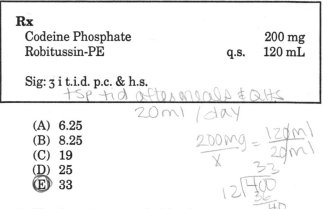

6. The directions intended for the patient on a prescription read "1 tbsp ac and hs for 10 days." What is the minimum volume the pharmacist should dispense?

    (A) 160 mL
    (B) 200 mL
    (C) 400 mL
    (D) 600 mL
    (E) 800 mL

15 ml x 3
45
15
600

7. The adult dose of a drug is 250 mg. What would be the approximate dose for a 6-year-old child? (Use Young's rule.)

    (A) 60 mg
    (B) 85 mg
    (C) 100 mg
    (D) 125 mg
    (E) 180 mg

$\left(\frac{6}{6+12}\right)(250mg) =$

$\frac{6}{18}$

8. What would be the appropriate dose for a child weighing 40 lb if the adult dose is 50 mg? (Use Clark's rule.)

    (A) 15 mg
    (B) 20 mg
    (C) 25 mg

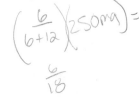

$\frac{Wt(lb) \times adult\ dose}{150}$

$\frac{40 \times 50}{150} = \frac{200}{150}$

(D) 30 mg
(E) 35 mg

9. The USP contains a nomogram for estimating body surface area for either children or adults. Which of the following measurements must be known in order to use this nomogram?

(A) age and height
(B) age and weight
(C) height and creatinine clearance
(D) height and weight
(E) weight and sex

10. The adult dose of a drug is 100 mg. What is an appropriate dose for a child whose body surface area is calculated to be .75 m²?

(A) 25 mg
(B) 40 mg
(C) 50 mg
(D) 75 mg
(E) 80 mg

11. Blood pressure measurements were made for 1 week on five patients with the following averages:

Patient #	1	2	3	4	5
B.P.	140/70	160/84	180/88	190/90	150/70

What is the median systole pressure?

(A) 80
(B) 83
(C) 84
(D) 160
(E) 164

12. After 1 month of therapy, all of the above patients had a systolic blood pressure reduction of 10 mm with a standard deviation of 5 mm. What percentage of patients had a reduction between 5 and 15 mm?

(A) 20
(B) 40
(C) 50
(D) 70
(E) 90

13. The concentration of sodium fluoride in a community's drinking water is 0.6 ppm. Express this concentration as a percentage.

(A) 0.00006%
(B) 0.0006%
(C) 0.006%
(D) 0.06%
(E) 0.6%

14. Directions for a prednisone 5-mg tablet prescription read "20 mg this PM then 15 mg b.i.d for 2 days then 10 mg b.i.d for 2 days, 5 mg t.i.d for 5 days, 5 mg b.i.d for 5 days, then 5 mg q.o.d for 6 days." The total number of tablets that should be dispensed is

(A) 42
(B) 46
(C) 48
(D) 52
(E) none of these

15. Lanoxin Pediatric Elixir contains 0.05 mg of digoxin per mL. How many micrograms (µg) are there in 3 mL of the elixir?

(A) 0.15
(B) 0.015
(C) 1.5
(D) 0.0015
(E) none of the above

16. What is the percentage of alcohol in a mixture of 300 mL of 95% V/V alcohol, 1000 mL of 70% V/V alcohol, and 200 mL of 50% V/V alcohol?

(A) 84%
(B) 72%
(C) 8.4%
(D) 7.2%
(E) 79%

17. What is the daily mg dose of pilocarpine hydrochloride in the following prescription? Assume that the dropper is calibrated to deliver 20 drops to the mL.

Rx
Pilocarpine HCl   4%
Pur. Water   q.s.   30 mL

Sig: gtt ii OU t.i.d.

(A) 12
(B) 24
(C) 60
(D) 120
(E) none of the above

18. A 20-mL vial of a biological solution is labeled "2.0 megaunits." How many units of drug are present in every mL of solution?

(A) 100
(B) 1000
(C) 2000
(D) 10,000
(E) 100,000

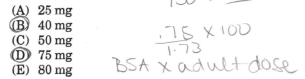

19. A pharmacist has 50 mL of 0.5% gentian violet solution. What will be the final ratio strength if he or she dilutes this solution to 1250 mL with purified water?

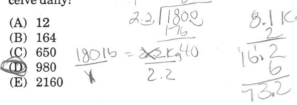

(A) 1:8
(B) 1:200
(C) 1:500
(D) 1:1000
(E) 1:5000

20. The adult IV dose of zidovudine is 2 mg/kg q 4 h six times daily. How many mg will a 180-lb patient receive daily?

(A) 12
(B) 164
(C) 650
(D) 980
(E) 2160

21. How many mL of a 0.5% gentian violet stock solution are needed to prepare 1 gallon of a 1:2000 solution?

(A) 47
(B) 94.5
(C) 200
(D) 378
(E) none of the above

22. For the following prescription, what is the approximate percentage strength of the diluted solution that the patient will use as a soak?

Rx
Potassium Permanganate Tab.   200 mg
Disp. #60

Sig: iii tab in pint of warm water. Use as soak.

(A) 0.06%
(B) 0.6%
(C) 0.13%
(D) 2.0%
(E) none of the above

23. How many grams of ammonia water (10% W/W) can be prepared from 1 lb of 28% W/W Strong Ammonia Solution?

(A) 84
(B) 162
(C) 280
(D) 1271
(E) 1400

24. How many mL of a 1:50 stock solution of ephedrine sulfate would be needed to prepare 30 mL of the following prescription?

Rx
Ephedrine Sulfate   0.25%
Normal Saline   q.s.   10 mL

(A) 1.25
(B) 3.75
(C) 4.0
(D) 7.5
(E) 12.5

25. How many mL of Sodium Hypochlorite Solution USP/NF will be needed to fill the following prescription? (Sodium Hypochlorite Solution USP/NF contains 5% W/V NaOCl.)

Rx
Sodium Hypochlorite Sol.
Purified Water   q.s.   120 mL

M & Ft sol. of such strength that 30 mL diluted to 1 pint contains 0.1% sodium hypochlorite.

(A) 2.4
(B) 9.5
(C) 37.8
(D) 75.6
(E) impossible to determine, since the amount of sodium hypochlorite solution was not specified in the prescription

26. A vial of a lyophilized drug is labeled "10,000 units: to reconstitute, add 17 mL of Sterile Water for Injection to obtain 500 units per mL." How many mL of SWFI must a pharmacist add if a 1000 unit/mL concentration is needed by the nurse?

(A) 7
(B) 8.5
(C) 10
(D) 17
(E) 20

27. An administration set delivers 60 drops to the mL. How many drops per minute are needed to obtain 20 units of heparin per minute if the IV admixture contains 15,000 units per 250 mL of normal saline?

(A) 20
(B) 40

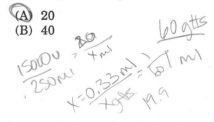

(C) 60
(D) 80
(E) 120

28. Determine the mg of drug to be administered to a patient if the physician requests a loading dose of 2 mg/lb of lean body mass. The 45-year-old male patient weighs 200 lb and is 5′ 10″ tall.

(A) 200
(B) 240
(C) 320
(D) 360
(E) 400

$$\frac{2mg}{1lb} = \frac{x}{200 lb}$$

$$x = 400$$

29. Dopamine (Intropin) 200 mg in 500 mL of normal saline at 5 µg/kg/min is ordered for a 155-lb patient. What is the final concentration of solution in µg/mL?

(A) 0.4
(B) 2.5
(C) 40
(D) 400
(E) 25

$$\frac{155 lb}{x kg} = \frac{2.2 kg}{1 lb} = 70.5$$

$$70.5 kg$$

$$352.5 \mu g \qquad \frac{.3525 mg}{x ml}$$

30. Referring to the previous question, at what rate (mL/min) should the solution be infused to deliver the desired dose of 5 µg/kg/min?

(A) 0.35
(B) 0.40
(C) 0.88
(D) 2.0
(E) 5.0

$$\frac{5}{min} \quad \frac{.4}{x}$$

31. A pharmacist adds 10 mL of potassium chloride injection labeled 2 mEq/mL to a 500-mL bottle of D5W injection. What is the concentration of potassium chloride expressed as mEq/mL in the final admixture?

(A) 0.02
(B) 0.04
(C) 0.06
(D) 0.08
(E) 2.0

32. A 250-mL infusion bottle contains 5.86 g of potassium chloride. How many milliequivalents of potassium chloride are present? (molecular weight of KCl = 74.6)

(A) 12.7
(B) 20
(C) 78.5
(D) 150
(E) none of the above

33. A solution contains 1.5 mEq of calcium per 100 mL. Express the solution's strength of calcium in terms of mg/L. (The atomic weight of calcium is 40.)

(A) 30
(B) 60
(C) 150
(D) 300
(E) 600

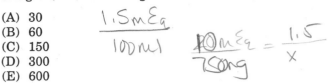

$$\frac{1.5 mEq}{100 ml}$$

$$20 mEq = \frac{1.5}{x}$$

$$750 mg$$

34. Calcium chloride ($CaCl_2$ • $2H_2O$) has a formula weight of 147. What weight of the chemical is needed to obtain 40 mEq of calcium? (Ca = 40.1; Cl = 35.5; H_2O = 18)

(A) 0.80 g
(B) 2.22 g
(C) 1.47 g
(D) 2.94 g
(E) 5.88 g

35. In changing a patient from U-40 to U-100 insulin, a pharmacist would instruct him to use _____ mL of U-100 if the previous dosage was 0.8 mL of U-40 per day.

(A) 0.32
(B) 0.40
(C) 0.50
(D) 0.80
(E) 2.0

$$\frac{.8 ml}{U-40} = \frac{x ml}{U-100}$$

36. Assuming that a 120-lb patient has a creatinine clearance rate of 40 mL/min, what maintenance dose should be administered if the normal maintenance dose is 2 mg/lb of body weight?

(A) 60 mg
(B) 100 mg
(C) 120 mg
(D) 160 mg
(E) 240 mg

$$240 mg$$

37. A TPN order requires 500 mL of D30W. How many mL of D40W should be used if the D30W is not available?

(A) 125
(B) 300
(C) 375
(D) 400
(E) 667

38. A physician requests 1 lb of bacitracin ointment containing 200 U of bacitracin per gram. How many grams of bacitracin ointment (500 U/g) must be used to make this ointment?

(A) 182
(B) 200
(C) 227
(D) 362
(E) none of the above

$$\frac{454 g}{200 U g} = \frac{x}{500}$$

39. A pharmacist repackages 10 lb of an ointment into jars to be labeled 2 oz (avoir.). How many jars can be filled?

(A) 73
(B) 80
(C) 83
(D) 88
(E) 100

$$10 \, lb = 4540 \, g$$
$$\frac{60 \, g}{1 \, jar} = \frac{4540 g}{x}$$

40. How many mL of glycerin would be needed to prepare 1 lb of an ointment containing 5% W/W glycerin? The density of glycerin is 1.25 g/mL.

(A) 1.2
(B) 18.2
(C) 22.7
(D) 24
(E) 28.4

41. A hospital clinic requests 2 lb of 2% hydrocortisone ointment. How many grams of 5% hydrocortisone ointment could be diluted with white petrolatum to prepare this order?

(A) 18.2
(B) 27.5
(C) 45.4
(D) 363
(E) 545

$$(908g)(2\%) = (x \, g)(5\%)$$

42. How many grams of pure hydrocortisone powder must be mixed with 60 g of 0.5% hydrocortisone cream if one wishes to prepare a 2.0% W/W preparation?

(A) .90
(B) .92
(C) .30
(D) 1.2
(E) 1.53

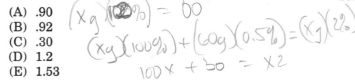

$$?g \, of \, 100\% \quad 2\%$$
$$60g \, of \, 0.5\%$$
$$(x g)(100\%) = 60$$
$$(xg)(100\%) + (60g)(0.5\%) = (x g)(2\%)$$
$$100x + 30 = x2$$

43. How much sodium chloride is needed to adjust the following prescription to isotonicity? (E value for zinc sulfate is 0.15.)

Rx	
Zinc Sulfate	1%
Sodium Chloride	q.s.
Purified Water	q.s. 60 mL

(A) 0.45 g
(B) 0.54 g
(C) 0.60 g
(D) 0.75 g
(E) 0.90 g

44. How much additional sodium chloride should be added to the following prescription to maintain isotonicity? Zincfrin is an isotonic solution.

Rx	
Zincfrin	15 mL
Sodium Chloride	q.s.
Sterile Water for Injection	60 mL

(A) 0.135 g
(B) 0.4 g
(C) 0.54 g
(D) 0.9 g
(E) none (since sterile water for injection is already isotonic)

45. Estimate the milliosmolarity, in terms of mOsm/L, for normal saline. (Na = 23; Cl = 35.5)

(A) 150
(B) 300
(C) 350
(D) 400
(E) 600

46. How many milliosmoles are present in a solution prepared by dissolving 1000 mg of sodium chloride in 100 mL D5W? (Na = 23; Cl = 35.5; hydrous dextrose = 198)

(A) 30
(B) 60
(C) 150
(D) 300
(E) 600

47. How many mL of Hydrochloric Acid USP are needed to prepare 4 L of Diluted Hydrochloric Acid USP? The label on the available hydrochloric acid bottle shows that the concentration of the acid is 36.8% W/W and the solution specific gravity is 1.19. The diluted acid is 10% W/V according to the official monograph.

(A) 147
(B) 400
(C) 913
(D) 1087
(E) 1294

48. How many grams of glacial acetic acid (99.9% W/W) must be added to 1 gallon of purified water to prepare an irrigation solution containing 0.25% W/V acetic acid?

$(X_{m})(99.9) = (3785ml)(0.25\%)$

(A) 1.2
(B) 9.5
(C) 12
(D) 20
(E) 95

49. A formula for Magnesium Citrate Solution requires 27.4 g of anhydrous citric acid (mol. wt. = 192). How many grams of citric acid monohydrate could be used as a replacement?

$192 + 18 = 210$

(A) 25.1
(B) 27.4
(C) 30.0
(D) 34.0
(E) 54.8

$\dfrac{210}{192} \times 27.4$

50. How much elemental iron is present in every 300 mg of ferrous sulfate ($FeSO_4 \cdot 7H_2O$)? 183
(Atomic weights are iron = 55.9; sulfur = 32.1; oxygen = 16.0; and hydrogen = 1.0. Iron has valences of +2 and +3.)

$\begin{array}{r} 55.9 \\ 32.1 \\ 64.0 \\ 1.0 \\ \hline 153.0 \\ \times 4 \\ \hline \end{array}$

183.

$\begin{array}{r} 55.9 \\ 32.1 \\ 80 \\ 14 \\ \hline 142.0 \end{array}$

$\dfrac{55.9}{142} \times 300$

$\dfrac{300mg \; FeS}{55.9 \; Fe} = \underline{\quad}$

(A) 30.2 mg
(B) 60.3 mg
(C) 110.3 mg
(D) 120.6 mg
(E) 164 mg

51. The USP states that 1 g of a chemical is soluble in 10 mL of alcohol. What is the percentage strength of a saturated solution of this chemical if alcohol has a sp.gr. of 0.80?

(A) 10.0% W/V
(B) 10.0% W/W
(C) 11.1% W/V
(D) 11.1% W/W
(E) 12.5% W/V

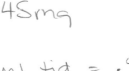

$\dfrac{1g}{10ml} \qquad \dfrac{1000mg}{1ml}$

$10\% = \dfrac{100mg}{1ml}$

52. Strong Iodine Solution USP contains 5% W/V iodine. How many mg of iodine are consumed daily if the usual dose is 0.3 mL t.i.d.?

(A) 7.5
(B) 15
(C) 22.5
(D) 45
(E) 90

$5\% = \dfrac{50mg}{mL}$

45mg

0.3ml tid = .9ml /day

$\dfrac{50mg}{1ml} = \dfrac{Xmg}{0.9ml}$

$\begin{array}{r} 50 \\ \times 9 \\ \hline 45.0 \end{array}$

$\dfrac{1g}{1g + 9g} = \dfrac{1}{9}$

Answers and Explanations

1. **(B)** Only the grain measurement is a common equivalent weight in both the apothecary and the avoirdupois systems. The apothecary ounce is 480 grains while the apothecary pound is 12 ounces (5760 grains). The avoirdupois ounce contains 437.5 grains; the pound contains 16 ounces (7000 grains). The use of apothecary weights for prescription compounding or concentration expressions is archaic and should be actively discouraged. Any expression in the apothecary system should be immediately converted to the metric system. The avoirdupois system is still used in the United States for the purchase and selling of bulk chemicals. *(23:58)*

2. **(D)** The prefix "nano" is used in the SI (Système International) measuring system, essentially an extension of the metric decimal system that has been adopted by most countries. The major prefixes in order of magnitude include:

Prefix	Magnitude	Example
kilo	$1000 \times$	kilogram
—	$1 \times$	gram
centi	$0.01 \times$	centigram
milli	$0.001 \times$	milligram
micro	$1 \times 10^{-6} \times$	microgram
nano	$1 \times 10^{-9} \times$	nanogram
pico	$1 \times 10^{-12} \times$	picogram
femto	$1 \times 10^{-15} \times$	femtogram
atto	$1 \times 10^{-18} \times$	attogram

(1:72)

3. **(C)** The USP contains a table of equivalents of weights and measures for the metric, avoirdupois, and apothecary systems. When converting specific quantities in pharmaceutical formulas, the exact equivalents must be used. For prescription compounding, the exact equivalents may be rounded to three significant figures. The metric equivalent of 1 grain is listed as 0.06480 g, which would then be expressed as 64.8 mg. Some sources use the value of 65 mg, which does not meet USP specifications. The value of 60 mg should not be used except for rough calculations in checking doses. *(18c:II/29)*

4. **(D)** The minimum weight that can be measured on any balance with a known sensitivity requirement (SR) in a given percent of error may be determined by the equation: SR = (min. amt that may be weighed) (x) (% permissible error)

$$6 \text{ mg} = (x \text{ mg})(5\%)$$
$$6 \text{ mg} = (x \text{ mg})(0.05)$$
$$x = 120 \text{ mg}$$

The USP specifies that pharmacists should not weigh quantities less than 120 mg mg on the Class A prescription balance in order to avoid errors of 5% or more. *(18c:II/26)*

5. **(E)** The symbol "ʒ i" represents 1 teaspoonful of medication. The directions read 1 teaspoonful three times a day after meals and at bedtime, for a total of four doses; this is equivalent to 20 mL since a teaspoonful is 5 mL.

$$\frac{200 \text{ mg Codeine P.}}{120 \text{ mL}} = \frac{x \text{ mg}}{20 \text{ mL}}$$
$$x = 33 \text{ mg}$$

(23:82)

(B) This is the correct amount of codeine phosphate per teaspoonful. The question asks for total daily dose. Choice D is obtained if one translates "ʒ i" as one fluidram, which is 3.75 mL. In modern medical practice the symbol ʒ i in a Sig refers to the teaspoonful dose (5 mL). The answer of 25 mg also applies if one assumes only three doses a day rather than four doses.

6. **(D)** One tablespoonful (tbsp) delivers 15 mL of liquid. In this prescription, the patient is receiving four doses per day for 10 days. Thus, $15 \text{ mL} \times 4 \times 10 = 600$ mL. *(23:80)*

7. **(B)** Young's rule states that:

$$\text{Child's dose} = \frac{\text{Age (yr)}}{\text{Age (yr)} + 12} \times \text{Adult dose}$$
$$\text{Child's dose} = \frac{6}{6 + 12} \times 250 \text{ mg}$$
$$\text{Child's dose} = 83.3 \text{ mg or } 85 \text{ mg}$$

(23:85)

8. **(A)** Clark's rule has been used to relate body weight to dosage. It states:

$$\text{Child's dose} = \frac{\text{Child's wt. (lb)}}{150} \times \text{Adult dose}$$

$$\text{Child's dose} = \frac{(40)}{150} \times (50 \text{ mg})$$

Child's dose = 13.3 mg or 15 mg

(23:85)

9. **(D)** The nomogram in the USP consists of three parallel, vertical lines. The left line is calibrated with height measurements in both centimeters and inches, while the right line lists weights in kilograms and pounds. Using data based upon the patient's measurements, one draws a line between the two outside parallel lines. The intercept on the middle line, which is calibrated in square meters of body surface area, allows one to estimate the patient's body surface area. *(23:86)*

10. **(B)** The average adult body surface area (BSA) is estimated to be 1.73m^2. A child's dose can be estimated by:

$$\frac{\text{BSA (child)}}{\text{BSA (adult)}} \times \text{Adult dose} = \text{Child dose}$$

$$\frac{0.75 \text{ m}^2}{1.73 \text{ m}^2} \times 100 \text{ mg} = 43 \text{ mg}$$

(1:91; 23:87)

11. **(D)** The median value in a series of numbers is that value in the middle (ie, the number of values lower than the median value is equal to the number of values higher than the median value). The median may not be the same as the average, which is obtained by adding all the values together and dividing by the number of values. *(23:254)*

12. **(D)** A standard deviation is mathematically calculated for experimental data. It allows one to picture the dispersion of numbers around the mean (average value). One standard deviation will include approximately 67% to 70% of all values, while two standard deviations will include approximately 97% to 98%.

(23:254)

13. **(A)** Since sodium fluoride is a solid, 0.6 ppm indicates a concentration of 0.6 grams of sodium fluoride per 1,000,000 mL of solution. Therefore, the grams present in every 100 mL will be:

$$\frac{0.6 \text{ g NaF}}{1,000,000 \text{ mL}} = \frac{x \text{ g NaF}}{100 \text{ mL}}$$

$$x = 0.00006 \text{ g or } 0.00006\% \text{ W/V}$$

(23:120)

14. **(D)** Calculate the total number of 5-mg tablets needed for each phase of therapy—day 1-4, days 2 & 3-12, days 4 & 5-8, days 6 through 10-15, days 11 through 15-10, days 16 through 21-3 (every other day)—for a total of 52. The answer can be checked by

determining the number of mg for each segment, totaling the amount and dividing by 5 mg (ie, 20 mg + 60 mg + 40 mg + 75 mg + 50 mg + 15 mg = 260 mg divided by 5-mg tablets = 42 tablets).

15. **(E)** 1 mg = 1000 micrograms (μg). Therefore 0.15 mg of digoxin (contained in 3 mL of the elixir) would be equivalent to 150 μg of drug. *(23:50)*

16. **(B)** The problem requires a "weighted average" calculation. The basic procedure is to multiply the volume of each product by the percentage strength of the labeled ingredient, sum up the total amount of pure ingredient, then divide that total by the total volume of the final mixture.

$$300 \text{ mL} \times 95\% = 285 \text{ mL (absolute alcohol)}$$
$$1000 \text{ mL} \times 70\% = 700 \text{ mL}$$
$$\underline{200 \text{ mL} \times 50\% = 100 \text{ mL}}$$
$$1500 \text{ mL (total)} \quad 1085 \text{ mL (total vol, of absolute alcohol)}$$

$$\frac{1085}{1500} = .723 \text{ or } 72.3\% \text{ V/V}$$

(23:157)

17. **(B)** The patient is placing two drops in each eye three times a day. The total number of drops is:

$$2 \text{ gtt} \times 2 \text{ eyes} \times 3 \text{ times} = 12 \text{ drops}$$

Since the dropper is calibrated at 20 gtt/mL:

$$\frac{20 \text{ gtt}}{1 \text{ mL}} = \frac{12 \text{ gtt}}{x \text{ mL}}$$

The amount of pilocarpine HCl present is:

$$0.6 \text{ mL} \times 0.04 = 0.024 \text{ g or } 24 \text{ mg}$$

(23:78)

18. **(E)** The prefix mega (M) represents one million in the SI system. A vial labeled 2 megaunits or 2 Munits contains a total of 2,000,000 units or 100,000 units per mL. *(1:72)*

19. **(E)** One can solve this problem by first determining how much pure (100%) gentian violet was originally present. The final ratio strength can then be determined by dividing the amount of chemical present by the final volume prepared.

(1) 50 mL of 0.5% contains 0.25 g
(2) 0.25 g is diluted to 1250 mL

$$\frac{0.25}{1250} = .0002 \text{ or } \frac{2}{10,000} = \frac{1}{5000} = 1:5000$$

Or by the equation: $(Q_1)(C_1) = (Q_2)(C_2)$

$$(1250 \text{ mL})(x) = (50 \text{ mL})(.05\%)$$
$$1250 x = 0.25$$
$$x = .0002, \text{ which converts to } 1:5000$$

(23:144)

20. (D) First, convert the pound weight to kilograms:

$$180 \text{ lb} \times \frac{1 \text{ kg}}{2.2 \text{ lb}} = 82 \text{ kg}$$

Second, determine total daily dose

$$82 \text{ kg} \times 2 \text{ mg} \times 6 \text{ doses} = 980 \text{ mg}$$

(23:83)

21. (D) Step 1. Determine the quantity of chemical in the final solution:

$$1 \text{ gallon} = 3785 \text{ mL; therefore,}$$
$$\frac{1 \text{ g}}{2000 \text{ mL}} = \frac{x \text{ g}}{3785 \text{ mL}}$$

Step 2. Determine the amount of the available solution needed to obtain the quantity of chemical determined in Step 1 (a 0.5% solution contains 0.5 g of chemical in 100 mL of solution):

$$\frac{0.5 \text{ g}}{100 \text{ mL}} = \frac{1.89 \text{ g}}{x \text{ mL}}$$
$$x = 378 \text{ mL}$$

(23:147)

22. (C) There are 473 mL of solution in 1 pint. Since three 200-mg tablets are dissolved in each pint:

$$\frac{0.6 \text{ g}}{473 \text{ mL}} \times 100 = 0.13\% \text{ W/V}$$

(23:120)

23. (D) One pound of Strong Ammonia Solution weighs 454 g. Since 28% of the 454 g is pure ammonia, there is present $454 \times 0.28 = 127.1$ g of pure ammonia. Since the new solution will contain 10 g of pure ammonia in every 100 g of solution, 127.1 g of pure ammonia will be present in every 1271 g of ammonia water. Or, by equation:

$$(Q_1)(C_1) = (Q_2)(C_2)$$
$$(x \text{ g})(10\% \text{ W/W}) = (454 \text{ g})(28\% \text{ W/W})$$
$$10\,x = 12712$$
$$x = 1271.2 \text{ g}$$

(23:146)

24. (B) The amount of pure ephedrine sulfate required is $30 \text{ mL} \times 0.25\% = 0.075$ g. The stock solution contains 1 g of ephedrine in every 50 mL of solution. Therefore:

$$\frac{1 \text{ g ephedrine sulfate}}{50 \text{ mL stock solution}} = \frac{0.075 \text{ g}}{x \text{ mL}}$$
$$x = 3.75 \text{ mL}$$

(23:147)

25. (C) One pint contains 473 mL. The final solution used by the patient will contain $473 \times 0.1\% = 0.473$ g of pure sodium hypochlorite. This amount is also present in each 30 mL of the prescription since the dilution process performed by the patient simply in-

volves the addition of water. If each 30 mL of the prescription contains 0.473 g of pure sodium hypochlorite, the total amount is:

$$0.473 \times \frac{120}{30} = 1.89 \text{ g}$$

The amount of Sodium Hypochlorite Solution required is:

$$\frac{5 \text{ g sodium hypochlorite}}{100 \text{ mL of official solution}} = \frac{1.89 \text{ g}}{x \text{ mL}}$$
$$x = 37.8 \text{ mL}$$

(23:148)

26. (A) When some drug powders are reconstituted, the volume occupied by the bulk powder in solution must be considered. In this example, the final volume of solution is:

$$\frac{500 \text{ units}}{1 \text{ mL}} = \frac{10,000 \text{ units}}{x \text{ mL}}$$
$$x = 20 \text{ mL}$$

Thus, the volume occupied by the powder is $20 - 17 = 3$ mL. Since a concentration of 1000 units/mL is desired, the total volume of solution that must be prepared will be:

$$\frac{1000 \text{ units}}{1 \text{ mL}} = \frac{10,000 \text{ units}}{x \text{ mL}}$$

Since 3 mL of this 10-mL volume represents the bulk volume of the dissolved drug, 7 mL of SWFI must be added.

(23:200)

27. (A) Step 1. Determine the drug concentration present in every mL:

$$\frac{15,000 \text{ units}}{250 \text{ mL}} = \frac{x \text{ units}}{1 \text{ mL}}$$
$$x = 60 \text{ units/mL}$$

Step 2. Determine the mL needed to obtain concentration requested:

$$\frac{60 \text{ units}}{1 \text{ mL}} = \frac{20 \text{ units}}{x \text{ mL}}$$

Step 3. Calculate the number of drops needed, based upon the administration set being used, to obtain the required volume:

$$\frac{60 \text{ drops}}{1 \text{ mL}} = \frac{x \text{ drops}}{0.33 \text{ mL}}$$
$$x = 19.8 \text{ or } 20 \text{ drops}$$

(23:207)

28. (C) One equation for estimating ideal body weight (IBW) or lean body mass (LBM) states:

IBW = 110 lb + 5 lb for every inch over 5 feet of height. In this problem:

$$IBW = 110 \text{ lb} + (5 \text{ lb} \times 10)$$
$$= 110 \text{ lb} + 50 \text{ lb}$$
$$= 160 \text{ lb}$$

Loading dose = 2 mg/lb × 160 lb = 320 mg

The ideal body weight equation for females is similar, except 100 lb is substituted for the 110-lb value

(23:236)

29. **(D)** 200 mg dopamine
500 mL solution = 0.4 mg/mL
1 mg = 1000 μg
0.4 mg = 400 μg
final concentration: 400 μg/mL

(23:132)

30. **(C)**

$$\frac{155 \text{ lb}}{2.2 \text{ lb/kg}} = 70.5 \text{ kg}$$

$$\frac{5 \text{ μg/kg}}{\text{minute}} \times 70.5 \text{ kg} = 352 \text{ μg/minute}$$

Since concentration of solution is 400 μg/mL, divide dosage rate by concentration of solution:

$$\frac{352 \text{ μg/minute}}{400 \text{ μg/mL}} = 0.88 \text{ mL/min}$$

(23:83,207)

31. **(B)**

$$10 \text{ mL KCl injection} \times \frac{2 \text{ mEq}}{1 \text{ mL}} = 20 \text{ mEq KCl}$$

$$\frac{20 \text{ mEq KCl}}{500 \text{ mL D5W}} = 0.04 \text{ mEq/mL}$$

32. **(C)** 1 equivalent weight of KCl = 74.6 g
1 milliequivalent (mEq) = 74.6 mg

$$\frac{1 \text{ mEq}}{74.6 \text{ mg}} = \frac{x \text{ mEq}}{5860 \text{ mg}}$$
$$74.6 \, x = 5860$$
$$x = 78.5 \text{ mEq}$$

Or by using the equation:

$$mg = \frac{(\text{mEq}) (\text{molecular wt.})}{(\text{valence}}$$
$$5860 \text{ mg} = \frac{(x) (74.6)}{(1)}$$
$$x = 78.5 \text{ mEq}$$

(23:190)

33. **(D)** Since the valence of calcium is + 2, one mEq equals 40 mg divided by 2 = 20 mg. Therefore, 1.5 mEq = 30 mg. If there are 30 mg/dL of solution, there will be 300 mg/L. By use of the equation:

$$mg/vol = \frac{(\text{mEq/vol}) (\text{atomic wt.})}{\text{valence}}$$
$$x \text{ mg/1000 mL} = \frac{1.5 \text{ mEq/100 mL} \, (40)}{(2)}$$
$$200 \, x = 60,000$$
$$x = 300 \text{ mg}$$

(23:189)

34. **(D)**
1 equivalent = 147/2 = 73.5 g
1 mEq = 73.5 mg
40 mEq = 2940 mg or 2.94 g of calcium chloride

Or, by equation:

$$mg = \frac{(\text{mEq}) (\text{formula wt.})}{(\text{valence})}$$
$$mg = \frac{(40) (147)}{(2)}$$
$$= 2940 \text{ mg or } 2.94 \text{ g of calcium chloride}$$

One must remember that 40 mEq of calcium combines with 40 mEq of chloride to form 40 mEq of calcium chloride. *(1:817; 23:205)*
(A–incorrect) This answer is obtained if one multiplies the 40 mEq desired by the atomic weight of calcium and then divides by the + 2 valence. The use of the atomic weight of calcium is incorrect since the official hydrated calcium chloride is being weighed to obtain the correct amount of calcium. The right answer can be obtained by adding this step:

$$\frac{0.80 \text{ g (calcium)}}{40 \text{ (atomic wt. Ca)}} = \frac{x \text{ g (hydrated calcium chloride)}}{147 \text{ (formula wt. hydrated salt)}}$$
$$x = 2.94 \text{ g hydrated calcium chloride}$$

(B–incorrect) The answer of 2.22 g is incorrect since it assumes that anhydrous calcium chloride (molecular weight of 111) was used. However, the problem specified that the official form, which contains two waters of hydration, was available.
(E–incorrect) The answer of 5.88 g is obtained if one ignores the + 2 valence of calcium. *(1:817; 23:205)*

35. **(A)** The number of units injected each day was:

$$\frac{40 \text{ units}}{1 \text{ mL}} = \frac{x}{0.8 \text{ mL}}$$
$$x = 32 \text{ units}$$

Since U-100 insulin contains 100 units per mL:

$$\frac{100 \text{ units}}{1 \text{ mL}} = \frac{32 \text{ units}}{x \text{ mL}}$$
$$x = 0.32 \text{ mL}$$

(23:216)

36. (B) The normal maintenance dose would be:

$$120 \text{ lb} \times 2 \text{ mg/lb} = 240 \text{ mg}$$

Since the normal creatinine clearance rate is 100 mL per minute:

$$\frac{40 \text{ mL/min}}{100 \text{ ml/min}} \times 240 \text{ mg} = 96 \text{ or } 100 \text{ mg}$$

(23:239)

37. **(C)** 500 mL of D30W will contain 150 g of dextrose. D40W contains 40 g of dextrose per 100 mL.

$$\frac{40 \text{ g dextrose}}{100 \text{ mL of solution}} = \frac{150 \text{ g dextrose}}{x \text{ of solution}}$$
$$x = 375 \text{ mL}$$

Or, this problem may be solved by using the equation:

$$(Q_1)(C_1) = (Q_2)(C_2)$$
$$(x \text{ mL})(40\%) = (500 \text{ mL})(30\%)$$

(23:151)

38. **(A)** One avoirdupois pound contains 454 g. The total number of bacitracin units required is 200 U × 454 g = 90,800 U. By proportion:

$$\frac{500 \text{ U}}{1 \text{ g}} = \frac{90,800 \text{ U}}{x \text{ g}}$$
$$500 x = 90,800$$
$$x = 181.6 \text{ g}$$

(23:216)

39. **(B)** Ten pounds contains 454 g/lb × 10 = 4540 g. Two ounces (av) consists of 28.4 g/oz × 2 = 56.8 g.

$$4540 \text{ g divided by } 56.8 = 80 \text{ jars}$$
$$\text{or}$$
$$16 \text{ av oz} = 1 \text{ lb}$$
$$16 \times 10 = 160 \text{ oz in 10 lb}$$
$$\frac{160 \text{ oz}}{2 \text{ oz jar}} = 80 \text{ jars}$$

(23:66)

40. **(B)** One pound of ointment = 454 g.

$$454 \text{ g} \times 5\% \text{ W/W} = 22.7 \text{ g of glycerin}$$
$$\text{Density} = \text{W/V}$$
$$1.25 = \frac{22.7 \text{ g}}{x \text{ mL}}$$
$$x = 18.2 \text{ mL}$$

(1:83)

41. **(D)** Two pounds would contain 454 × 2 = 908 g of ointment. The final preparation would contain 908 g × 2% = 18.18 g of pure hydrocortisone. Since the available hydrocortisone ointment is 5% strength, one would use:

$$\frac{5 \text{ g}}{100 \text{ g}} = \frac{18.6 \text{ g}}{x \text{ g}}$$
$$x = 363.2 \text{ g of the 5\% ointment}$$

Or, by equation: $(Q_1)(C_1) = (Q_2)(C_2)$

$$(908 \text{ g})(2\% \text{ W/W}) = (x \text{ g})(5\% \text{ W/W})$$
$$x = 363.2 \text{ g}$$

(23:155)

(A) This is the amount of pure hydrocortisone needed to prepare 2 lb of 2% ointment. Choice E (incorrect) is the amount of ointment diluent that would be added to the 5% hydrocortisone ointment.

42. **(B)** Since the amount of 0.5% hydrocortisone cream is exactly 60 g, the final weight of the cream will be greater when the hydrocortisone powder is added. Therefore, solve the problem by alligation alternate method or by simple algebra.

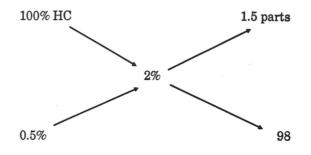

$$\frac{98 \text{ parts (.5\%)}}{60 \text{ g}} = \frac{1.5 \text{ parts (100\%)}}{x \text{ g}}$$
$$x = .92 \text{ g}$$

Or, by algebra, let x = wt. of 100% HC powder

$$(x \text{ g})(100\%) + (60 \text{ g})(.5\%) = (60 + x \text{ g})(2\%)$$
$$x + .3 = 1.2 + .02 x$$
$$x - .02 x = 1.2 - .3$$
$$.98 x = 0.9$$
$$x = .92 \text{ g}$$

(23:59)

43. **(A)** If only sodium chloride was being used to render the 60 mL isotonic: 60 mL × 0.9% = 0.54 g or 540 mg would be needed. However, the zinc sulfate will contribute toward making the solution isotonic. The E value for zinc sulfate is 0.15, which indicates that 1 g of zinc sulfate has the same effect on isotonicity as 150 mg of sodium chloride. The effect of zinc sulfate may be calculated as: (1) 60 mL × 1% = 0.60 g or 600 mg of zinc sulfate required to fill the prescription. (2) This 600 mg is equivalent to 600 × 0.15 = 90 mg of sodium chloride. Therefore, the amount of sodium chloride needed is equal to:

$$540 \text{ mg} - 90 \text{ mg} = 450 \text{ mg}$$

(1:1490,1497)

44. **(B)** Only 45 mL of the prescription must be adjusted to isotonicity, since the 15 mL of Zincfrin is already isotonic. An isotonic solution of sodium chloride contains 0.9% sodium chloride:

$$45 \text{ mL} \times 0.009 = 0.4 \text{ g}$$

(1:1490)

45. **(B)** One liter of normal saline contains 0.9% NaCl or 9 g. To calculate the milliosmolarity of the solution:

Step 1. Determine the moles present

$$\frac{\text{Wt. of chemical}}{\text{Mol. wt.}} = \frac{9\text{ g}}{58.5} = .154 \text{ moles or } 154 \text{ millimoles}$$

Step 2. Multiply the millimoles by the "i" value (the "i" value is the theoretical number of ions or particles formed by one molecule of chemical assuming complete ionization)

$$154 \text{ millimoles} \times 2 = 308 \text{ mOsm/L}$$

(23:194)

46. **(B)** Unlike the above problem, this question asks for mOsm/100 mL and there are two chemicals present.

$$\text{NaCl } \frac{1000\text{ mg}}{58.5} = 17.09 \text{ mmol} \times 2 = 34.2 \text{ mOsm}$$

$$\text{Dextrose } \frac{5000\text{ mg}}{198} = 25.3 \text{ mmol} \times 1 = 25.3 \text{ mOsm}$$

$$\text{total} = 59.5 \text{ mOsm}$$

47. **(C)** Step 1. If pure HCl were available, how much would be needed? Since diluted HCl is 10% W/V, 4000 mL × 10% = 400 g of pure HCl needed.

Step 2. How much of the available 36.8% W/W solution would be needed to obtain 400 g of pure HCl? By definition, a 36.8% W/W solution contains 36.8 g in 100 g of solution.

$$\frac{36.8\text{ g}}{100\text{ g}} = \frac{400\text{ g}}{x\text{ g}}$$
$$x = 1087 \text{ g}$$

Step 3. What is the volume of 1087 g of concentrated acid if its specific gravity is 1.19? 100 mL of acid weighs 119 g.

$$\frac{100\text{ mL}}{119\text{ g}} = \frac{x\text{ mL}}{1087\text{ g}}$$
$$x = 913 \text{ mL}$$

Thus, 4 L of diluted hydrochloric acid is prepared by measuring 913 mL of Hydrochloric Acid USP and diluting it with sufficient purified water to measure 4000 mL. *(23:153)*

48. **(B)** One gallon contains 3785 mL.

$$3785 \text{ mL} \times 0.25\% \text{ W/V} = 9.46 \text{ or } 9.5 \text{ g}$$

Since the volume contributed by the acetic acid is insignificant when compared to 3785 mL, it does not enter into the calculation of final volume.

(1:1317; 23:153)

49. **(C)** More hydrous citric acid than anhydrous citric acid would be needed. The molecular weight of monohydrated citric acid would be: 192 + 1 water (18) = 210.

$$\frac{210}{192} \times 27.4 \text{ g} = 30.0 \text{ g}$$

(1:786; 23:329)

50. **(B)** The formula weight of ferrous sulfate is 278. The amount of iron present in 300 mg of the chemical will be:

$$\frac{55.9}{278} \times 300 \text{ mg} = 60.3 \text{ mg}$$

(23:326)

Choices A and D would be obtained if the correct answer were either doubled or halved to reflect the + 2 valence of iron. The valence of iron has no significance in this type of problem since only one atom of iron is present in each molecule of ferrous sulfate. Choice C assumes that the ferrous sulfate is anhydrous, with a molecular weight of 152. This is incorrect, since the 300-mg weight is based upon a chemical formula containing 7 waters of hydration. Choice E is the amount of anhydrous ferrous sulfate present in each 300 mg. The question asks for iron (Fe) only.

51. **(D)** A saturated solution of the chemical consists of 1 g of chemical plus 10 mL of alcohol. The exact volume of this solution is unknown since the volume occupied by 1 g of the chemical when dissolved cannot be determined. Therefore, the concentration of the saturated solution must be calculated as a % W/W, not a % W/V. The weight of alcohol present will be 8 g since its specific gravity is 0.80.

$$\frac{\text{solute}}{\text{solute} + \text{solvent}} = \frac{1\text{ g}}{1\text{ g} + 8\text{ g}}$$
$$= \frac{1\text{ g}}{9\text{ g}}$$
$$= 11.1\% \text{ W/W}$$

(23:296)

52. **(D)** The daily dose is 0.3 mL × 3 doses = 0.9 mL.

$$0.9 \text{ mL} \times 5\% = 0.045 \text{ g or } 45 \text{ g}$$

(1:94)

CHAPTER 3

Pharmacy

Traditionally, pharmacy has been defined as the art of preparing and dispensing drugs. Today, pharmacy encompasses all aspects of drug preparation and dispensing, as well as evaluation of therapeutic effects in patients. The term "pharmaceutical care" is being used to stress the duty of the pharmacist to ensure that drug therapy produces maximum beneficial outcomes. This chapter includes basic material that a practicing pharmacist must know in order to successfully dispense drug products. This includes knowledge of the manufacture and characteristics of the dosage form, tradenames and generic names, drug strengths and commercial dosage forms, packaging and dispensing advice, and selection of over-the-counter products. Subsequent chapters will stress the actions of drugs within the body, the selection of specific drugs to treat various diseases, and the evaluation of therapeutic outcomes.

Questions

DIRECTIONS (Questions 1 through 201): Each of the numbered items or incomplete statements in this section is followed by answers or by completions of the statement. Select the ONE lettered answer or completion that is BEST in each case.

1. The USP describes several tests for evaluating prescription balances. These tests include all of the following EXCEPT

   (A) arm ratio
   (B) rest point
   (C) rider and graduated beam
   (D) sensitivity requirement
   (E) shift

2. Weights are classified by an alphabetical system. For prescription work, the pharmacist should use which class (or better) weights?

   (A) A
   (B) C
   (C) P
   (D) Q
   (E) T

   P - Most sensitive (do tests)
   Q - Rx work

3. According to the USP, the instruction "protect from light" in a monograph indicates storage in a

   (A) dark place
   (B) amber glass bottle
   (C) light-resistant container
   (D) hermetic container
   (E) tight glass container

   290 - 450 nm
   glass or plastic

4. According to the National Bureau of Standards (NBS), the initial calibration mark on a 100-mL graduate should be

   (A) 5 mL
   (B) 10 mL
   (C) 15 mL
   (D) 20 mL
   (E) 30 mL

   1st mark not less 1/5
   not more than 1/4

5. The pharmacist may suggest Riopan Plus in place of Riopan when the patient desires

   (A) a chewable tablet
   (B) relief from gas
   (C) greater antacid capacity
   (D) lower sodium levels
   (E) a mixture of two antacids

6. According to USP standards, a refrigerator can be used to store pharmaceuticals that specify storage in a

   (A) cold place *2-8 not more than 8°C*
   (B) cool place *8-15* *46°F*
   (C) controlled room temperature *15-30*
   (D) dark place
   (E) both B and C

   refrig 2-8

7. Liquifilm is a vehicle used in preparing

   (A) topical gels
   (B) ophthalmic solutions
   (C) topical aerosols
   (D) otic solutions
   (E) none of the above

   polyvinyl alcohol
   ↑ viscosity & prolonging contact w/ corneal surface

8. The solubility of a chemical in a given solvent is influenced by many factors. All of the following physicochemical constants may be useful in predicting the solubility of a chemical EXCEPT

   (A) dielectric constants
   (B) pH of solution
   (C) pKa of the chemical
   (D) solubility parameters
   (E) valence of the chemical

9. Descriptions of the Federal Controlled Substances Act, Approved Drug Products with Therapeutic Equivalence Evaluations, and USP/NF dispensing requirements may be found in

   (A) *USP DI* Volume I
   (B) *USP DI* Volume II

(C) *USP DI* Volume III
(D) *Facts and Comparisons*
(E) *PDR*

10. Prescription drug descriptions most useful as handouts for patients may be photocopied from the

(A) *USP DI* Volume I — for health prof
(B) *USP DI* Volume II — for pt
(C) *USP DI* Volume III — therp. Equiv
(D) *Facts and Comparisons*
(E) *Remington's Pharmaceutical Sciences*

11. Solubility of a substance may be expressed in several ways. When a quantitative statement of solubility is given in the USP, it is generally expressed as

(A) g of solute soluble in 1 mL of solvent
(B) g of solute soluble in 100 mL of solvent
(C) mL of solvent required to dissolve 1 g of solute
(D) mL of solvent required to dissolve 100 g of solute
(E) mL of solvent required to prepare 100 mL of saturated solution

12. If a bottle of tablets has an expiration date of "Jan 1997," the pharmacist may

(A) continue to dispense the product if he has already opened the container
(B) dispense the tablets only until January 1, 1997
(C) dispense the tablets through January 15, 1997
(D) dispense the tablets through January 31, 1997
(E) dispense the tablets if he informs the patient to discard unused tablets in 6 months

13. The expiration date on a pharmaceutical container states "Expires July 1997." This statement means that by that expiration date, the product may have lost

(A) 5% of its activity
(B) 10% of its activity
(C) 20% of its activity
(D) 50% of its activity
(E) sufficient activity to be outside USP monograph requirements

14. Which of the following agents is/are available in a sublingual dosage form?
   I. isorbide dinitrate (Isordil) } coronary vasodilators
   II. nitroglycerin
   III. hydrogenated ergot alkaloids (Hydergine) Senile dementia

(A) I only
(B) III only
(C) II and III only
(D) I and III only
(E) I, II, and III

15. A chelate must always contain a(n)

(A) multivalent metal
(B) amine group
(C) triple bond
(D) ethylenediamine group
(E) polyoxyethylene chain

16. Which of the following is a chelating agent?

(A) cyanocobalamin (vitamin B_{12})
(B) hydroquinone
(C) edetate — toad
(D) sulfobromophthalein sodium
(E) fluorescein sodium

17. Official forms of water include
   I. Water for Injection
   II. Bacteriostatic Water for Injection
   III. Sterile Water for Inhalation

Sterile H2O for Irrigation

(A) I only
(B) III only
(C) I and II only
(D) II and III only
(E) I, II, and III

18. Which is true for alcohols?

(A) Water solubility increases as the molecular weight of the alcohol increases.
(B) Water solubility increases with an increase in the number of hydroxyl groups.
(C) Water solubility decreases with branching of the carbon chain of the alcohol.
(D) For a given carbon chain, the boiling point is decreased as the number of hydroxyls is increased.
(E) Polarity decreases with increase in the number of hydroxyl groups.

19. An early sign of a decomposing epinephrine solution is the presence of a

(A) brown precipitate 1st sign pink color
(B) pink color   then it darkens
(C) white precipitate to form brown ppt
(D) crystal
(E) odor

20. Upon exposure to air, aminophylline solutions may develop

(A) crystals of theophylline
(B) a gas
(C) a precipitate of aminophylline
(D) a precipitate of ethylenediamine
(E) a straw color

21. The process of grinding a substance to a very fine powder is termed

    (A) levigation
    (B) sublimation
    (C) trituration
    (D) percolation
    (E) maceration

22. The term "impalpable" refers to a substance that is

    (A) bad tasting
    (B) not perceptible to the touch
    (C) greasy
    (D) nongreasy
    (E) tasteless

23. Micromeritics refers to the study of

    (A) metric systems of measurement
    (B) microscopes
    (C) microscopic ocean life
    (D) dimensions of microorganisms
    (E) small particles

24. Dosage forms of cafergot include
    I. oral tablets
    II. rectal suppositories
    III. parenteral solution

    (A) I only
    (B) III only
    (C) I and II only
    (D) II and III only
    (E) I, II, and III

25. Different crystalline forms (polymorphs) of the same drug exhibit different
    I. metabolism rates
    II. melting points
    III. solubilities

    (A) I only
    (B) III only
    (C) I and II only
    (D) II and III only
    (E) I, II, and III

26. Benzalkonium chloride is a germicidal surfactant that is rendered inactive in the presence of

    (A) organic acids
    (B) gram-negative organisms
    (C) cationic surfactants
    (D) soaps
    (E) inorganic salts

27. The shrinkage that occurs when alcohol and purified water are mixed is primarily due to

    (A) attractive van der Waals forces
    (B) covalent bonding
    (C) hydrogen bonding

    (D) ionic bonding
    (E) temperature changes

28. The type of flow in which the viscosity of a liquid increases with agitation is

    (A) plastic
    (B) dilatant
    (C) pseudoplastic
    (D) thixotropic
    (E) Newtonian

29. According to the Poiseuille equation, the factor that has the relatively greatest influence on the rate of flow of liquid through a capillary tube is the

    (A) length of the tube
    (B) viscosity of the liquid
    (C) pressure differential on the tube
    (D) radius of the tube
    (E) temperature of the liquid

30. Patients following low-sodium diets may resort to the use of sodium-free salt substitutes such as Co-Salt (U.S.V.). The major ingredient in these products is

    (A) ammonium chloride
    (B) calcium chloride
    (C) potassium chloride
    (D) potassium iodide
    (E) none of these

31. Potassium supplements are administered in all of the following manners EXCEPT

    (A) IV infusion
    (B) IV bolus
    (C) elixirs, p.o.
    (D) effervescent tablets
    (E) slow-release tablets, p.o.

32. Which of the following statements concerning fluorouracil is NOT true?

    (A) Its chemical structure is a modified pyrimidine similar to uracil and idoxuridine.
    (B) It is effective only when administered by injection.
    (C) Anorexia or nausea and vomiting are very common side effects.
    (D) The drug interferes with the synthesis of ribonucleic acid.
    (E) Major clinical toxic effect is leukopenia.

33. Which one of the following liquid products is NOT a source of potassium?

    (A) Isoclor
    (B) Kaochlor
    (C) Kaon
    (D) Kay Ciel
    (E) all of the above products are potassium supplements

34. Slow release of potassium salts from dosage forms have been accomplished by

   (A) using the slowly dissolving carbonate salt
   (B) enteric coating of successive layers of KCl
   (C) using a wax matrix tablet core from which the potassium slowly dissolves
   (D) using an outer layer of rapidly dissolving KCl and an inner core of slowly dissolving potassium gluconate
   (E) a series of enteric coated granules of KCl that have been compressed into tablet form

35. A comparison of individual amino acids present in commercial amino acids injection solutions may be found in
   I.   *Facts and Comparisons*
   II. *Trissel's Handbook on Injectable Drugs*
   III. *Remington's Pharmaceutical Sciences*

   (A) I only
   (B) III only
   (C) I and II only
   (D) II and III only
   (E) I, II, and III

36. Insulin preparations are usually administered by

   (A) intradermal injection
   (B) intramuscular injection
   (C) intravenous bolus
   (D) intravenous infusion
   (E) subcutaneous injection

37. Which one of the following needles is most suited for the administration of insulin solutions?

   (A) 16G 5/8″
   (B) 21G 1/2″
   (C) 21G 5/8″
   (D) 25G 5/8″
   (E) 25G 1″

38. "Winged" needles are most closely associated with which type of injections?

   (A) intradermal
   (B) intramuscular
   (C) intrathecal
   (D) intravenous
   (E) subcutaneous

39. Hypodermic needle sizes are expressed by gauge numbers. The gauge number refers to the

   (A) bevel size
   (B) external diameter of the cannula — *gauge*
   (C) internal diameter of the cannula
   (D) length of the needle
   (E) size of the lumen opening

   larger the gauge smaller the diameter

40. The Busher Injector is

   (A) an automatic device for self-injecting
   (B) a disposable syringe and needle system
   (C) a device used to start an intravenous injection
   (D) a prefilled syringe unit
   (E) Wyeth's cartridge injection system.

41. The quantities of all ingredients present in parenteral solutions must be specified on the label EXCEPT for
   I.   antimicrobial preservatives *Must label*
   II. isotonicity adjustors
   III. pH adjustors

   (A) I only
   (B) III only
   (C) I and II only
   (D) II and III only
   (E) I, II, and III

42. Which of the following commonly available large-volume dextrose solutions for intravenous use is isotonic?

   (A) 2.5%
   (B) 5.0%   *5 or 5.5%*
   (C) 10%
   (D) 20%
   (E) 50%

43. The term venoclysis is most closely associated with

   (A) intravenous injections
   (B) intrathecal injections
   (C) intravenous infusions
   (D) intrapleural withdrawals
   (E) peritoneal dialysis

44. The designation "minibottles" refers to

   (A) partially filled parenteral bottles with 50- to 150-mL volumes
   (B) any parenteral bottle with a capacity of less than 1 L
   (C) 10- to 30-mL glass vials
   (D) prescription bottles with capacities of 4 oz or less
   (E) vials with a capacity of less than 10 mL

45. The term piggyback is most commonly associated with

   (A) intermittent therapy
   (B) intrathecal injections
   (C) intravenous bolus
   (D) slow intravenous infusions
   (E) total parenteral nutrition

46. What is the approximate maximum volume of fluid that should be administered daily by intravenous infusion to a stabilized patient?

    (A) 1 L
    (B) 4 L
    (C) 8 L
    (D) 12L
    (E) 16 L

47. Which one of the following injectable solutions may result in a precipitate when added to D5W or NS?

    (A) diazepam (Valium)
    (B) folic acid (Folvite)
    (C) furosemide (Lasix)
    (D) gentamicin sulfate (Garamycin)
    (E) succinylcholine chloride (Anectine)

48. Becton Dickinson supplies packages of insulin syringes and needles. Which one of the following statements concerning these products is NOT true?

    (A) Syringes are available for U-40 and U-100 insulins.
    (B) Syringes are color coded and calibrated according to the insulin strengths available.
    (C) The syringes are available either individually wrapped or in bags of 10 each.
    (D) The syringes have 26-gauge needles.
    (E) The smallest volume syringe available is 1.0 mL.

49. The method of preparation must be indicated on labels for

    (A) Bacteriostatic Water for Injection USP
    (B) Milk of Magnesia USP
    (C) Purified Water USP
    (D) Sterile Water for Injection USP
    (E) Water for Injection USP

50. Of the following vehicles, which is the most appropriate for an IV admixture of ampicillin (500 mg/50 mL)?

    (A) dextrose 5% injection
    (B) dextrose 5% and sodium chloride 0.9% injection
    (C) dextrose 2.5% and sodium chloride 0.45% injection
    (D) sodium chloride 0.9% injection
    (E) all of the above

51. The usual expiration dating that should be placed on a parenteral admixture prepared in a hospital pharmacy is

    (A) 1 hour
    (B) 24 hours
    (C) 48 hours
    (D) 72 hours
    (E) 1 week

52. Which one of the following injection solutions will have an alkaline pH?

    (A) Folvite
    (B) Reglan
    (C) Numorphan
    (D) Sandostatin
    (E) Zantac

53. Although isotonicity is desirable for almost all parenterals, it is particularly critical for which injections?

    (A) intra-articular
    (B) intradermal
    (C) intramuscular
    (D) intravenous
    (E) subcutaneous

54. The osmotic pressure of a 0.1 molar dextrose solution will be approximately how many times that of a 0.1 molar sodium chloride solution?

    (A) 0.5
    (B) 1
    (C) 2
    (D) 3
    (E) 4

55. Parenteral solutions that are isotonic with human red blood cells have an osmolality of approximately how many mOsm/L?

    (A) 20
    (B) 40
    (C) 50
    (D) 150
    (E) 300

56. The form of water most commonly used as a solvent during the manufacture of parenterals is

    (A) Bacteriostatic Water for Injection USP
    (B) Deionized Water
    (C) Distilled Water
    (D) Sterile Water for Injection USP
    (E) Water for Injection USP

57. A suspension is NOT a suitable dosage form for what type of injection?

    (A) intra-articular
    (B) intradermal
    (C) intramuscular
    (D) intravenous
    (E) subcutaneous

58. Which one of the following parenteral solutions is considered to most closely approximate the extracellular fluid of the human body?

(A) dextrose 2 1/2% and sodium chloride 0.45% injection
(B) lactated Ringer's injection
(C) Ringer's injection
(D) sodium chloride injection
(E) sodium lactate injection

59. Even distribution of a drug into the blood after an IV bolus injection can be expected within _____ minutes.

(A) 1
(B) 4
(C) 10
(D) 30
(E) 60

Bolus

60. Which one of the following routes of administration is NOT considered suitable for Heparin Sodium Injection USP?

(A) continuous IV infusion
(B) intermittent IV infusion
(C) intramuscular —painful
(D) subcutaneous
(E) all are suitable

localized hematoma

61. The IV fluid systems that use glass bottles may be divided into two types according to the

(A) presence or absence of a vacuum in the bottle
(B) presence or absence of an airway tube in the bottle
(C) type of closure utilized (ie, screw cap vs rubber plug)
(D) size (volume) of the available solutions
(E) presence or absence of pressure in the bottle

62. Which one of the following facts concerning the pharmacokinetics of insulin is NOT true?

degrades in the liver

(A) degradation occurs only in the liver
(B) insulin has a short plasma half-life
(C) insulin has a large volume of distribution
(D) insulin undergoes the first-pass effect in the liver *50% destroyed*
(E) insulin is well absorbed from subcutaneous injection sites.

Kidneys

63. The approximate time for onset of action of the intermediate-acting insulins is _____ hours.

(A) 2
(B) 4
(C) 5 *long*
(D) 6
(E) 8 *none*

① Fast Acting Prompt <1 hr
② Isophane Zinc 1-2 hrs.
③ protamine Zinc 4-6 hrs.

64. Which one of the following parenteral antibiotics is the most stable in aqueous solution?

(A) gentamicin sulfate — 2yrs @ room temp
(B) methicillin sodium
(C) oxacillin sodium
(D) tetracycline hydrochloride
(E) vancomycin hydrochloride

65. Which of the following vitamins possess antioxidant properties?

I. ascorbic acid *vit C*
II. ergocalciferol *Calcium Vit D*
III. vitamin A

(A) I only
(B) III only
(C) I and III
(D) II and III
(E) I, II, and III

Vit C C
Vit E ✗ antioxidant prevent from rancidity or from breakdown of vitamins

66. Naturally occurring vitamin K_1 is also called

(A) menadione - Synthesized
(B) phytonadione
(C) tocopherol
(D) dihydrotachysterol
(E) biotin

67. Which of the following is likely to have the greatest water solubility?

(A) butane
(B) tertiary butanol
(C) tertiary pentanol
(D) n-butanol
(E) n-pentanol

68. Methylparaben is an ester of

(A) benzoic acid
(B) p-hydroxybenzoic acid
(C) para-aminosalicylic acid
(D) propionic acid
(E) benzyl alcohol

Preservative to protect against Mold & yeast

69. Biologicals can be used to obtain either active or passive immunity. Which one of the following pairs is NOT correct?

(A) antiserum, passive immunity
(B) antitoxin, passive immunity
(C) human immune serum, active immunity
(D) toxoid, active immunity
(E) vaccine, active immunity

toxons → active

70. The Schick test is used to determine susceptibility to

(A) diphtheria
(B) measles
(C) polio
(D) TB
(E) typhoid fever

71. All of the following biologicals are used for active immunization EXCEPT

(A) bacterial vaccines
(B) bacterial antigens
(C) human immune sera *passive*
(D) multiple antigen preparations
(E) toxoids

72. Immune serum globulin (gamma globulin) is usually administered by what type of injection?

(A) intradermal
(B) intramuscular
(C) intravenous
(D) subcutaneous
(E) any of the usual methods of injection

73. The Mantoux test uses

for TB. Mantoux & tuberculin fine

(A) diagnostic diphtheria toxin
(B) DPT toxin
(C) mumps skin test antigen
(D) old tuberculin
(E) scarlet fever streptococcus toxin

74. The intermediate tuberculin skin test (intermediate strength PPD) contains

1 or 5 units

(A) 2 tuberculin units
(B) 5 tuberculin units
(C) 25 tuberculin units
(D) 250 tuberculin units
(E) 500 tuberculin units

75. All of the following are used for the prophylaxis or treatment of diseases EXCEPT

avail 6, or 25%

(A) antitoxins
(B) antivenins
(C) globulins
(D) serums
(E) serum albumin *protein in plasma that controls blood volume*

76. The usual storage condition specified for biologicals is

(A) below 2° C
(B) 2 to 8° C — *refrigeration*
(C) a cool place
(D) 8 to 15° C *(cool place)*
(E) room temperature *(15-30)*

77. All of the following statements concerning toxoids are true EXCEPT

(A) toxoids are detoxified toxins
(B) toxoids are antigens
NO (C) toxoids produce permanent immunity
(D) toxoids are often available in a precipitated or adsorbed form
(E) toxoids produce artificial active immunity

78. The capacity of the syringe commonly known as the tuberculin syringe is

(A) 0.1 mL
(B) 0.5 mL
(C) 1.0 mL *Terb 1.0ml*
(D) 2.0 mL
(E) 5.0 mL

79. All of the following are viral infections EXCEPT

(A) influenza *viral*
(B) measles *viral*
(C) mumps *viral*
(D) hepatitis *viral*
(E) typhoid fever *bacterial*

80. All of the following are bacterial infections EXCEPT

(A) cholera *bacteria*
(B) plague *bacteria*
(C) rabies *viral*
(D) pertussis *bacteria*
(E) tuberculosis *bacteria*

81. The route of administration for toxoids in the prophylactic treatment of tetanus would be

(A) intramuscular
(B) intravenous
(C) intradermal
(D) subcutaneous
(E) either subcutaneous or intramuscular

82. Which of the following preparations will induce passive rather than active immunity?

(A) tetanus toxoid *active*
(B) botulism antitoxin *passive*
(C) typhoid vaccine
(D) mumps virus vaccine, attenuated
(E) cholera vaccine

*toxoid — active
antitoxin - passive
attenuated live } active
killed*

83. Which of the following is considered effective in the treatment of accidental drug poisoning?
    I. activated charcoal
    II. ipecac syrup
    III. "universal antidote"

    (A) I only
    (B) III only
    (C) I and II only
    (D) II and III only
    (E) I, II, and III

84. Which one of the following compounds is NOT adsorbed by activated charcoal?

    (A) acetaminophen
    (B) cyanide
    (C) phenothiazines
    (D) propoxyphene
    (E) tricyclic antidepressants

85. A cough syrup is labeled as containing 20% alcohol by volume. Which of the following statements is(are) true?
    I. Each 100 mL of syrup contains exactly 20 mL Alcohol USP.
    II. There is the equivalent of 20 mL of absolute alcohol present in every 100 mL of syrup.
    III. The proof strength of this product is 40.

    (A) I only
    (B) III only
    (C) I and II only
    (D) II and III only
    (E) I, II, and III

86. Bactrim and Septra are trade names for a synergistic combination of

    (A) sulfamethoxazole and trimethoprim
    (B) sulfamethizole and trimethizole
    (C) sulfamethoxazole and trimethadione
    (D) sulfadiazine and phenazopyridine
    (E) sulfisoxazole and methenamine

87. Atropine sulfate is included in the Lomotil formulation in order to

    (A) enhance the laxative action of diphenoxylate
    (B) diminish the unpleasant side effects of diphenoxylate
    (C) enhance the antidiarrheal action of diphenoxylate
    (D) minimize the abuse potential for Lomotil
    (E) diminish the output of gastric secretions

88. Colostomy pouches are classified by
    I. an open vs closed design
    II. size of stoma
    III. whether for a male or female

    (A) I only
    (B) III only
    (C) I and II only
    (D) II and III only
    (E) I, II, and III

89. The most hygroscopic of the following liquids is

    (A) acetone
    (B) alcohol
    (C) glycerin
    (D) mineral oil
    (E) PEG 400

90. Glass used to make pharmaceutical containers is designated as Types I, II, III, and NP. All of these glasses are composed of soda-lime EXCEPT

    (A) Type I
    (B) Type II
    (C) Type III
    (D) Type NP
    (E) Types II and III

91. The containers used to package drugs may consist of several components and/or be composed of several materials. The release of an ingredient from packaging components into the actual product is best described by the term

    (A) adsorption
    (B) diffusion
    (C) leaching
    (D) permeation
    (E) porosity

92. Techniques used in the development of "biotechnological drugs" include

    I. gene splicing
    II. preparation of monoclonal antibodies
    III. lyophilization

    (A) I only
    (B) III only
    (C) I and II only
    (D) II and III only
    (E) I, II, and III

93. Which one of the following drugs is **NOT** prepared by recombinant DNA technology?

    (A) humulin
    (B) interferon
    (C) erythropoietin
    (D) Protropin
    (E) urokinase

94. Which of the following home diagnostic tests incorporate monoclonal antibodies into the testing procedure?

    I. fecal occult blood
    II. ovulation prediction
    III. pregnancy determination

    (A) I only
    (B) III only
    (C) I and II only
    (D) II and III only
    (E) I, II, and III

95. All of the following topical products contain benzoyl peroxide as the active ingredient EXCEPT

    (A) Uticort Gel (Parke-Davis)
    (B) Benzagel (Dermik)
    (C) Desquam X (Westwood Pharmaceuticals)
    (D) Persa-Gel (Ortho-Derm)
    (E) all contain benzoyl peroxide

96. The HLB system is most applicable for the classification of which surfactants?

    (A) anionic
    (B) ampholytic
    (C) cationic
    (D) nonionic
    (E) either anionic or cationic

97. An example of a nonionic surfactant would be

    (A) ammonium laurate
    (B) cetylpyridinium chloride
    (C) dioctyl sodium sulfosuccinate
    (D) sorbitan monopalmitate
    (E) triethanolamine stearate

98. A vehicle for nasal medication should possess all of the following properties EXCEPT

    (A) an acid pH
    (B) isotonicity
    (C) high buffer capacity
    (D) ability to resist growth of microorganisms
    (E) all of the above are important properties; no exceptions

99. All of the following laxatives contain mineral oil EXCEPT

    (A) Agoral
    (B) Kondremul

(C) Neoloid
(D) Haley's M-O
(E) Neo-Cultol

100. Which one of the following statements concerning bisacodyl is NOT true?

    (A) Laxative action occurs within 6 hours after oral administration.
    (B) Action of suppositories occurs within 1 hour of insertion.
    (C) Suppositories may cause rectal irritation with continued administration.
    (D) Tablets should be swallowed whole.
    (E) Tablets should be administered with milk to avoid gastric irritation.

101. Iron salts are usually administered orally. A commercially available parenteral product is

    (A) Chel-Iron
    (B) Feosol
    (C) Simron
    (D) InFeD
    (E) Troph-Iron

102. Which one of the following chemicals is an effective and safe drug in the treatment of either diarrhea or constipation?

    (A) activated charcoal
    (B) bismuth salts
    (C) kaolin
    (D) attapulgite
    (E) polycarbophil

103. All of the following OTC laxative products contain phenolphthalein EXCEPT

    (A) Agoral (Warner Chilcott)
    (B) Alophen (Parke-Davis)
    (C) Perdiem (Rhone-Poulenc Rorer)
    (D) Correctol (Plough)
    (E) Phenolax (Upjohn)

104. Not only are the insoluble bismuth salts adsorbent, but they also possess useful astringent and protective properties. A commercial product containing a bismuth compound is

    (A) Bisodol (Whitehall)
    (B) Donnagel (Robins)
    (C) Kaopectate (Upjohn)
    (D) Pepto-Bismol (Norwich)
    (E) Rheaban (Leeming)

105. Which of the following antidiarrheal products contains the adsorbent clay attapulgite?

    (A) Donnagel
    (B) Kaopectate suspension
    (C) Bacid

(D) Parepectolin   *Kaolein pectin paregoric*
(E) Kaopectate tablets   *750 mg*

106. Which of the following statements concerning vitamin E is NOT true?   *↓ absorption of iron & ca*

(A) appears to be compatible with mineral supplements such as calcium and iron
(B) can be taken in large doses without toxic effects
(C) consists mainly of α tocopherol
(D) deficiency is not common in the general population
(E) is an antioxidant

107. A sympathomimetic often present in OTC appetite suppressants is

(A) ephedrine
(B) phenylephrine
(C) phenylpropanolamine
(D) pseudoephedrine
(E) caffeine

108. The active ingredient in Bacid is best described as a(n)   *Lactobacillus   24–48 Hrs for diarrhea*

(A) antacid
(B) astringent
(C) clay
(D) demulcent
(E) microorganism

109. All of the following products contain buffered aspirin EXCEPT

(A) Ascriptin
(B) Cope
(C) Arthritis Strength Bufferin
(D) Excedrin   *ASA, caffeine, ASA no buffer*
(E) Vanquish

110. Which one of the following OTC internal analgesics contains magnesium salicylate?

(A) Bromo-Seltzer
(B) Doan's Original   *Mag Salicylate*
(C) Ecotrin
(D) Pamprin
(E) Sinarest

111. Advantages of dextromethorphan as a cough suppressant include all of the following EXCEPT   *120mg/day*

(A) as effective as codeine on a weight/weight basis
(B) does not cause respiratory depression
(C) is nonaddicting
(D) doses of 10 to 15 mg suppress coughing for at least 4 hours
(E) maximum daily adult dose is 30 mg   *Max 120mg*

112. Which of the following statements is NOT true about the liquid product Emetrol?

(A) contains both levulose and dextrose
(B) is manufactured by Rorer

(C) may be dispensed without a prescription
(D) should be either diluted or administered with water or other fluids   *NO*
(E) has a dosage limit of 15 to 30 mL every 15 minutes for not more than five doses   *30ml Q15min ×5doses*

113. Disadvantages of calcium carbonate as an antacid include all of the following EXCEPT

(A) some patients may develop hypercalcemia   *very good*
(B) capacity for acid neutralization is poor
(C) may cause constipation
(D) may induce gastric hypersecretion
(E) prolonged use may induce renal calculi and decreased renal function

114. Which one of the following antacid products is a chemical combination of aluminum and magnesium hydroxides?

(A) Gelusil
(B) Maalox   *Riopan*
(C) Mylanta   *Al Mg*
(D) Riopan
(E) Tums   *NO*

115. Which one of the following antacids is CONTRAINDICATED for individuals on a low-sodium diet?

(A) Chooz tablets
(B) Digel tablets
(C) Mylanta tablets
(D) Milk of Magnesia tablets
(E) Rolaids tablets   *53mg Na per tab*

116. Aminobenzoic acid is included in topical preparations as a(n)

(A) antiacne agent
(B) anti-infective
(C) antimicrobial preservative
(D) local anesthetic
(E) sunscreen

117. Poorly manufactured tablets may result in splitting off of the upper surface of the tablet. This phenomenon is known as

(A) capping
(B) cracking
(C) impacting
(D) mottling   *uneven color*
(E) picking   *splitting of upper surface of tab*

118. Picking of tablets can be caused by all of the following EXCEPT

(A) excessive compression pressure
(B) a granulation that is too damp
(C) scratched punches
(D) static charges on the powder
(E) unsatisfactory lubricant

119. Which of the following is NOT used primarily as a diluent in tablet formulations?

    (A) magnesium stearate — *stearates are lubricants*
    (B) dicalcium phosphate
    (C) lactose
    (D) mannitol
    (E) starch

120. Which of the following is NOT a function of the lubricant in a tablet formulation?

    (A) improving flow properties of granules
    (B) reducing powder adhesion onto the dies and punches
    (C) improving tablet wetting in the stomach
    (D) reducing punch and die wear
    (E) facilitating tablet ejection from the die

121. An ingredient that is added to a tablet formula to improve flow properties into a die for compression is known as a(n)

    (A) disintegrant   *potato or corn starch*
    (B) glidant
    (C) lubricant
    (D) surfactant
    (E) emollient
        → powder not cohesive

122. The capping of a tablet may be the result of any of the following EXCEPT

    (A) excessive lubricant
    (B) excessive pressure of compression
    (C) excessive fine powder
    (D) insufficient binder
    (E) too dry a granulation

123. All of the following ingredients have been commonly used as the coating agents for film coating EXCEPT

    (A) carnauba wax — *sugar coating*
    (B) cellulose acetate phthalate
    (C) starch
    (D) sodium carboxymethylcellulose
    (E) castor oil

124. Which of the following trademarked dosage forms is enteric coated?

    (A) Enduret *SA*
    (B) Enseal
    (C) Extentab
    (D) Filmtab
    (E) all of the above

125. A sweetener that is widely employed in chewable tablet formulas is

    (A) cyclamate sodium
    (B) glucose

    (C) lactose
    (D) mannitol
    (E) sucrose

126. Mannitol may be included in lyophilized products as a

    (A) buffer
    (B) bulking agent   *↳ Freezedried*
    (C) preservative
    (D) sweetener
    (E) tonicity adjustor

127. Benzyl alcohol is present in some parenteral solutions as a(n)

    (A) antimicrobial preservative
    (B) antioxidant
    (C) chelating agent
    (D) buffering agent
    (E) tonicity adjustor

128. Which of the following properties is desirable in a pharmaceutical suspension?

    No I. caking *hard cake at bottom of susp.*
    II. pseudoplastic flow *flow when shaken*
    III. thixotropy — *flow better when shaken*

    (A) I only
    (B) III only
    (C) I and II only
    (D) II and III only
    (E) I, II, and III

129. Characteristics of inhalation aerosol dosage forms include

    I. avoid first pass effect
    II. rapid onset of action
    III. can administer large amounts of drug to intended site

    (A) I only
    (B) III only
    (C) I and II only
    (D) II and III only
    (E) I, II, and III

130. Which of the following ingredients is(are) available in OTC aerosol asthmatic products?

    I. epinephrine *primalene*
    II. ephedrine *Rx*
    III. metaproterenol *Rx*

    (A) I only
    (B) III only
    (C) I and II only
    (D) II and III only
    (E) I, II, and III

131. Which of the following commercially available thyroid preparations contains both liothyronine (T_3) and thyroxine (T_4) in roughly the same ratio in which they are secreted by the thyroid gland?

    (A) Proloid
    (B) Synthroid
    (C) Thyrolar
    (D) Levothroid
    (E) Cytomel

132. Which of the following narcotics may NOT be used for medicinal purposes in this country?

    (A) diacetylmorphine
    (B) ethylmorphine
    (C) dihydrocodeinone
    (D) methylmorphine
    (E) all are permitted

133. Burns are classified according to relative severity. Characteristics of a first-degree burn are

    (A) erythema, pain, no blistering
    (B) erythema, pain, blistering
    (C) blisters, pain, skin will regenerate
    (D) no blisters, leathery appearance of skin, skin grafting necessary
    (E) blackened skin, danger of deep infection

134. The local anesthetic most commonly used in OTC burn remedies is

    (A) benzocaine
    (B) butamben picrate
    (C) lidocaine
    (D) phenol
    (E) tetracaine

135. Which one of the following statements concerning dextranomer (Debrisan by Johnson & Johnson) is NOT correct?

    (A) aids in the removal of wound exudates
    (B) can be used to treat decubitus ulcers
    (C) consists of spherical hydrophilic beads
    (D) is effective in the healing of both secreting and nonsecreting wounds
    (E) must be physically removed after treatment

136. For effectiveness as a local anesthetic, the level of benzocaine in a topical preparation should be AT LEAST

    (A) 0.1%
    (B) 35%
    (C) 1.0%
    (D) 2.0%
    (E) 5.0%

137. Rectal clinical thermometers differ from oral thermometers in

    (A) bulb shape
    (B) stem length
    (C) distance between graduation marks on the stem
    (D) standards for accuracy
    (E) stem shape

138. A basal thermometer is

    (A) a rectal thermometer
    (B) used to estimate time of ovulation
    (C) used to determine basal metabolic rate
    (D) graduated only in Celsius degrees
    (E) used vaginally

139. The scale most commonly used in this country for denoting catheter sizes is the

    (A) American
    (B) English
    (C) French
    (D) Stubbs
    (E) Foley

140. Which one of the following statements concerning allergic reactions to insect bites and stings is NOT true?

    (A) cross-sensitization to bites of different insects (ants, wasps, bees, etc) can be expected
    (B) death may occur due to anaphylactic reaction
    (C) the initial systemic reaction will usually occur within 20 minutes of the time of the bite
    (D) the toxicity of the venom is the prime cause of the severe reaction or death
    (E) subsequent sting episodes usually cause more severe reactions than the earlier ones do

141. Emergency insect sting and bite kits usually contain all of the following except

    (A) antiseptic pads
    (B) antihistamines
    (C) epinephrine HCl injection
    (D) tourniquet
    (E) tweezers

142. The properties of the ointment base, Eucerin, are most similar to

    (A) hydrophilic ointment
    (B) cold cream
    (C) Jelene
    (D) polyethylene glycol ointment
    (E) Unibase

143. Ingredients in Debrox Drops include
     I. alcohol
     II. carbamide peroxide
     III. glycerin

     (A) I only
     (B) III only
     (C) I and II only
     (D) II and III only
     (E) I, II, and III

144. Which one of the following procedures would NOT improve the absorption of a drug into the skin?

     (A) applying the ointment and covering the area with an occlusive bandage or Saran wrap
     (B) incorporating an oil-soluble drug in polyethylene glycol ointment rather than white ointment
     (C) applying the medicated ointment on the back of the hand rather than on the palms
     (D) increasing the concentration of the active drug in the ointment bases
     (E) using an ointment base in which the active drug has excellent solubility

145. Aqueous solutions can be directly incorporated into all of the following ointment bases EXCEPT

     (A) Aquaphor
     (B) lanolin
     (C) Polysorb
     (D) Unibase
     (E) white ointment

146. Most commercial emulsion bases are O/W emulsion systems. An exception, which is a W/O emulsion, is

     (A) Allercreme Skin Lotion
     (B) Cetaphil
     (C) Keri lotion
     (D) Neobase
     (E) Polysorb Hydrate

147. Alphosyl cream contains allantoin, which is present as a(n)

     (A) antibacterial agent
     (B) antifungal agent
     (C) antipruritic
     (D) emollient
     (E) healing agent

148. A synonym for Cold Cream USP is

     (A) Galen's cerate
     (B) petrolatum rose water ointment
     (C) rose water ointment
     (D) wool fat emulsion
     (E) vanishing cream

149. Characteristics of rectal drug administration include all of the following EXCEPT

     (A) neutral pH of colon fluids lessens possible drug inactivation by stomach acidity
     (B) drugs may avoid first-pass hepatic inactivation
     (C) drugs intended for systemic activity can be administered
     (D) the release and absorption of drugs is predictable
     (E) irritating drugs have less effect on the rectum than on the stomach

150. Most commercial vaginal suppositories use a base of

     (A) beeswax
     (B) cocoa butter
     (C) glycerin
     (D) glycerinated gelatin
     (E) polyethylene glycols

151. An excellent choice of diluent for a compressed vaginal tablet formulation would be

     (A) lactose
     (B) starch
     (C) sucrose
     (D) talc
     (E) all are equally effective

152. Norforms suppositories may be used as a(n)

     (A) antitrichomonal agent
     (B) contraceptive
     (C) deodorant
     (D) mild laxative
     (E) tampon

153. Certain vaginal products must be refrigerated for greater stability. The pharmacist should attach a "store in the refrigerator" label on which one of the following products?

     (A) Betadine Vaginal Gel
     (B) Monistat Cream
     (C) Sultrin Cream
     (D) Lotrimin Cream
     (E) Mycostatin Tablets

154. Which of the following comments concerning dextran is NOT true?

     (A) available in two types—Dextran 40 and 75
     (B) administered by intravenous injection
     (C) useful in emergency treatment of shock
     (D) used as a blood substitute
     (E) may be used in relieving edema of nephrosis

155. The colligative properties of a solution are related to the

(A) total number of solute particles
(B) pH
(C) number of ions
(D) number of unionized molecules
(E) the ratio of the number of ions to the number of molecules

156. Colligative properties are useful in determining

(A) tonicity
(B) pH
(C) solubility
(D) sterility
(E) stability

157. All of the following properties are classified as colligative properties EXCEPT

(A) elevation of boiling point
(B) osmotic pressure
(C) increase in conductivity
(D) lowering of freezing point
(E) lowering of vapor pressure

158. An isotonic solution has the same

(A) salt content as blood
(B) pH as blood
(C) fluid pressure as blood
(D) osmotic pressure as blood
(E) specific gravity as blood

159. All of the following substances readily permeate the red blood cell, causing hemolysis, EXCEPT

(A) boric acid
(B) glucose
(C) glycerin
(D) propylene glycol
(E) urea

160. Mixing a hypertonic solution with red blood cells will cause _____ of the red blood cells.

(A) bursting
(B) chelating
(C) crenation
(D) hemolysis
(E) hydrolysis

161. Sodium chloride equivalents are used to estimate the amount of sodium chloride needed to render a solution isotonic. The sodium chloride equivalent or "E" value may be defined as the

(A) amount of sodium chloride that is theoretically equivalent to 1 g of a specified chemical
(B) amount of a specified chemical theoretically equivalent to 1 g of sodium chloride

(C) milliequivalents of sodium chloride needed to render a solution isotonic
(D) weight of a specified chemical that will render a solution isotonic
(E) percent sodium chloride needed to make a solution isotonic

162. A second method for adjusting solution to isotonicity is based upon

(A) boiling point elevation
(B) blood coagulation time
(C) freezing point depression
(D) milliequivalent calculation
(E) refractive index

163. All aqueous solutions that freeze at −0.52° C are isotonic with red blood cells. They are also isoosmotic with each other. Which of the following apply?

(A) Both statements are true.
(B) Both statements are false.
(C) The first statement is true but the second is false.
(D) The second statement is true but the first is false.
(E) There is no correlation between freezing points and osmotic pressures of solutions.

164. One disadvantage in calculating isotonicity adjustments using either the sodium chloride equivalent or freezing point depression methods is

(A) D values are not accurate
(B) E values are not accurate
(C) it is difficult to locate the values in the literature
(D) only sodium chloride can be used for tonicity adjustments
(E) the adjusted solution will be isoosmotic but may not be isotonic

165. Methylcellulose and similar agents are used in ophthalmic solutions to

(A) increase drop size
(B) increase ocular contact time
(C) reduce inflammation of the eye
(D) reduce tearing during instillation of the drops
(E) reduce drop size

166. The presence of *Pseudomonas aeruginosa* would be of particular danger in an ophthalmic solution of

(A) atropine sulfate
(B) fluorescein sodium
(C) pilocarpine hydrochloride
(D) silver nitrate
(E) zinc sulfate

167. The most popular commercial combination of preservatives that appears to be effective for ophthalmic use is

(A) benzalkonium chloride and EDTA
(B) benzalkonium chloride and chlorobutanol
(C) chlorobutanol and EDTA
(D) methyl and propyl paraben
(E) phenylmercuric nitrate and phenylethyl alcohol

168. Which one of the following ophthalmic solutions does NOT require storage in the refrigerator?

(A) Chloroptic
(B) Eppy
(C) Ophthochlor
(D) Sodium Sulamyd
(E) all require refrigeration

169. Which one of the following anesthetics is available as an ophthalmic solution?

(A) dibucaine hydrochloride
(B) hexylcaine hydrochloride
(C) lidocaine hydrochloride
(D) procaine hydrochloride
(E) tetracaine hydrochloride

170. All of the following viscosity builders have been used in ophthalmic solutions EXCEPT

(A) hydroxypropylmethylcellulose
(B) polyvinyl alcohol
(C) polyvinylpyrrolidone
(D) methylcellulose
(E) veegum

171. The function of papain in a soft contact lens product is to

(A) remove oil films
(B) disinfect
(C) keep the lens soft
(D) remove proteinaceous residues
(E) prevent dehydration of the lens

172. The presence of sodium bisulfite in a drug solution implies that the drug

(A) has poor water solubility
(B) is heat labile
(C) is susceptible to oxidation
(D) requires an alkaline media
(E) will sustain growth of microorganisms

173. Which of the following side effects occur in some individuals who are sensitive to bisulfites?

(A) difficulty in breathing
(B) a dry cough
(C) diarrhea
(D) dizziness
(E) loss of body hair

174. Which of the following would be most irritating to the eye?

(A) purified water
(B) 0.7% sodium chloride solution
(C) 0.9% sodium chloride solution
(D) 1.2% sodium chloride solution
(E) either .7% or 1.2% sodium chloride solution

175. Which layer of the human cornea is LEAST lipophilic?

(A) sclera
(B) conjunctiva
(C) corneal endothelium
(D) corneal epithelium
(E) stroma

176. The capacity of the human eye for instilled ophthalmic drops is approximately

(A) 0.01 to 0.05 mL
(B) 0.1 mL
(C) 0.5 mL
(D) 1.0 mL
(E) 2.0 mL

177. pH is mathematically

(A) the log of the hydroxyl ion concentration
(B) the negative log of the hydroxyl ion concentration
(C) the log of the hydronium ion concentration
(D) the negative log of the hydronium ion concentration
(E) none of the above

178. The pH of a buffer system can be calculated by using the

(A) pH partition theory
(B) Noyes-Whitney Law
(C) Henderson-Hasselbalch equation
(D) Michaelis-Menten equation
(E) none of the above

179. pH is equal to pKa at

(A) pH 1
(B) pH 7
(C) the neutralization point
(D) the end point
(E) the half-neutralization point

180. Units for expressing radioisotope decay include the
  I. rad
  II. curie
  III. becquerel

(A) I only
(B) III only
(C) I and II only
(D) II and III only
(E) I, II, and III

181. Which of the following radioisotopes is used in therapeutic doses to treat polycythemia vera?

    (A) gold (^{198}Au)
    (B) iridium (^{192}Ir)
    (C) yttrium (^{90}Y)
    (D) sodium phosphate (^{32}P)
    (E) sodium iodide (^{131}I)

182. A radioisotope generator is a(n)

    (A) pharmaceutical product labeled with a radioactive substance
    (B) ion-exchange column upon which a nuclide has been adsorbed
    (C) ionization chamber
    (D) high-energy–yielding radioactive isotope that produces one or more isotopes emitting low-energy radiation
    (E) apparatus in which radioactive isotopes are incorporated into biological molecules

183. Which of the following widely used radioisotopes is considered to be an almost ideal isotope for medical applications and is commercially available as a radioisotope generator?

    (A) ^{131}I (iodine)
    (B) ^{99m}TC (technetium)
    (C) ^{32}P (phosphorus)
    (D) ^{59}Fe (iron)
    (E) ^{198}Au (gold)

184. Isotopes are atomic species having the same number of

    (A) protons and neutrons
    (B) protons and electrons
    (C) protons but a different number of electrons
    (D) neutrons but a different number of protons
    (E) protons but a different number of neutrons

185. The decay of radioactive atoms occurs

    (A) at a constant rate
    (B) as a first-order reaction
    (C) as a zero-order reaction
    (D) as a second-order reaction
    (E) at constantly increasing rates

186. Which one of the following forms of radiation has the greatest penetrating power?

    (A) alpha radiation
    (B) beta radiation
    (C) gamma radiation
    (D) x-rays
    (E) ultraviolet radiation

187. Which of the following is(are) true of the ergot alkaloids?
    I. natural source is a fungus
    II. their salts would be compatible with acids

III. used as oxytocic or antimigraine drugs

    (A) I only
    (B) III only
    (C) I and II only
    (D) II and III only
    (E) I, II, and III

188. Surfactants are characterized by the presence of

    (A) water-solubilizing groups
    (B) negative charges
    (C) positive charges
    (D) fat-solubilizing groups
    (E) water-solubilizing and fat-solubilizing groups in the same molecule

189. Which one of the following general characteristics is NOT true for alkaloids?

    (A) contain nitrogen in the molecule
    (B) have good alcohol solubility
    (C) have pKa's less than 7
    (D) often exhibit stereoisomerism
    (E) have poor water solubility

190. The agency in the United States responsible for selecting appropriate nonproprietary names for drugs is the

    (A) AMA
    (B) APhA
    (C) FDA
    (D) USAN
    (E) USP

191. The product inserts for many drug products contain cautionary statements. Which one of the following sequences lists the three types of cautions in the order of least serious to most serious?

    (A) contraindication, precaution, warning
    (B) precaution, warning, contraindication
    (C) warning, contraindication, precaution
    (D) warning, precaution, contraindication
    (E) contraindication, warning, precaution

192. The degree of dissociation of acids is often expressed in terms of pKa. A pKa for an acid is

    (A) directly measured by titration of the acid with sodium hydroxide
    (B) calculated by determining the acid's buffer capacity
    (C) directly determined by conductivity measurements
    (D) the natural log of the acid's dissociation constant
    (E) the reciprocal log of the dissociation constant

Questions 193 through 195

Answer questions 193 through 195 by referring to the following table as necessary.

TABLE OF pKa VALUES FOR ACIDS

Acid	pKa
acetic	4.76
acetylsalicylic	3.49
boric	9.24
lactic	3.86
salicylic	2.97

193. Which one of the following acids would have the greatest degree of ionization in water?

(A) acetic
(B) boric
(C) hydrochloric
(D) lactic
(E) salicylic

Strongest acid the More ionization close to Ø ∴ strongest acid

194. Which one of the following acids would be considered the weakest (with the least amount of ionization) in water?

(A) acetic
(B) acetylsalicylic
(C) boric
(D) lactic
(E) salicylic

195. To prepare a buffer system with the greatest buffer capacity at a pH of 4.0, one would use which one of the following acids?

(A) acetic
(B) acetylsalicylic
(C) boric
(D) lactic
(E) salicylic

pKa = 3.86

196. Ibuprofen has a pKa of 5.5. If the pH of a patient's urine is 7.5, what would the ratio of dissociated to undissociated drug be?

(A) 2:1
(B) 100:1
(C) 20:1
(D) 1:2
(E) 1:100

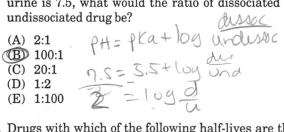

pH = pKa + log dissoc/undissoc

7.5 = 5.5 + log du/und

2 = log d/u

197. Drugs with which of the following half-lives are the best candidates for oral <u>sustained</u> release dosage formulations?

(A) <1 hour
(B) 1 to 2 hours
(C) 2 to 8 hours

(D) 8 to 12 hours
(E) 12 hours

Questions 198 through 201

MATCH the lettered dosage strength which is NOT commercially available under each of the following numbered drug brand names.

198. Inderal

(A) 5 mg
(B) 10 mg
(C) 20 mg
(D) 40 mg
(E) 80 mg

199. Coumadin

(A) 2 mg
(B) 5 mg
(C) 10 mg
(D) 20 mg
(E) all are available

200. Theo-Dur

(A) 100 mg
(B) 200 mg
(C) 250 mg
(D) 300 mg
(E) 450 mg

201. Valium (diazepam) is available in which of the following dosage forms?

   I. elixir
   II. injection solution
   III. tablet

(A) I only
(B) III only
(C) I and II only
(D) II and III only
(E) I, II, and III

DIRECTIONS (Questions 202 through 309): Each group of items in this section consists of lettered headings followed by a set of numbered words or phrases. For each numbered word or phrase, select the ONE lettered heading that is most closely associated with it. Each lettered heading may be selected once, more than once, or not at all.

Questions 202 through 217

MATCH the lettered manufacturer with the associated numbered trademarked dosage form.

(A) Robins
(B) Abbott
(C) Parke-Davis

(D) Schering
(E) Sandoz

202. Filmtab ~~B~~ Abbott

203. Kapseal C Parke-Davis

204. Extentab A Robins

205. Spacetab E Sandoz

(A) Wyeth
(B) Lilly
(C) Schering
(D) Winthrop
(E) Abbott

206. Chronotab C Shering

207. Caplet D Winthrop

208. Wyseal A Wyeth

209. Enseal B Lilly

(A) Smith Kline & French
(B) Wyeth
(C) Ciba
(D) Parke-Davis
(E) Schering

210. Filmseal D

211. Repetab A

212. Spansule A

213. Transderm C

(A) Schering
(B) Abbott
(C) Ciba
(D) Lakeside
(E) Parke-Davis

214. Gradumet B Abbott

215. Infatab E Parke

216. Dospan A Schering

217. Oros D Lakeside

Questions 218 through 227

MATCH the lettered dosage strength with its most closely corresponding numbered drug brand name.

(A) 5 mg
(B) 25 mg
(C) 40 mg

(D) 150 mg
(E) 300 mg

218. Orudis C

219. Micronase A

220. Cleocin D

221. Lopid E

222. Indocin B

(A) 1 mg
(B) 10 mg
(C) 50 mg
(D) 60 mg
(E) 250 mg

223. Aldomet E

224. Hygroton C

225. Hismanal B

226. Tenex A

227. Sudafed D

Questions 228 through 242

MATCH the lettered generic name most closely corresponding to the numbered drug brand name.

(A) nizatidine
(B) verapamil
(C) metronidazole
(D) propranolol
(E) triamterene

228. Inderal D

229. Axid A

230. Dyazide E

231. Isoptin B

232. Flagyl C

(A) diazepam
(B) diphenhydramine
(C) methyldopa
(D) atenolol
(E) phenytoin

233. Benadryl B

234. Valium A

235. Tenormin D

236. Dilantin E

237. Aldomet C

(A) nifedipine
(B) enalapril
(C) diflunisal
(D) clofibrate
(E) dipyridamole

238. Dolobid C

239. Procardia A

240. Persantine E

241. Atromid-S D

242. Vasotec B

Questions 243 through 251

MATCH the lettered drug brand name having the same active therapeutic ingredient as the numbered drug brand name.

(A) Procan SR
(B) Calan
(C) Esidrix
(D) Sorbitrate
(E) Ventolin

243. Pronestyl A

244. HydroDIURIL C

245. Isordil D

246. Proventil E

247. Isoptin B

(A) ERYC
(B) Nilstat
(C) Larobec
(D) Erythrocin - Ethyl
(E) Lithane

248. Pediamycin D

249. Eskalith E

250. E-Mycin A

251. Mycostatin B

Questions 252 through 256

MATCH the lettered trade name with the related numbered nonproprietary name.

(A) Afrin
(B) Privine
(C) Neo-Synephrine
(D) Triaminicin
(E) Otrivin

252. phenylephrine C

253. phenylpropanolamine D

254. oxymetazoline A

255. naphazoline B

256. xylometazoline E

Questions 257 through 259

MATCH each lettered nonproprietary name with the corresponding numbered tradename for an ophthalmic solution.

(A) demecarium bromide
(B) echothiophate iodide
(C) isoflurophate
(D) neostigmine bromide
(E) physostigmine salicylate

257. Floropryl C

258. Humorsol A

259. Phospholine B

Questions 260 through 263

MATCH the lettered brand name with the numbered nonproprietary name most closely related to it.

(A) Marcaine
(B) Carbocaine
(C) Novocaine
(D) Xylocaine
(E) Tronothane

260. lidocaine D

261. pramoxine E

262. bupivacaine A

263. procaine C

Questions 264 through 268

MATCH the lettered antacid ingredients with the corresponding numbered commercial antacid product.

(A) aluminum hydroxide
(B) mixture of aluminum and magnesium hydroxides
(C) mixture of aluminum hydroxide, magnesium trisilicate, and sodium bicarbonate
(D) calcium carbonate
(E) sodium bicarbonate

264. Amphojel *A*

265. Gaviscon *E* algenicaaa Al, Mg S Bicarb

266. Mylanta *B* Al Mg

267. Titralac *D* Al Mg SbCC

268. Maalox *B*

Questions 269 through 275

MATCH the lettered manufacturer with the associated numbered syringe or parenteral container system.

(A) Wyeth
(B) Roche
(C) Squibb
(D) Winthrop
(E) Pfizer

269. Unimatic *C* Squibb

270. Isoject *E* Pfizer

271. Carpuject *D* Winthrop

272. Tubex *A* Wyeth

(A) Abbott
(B) Baxter
(C) Lilly
(D) McGaw
(E) Wyeth

273. Accumed *D*

274. Lifecare *A*

275. Viaflex *B*

Questions 276 through 279

MATCH the lettered nonproprietary name with the associated numbered B complex vitamin.

(A) cyanocobalamin
(B) pyridoxine
(C) thiamine
(D) riboflavin
(E) pantothenic acid   *S*

276. B₁ *C* thiamine B1

277. B₂ *D* riboflavin B2

278. B₆ *B* pyridoxine B6

279. B₁₂ *A* cyanocobalamin B12

Questions 280 through 282

Alcohol has many pharmaceutical uses and is available in several concentrations. MATCH the lettered concentration (% V/V) with the associated numbered official product.

(A) 49%
(B) 70% — rubbing
(C) 92%
(D) 95%
(E) 100%

280. Alcohol *D*

281. Diluted Alcohol *A*

282. Rubbing Alcohol *B*

Questions 283 through 286

MATCH the lettered term concerning hypodermic needles with the associated numbered description.

(A) bevel
(B) cannula
(C) hub
(D) heel of bevel
(E) lumen

283. extension of needle that fits onto the syringe *C* hub

284. portion of needle that is ground for sharpness *A*

285. shaft portion of the needle *B*

286. the needle hole *E*

Questions 287 through 290

As a pharmacist you may be asked for advice in selecting a suitable product for a skin condition. MATCH the lettered OTC ointment with the most appropriate numbered request.

(A) calamine
(B) Butesin
(C) coal tar
(D) ichthammol
(E) sulfur

287. to treat inflammation and boils *D*

288. an astringent/protective *A*

289. to treat a mild case of scabies *E*

290. to treat a mild eczematic condition *C*

Questions 291 through 294

It is often desirable to formulate a dosage form so that its pH approximates that of the area to which it is administered. MATCH the lettered pH value that is nearest to the pH usually found in the numbered body areas. Answers may be used once, more than once, or not at all.

(A) 4.0–4.5
(B) 5.5
(C) 6.4
(D) 7.0
(E) 7.4

291. blood *E*

292. eye *E*

293. skin *B*

294. vagina *A*

Blood, Eye pH 7.4
Skin 5.5
Vagina 3-4

Questions 295 through 300

MATCH the lettered route(s) of administration with the numbered anesthetic. Letters may be used once, more than once, or not at all.

(A) intravenous and local injection
(B) local injection
(C) topical
(D) topical and local injection
(E) topical, local injection, and intravenous injection

295. cocaine *C*

296. lidocaine (Xylocaine) *E*

297. mepivacaine (Carbocaine) *B*

298. bupivacaine (Marcaine) *B*

299. ketamine (Ketalar) *A*

300. tetracaine (Pontocaine) *D*

Questions 301 through 305

Select the lettered formulation design that best describes the mechanism of release for each of the following numbered drug products.

(A) complexation
(B) pellets in a tablet
(C) repeat action
(D) slow erosion core
(E) slow erosion core with an initial dose

301. Triaminic Tablets *repeat action*

302. Dimetapp Extentabs *slow erosion core w/ initial dose*

303. Isordil Tembids Tablets *pellets in tabs*

304. Rynatan Tablets *complexation*

305. Tenuate Dospan *slow erosion*

Questions 306 through 309

MATCH the numbered sustained-action principle with the corresponding lettered drug product.

(A) Ornade (SKB)
(B) Ionamin (Pennwalt)
(C) Desoxyn (Abbott)
(D) Demazin (Schering)
(E) Medrol Medules (Upjohn)

306. ion-exchange resin *B*

307. microencapsulated drug *D*

308. pellet form in capsule *A*

309. leaching from insoluble matrix *C*

Answers and Explanations

1. (B) The rest point is simply the point at which the balance indicator pointer stops. It may be easily shifted by adjusting the leveling screws of the balance. Most operators simply observe the equidistant swing of the indicator to confirm equilibrium.

(A–incorrect) This test confirms that the two arms of the balance are equal in length.

(C–incorrect) The rider test confirms the accuracy of the calibrated beam or dial at both the 500-mg and 1-g position.

(D–incorrect) The sensitivity is reflected by the minimum weight that will shift the indicator point one unit or mark on the indicator plate. This shift is considered the smallest change that an operator can consistently observe. Therefore, it is the smallest discernible weighing error. The sensitivity requirement (S.R.) for Class A prescription balances is 6 mg. For the less precise Class B prescription balance, the S.R. is 30 mg. *(1:77; 18c:II–25)*

(E–incorrect) The shift tests check the balance construction, especially the arm and lever components.
(1:77; 18c:II–25)

2. (D) The accuracy of weights is expressed in tolerances that are + or – deviations from the stated weight. The Class Q weights have lower tolerances than the sensitivity requirement of the Class A prescription balance. *(18c:II–26)*

(C–incorrect) The Class P weights are more accurate than Class Q and are suggested for performance of the balance tests and to check other weights.
(18c:II–26)

3. (C) A container that reduces light transmission in the range between 290 and 450 nanometers to the level specified in the USP may be considered light resistant and suitable protection from light. The container may be constructed of glass or plastic. Although amber units are most common, other colored or opaque containers may meet the official requirements. *(18c:II–22)*

4. (D) The NBS specifications state that a graduate shall have an initial interval of not less than one fifth nor more than one fourth of the capacity of the graduate. Therefore, a 100 mL graduate would prob-ably have either a 20 or 25 mL calibration mark as the initial calibration. This regulation is intended to discourage small-volume measurements in large graduates when a smaller graduate should be used. For some measurements, the conical graduate is less accurate than the cylindrical graduate. NBS specifications state that graduates holding 10 mL or less must be cylindrical. Whatever the shape and size of the graduate, one should not attempt to measure volumes less than one fourth to one fifth of the total capacity. *(1:81)*

5. (B) Riopan Plus differs from Riopan by having an additional ingredient, simethicone. Simethicone is included in some antacid products as an antifoaming agent. It is used as adjunctive therapy in patients with postoperative gaseous distention, air swallowing, functional dyspepsia, and peptic ulcers. The agent does not have any antacid properties. *(1:776)*

6. (A) A cold place indicates a temperature not exceeding 8° C (46° F). A refrigerator is a cold place in which the temperature is maintained between 2 and 8° C (36 to 46° F).

(B–incorrect) A cool place indicates temperatures between 8 and 15° C (46 to 59° F).

(C–incorrect) Controlled room temperature is 15 to 30° C (59 to 86° F). *(18c:II–4; 24:113)*

7. (B) Liquifilm is a name used for an ophthalmic vehicle containing polyvinyl alcohol. The polyvinyl alcohol increases the viscosity of the ophthalmic solutions, thereby prolonging the contact with the corneal surface. A second viscous vehicle (Isopto) contains hydroxypropylmethylcellulose. *(33:568)*

8. (E) Valences of atoms do not reflect the solubility characteristics of a chemical. *(12:228)*

(A–incorrect)(D–incorrect)

Both dielectric constants and solubility parameters of solutes and solvents reflect relative polarities. The closer the solute and solvent values, the greater the potential solubility. *(12:279,284)*

(B–incorrect)(C–incorrect)

The pKa of a weak acid or base and the pH of the final solution will determine the species of chemical that will be present and the corresponding degree or extent of solubility.   *(12:296)*

9. **(C)** Federal drug laws and regulations are described in the *USP DI volume III*, which also contains listings of therapeutic equivalent drugs and drugs that are biologically inequivalent. The latter information is from the FDA's "Orange Book".   *(18c)*

10. **(B)** Volume II of the *USP DI* contains drug monographs written for the layperson. Pharmacists have permission to photocopy individual drug descriptions for distribution to the patient when dispensing the drug. Volume I of the *USP DI* contains drug information for the health professional. It contains more detailed and more scientific information than Volume II.   *(18a; 18b)*

11. **(C)** For example, boric acid 1:18 in water indicates that 1 g of boric acid is soluble in 18 mL of water. In extemporaneous compounding, it is advisable to use excess solvent since saturated solutions are difficult to prepare and their concentrations are usually temperature dependent.   *(1:207)*

12. **(D)** When expiration dates are expressed only in terms of month and year, the intended expiration date is the last day of the stated month.   *(18c:II–4)*

13. **(E)** The expiration date for a pharmaceutical is based on the length of time during which the product should continue to meet the specified monograph requirements. Requirements are stated in terms of amount of active ingredient that is present as determined by suitable assay. Most drug products are considered usable until approximately 10% of drug or drug activity has been lost. However, some monographs specify other ranges. For example, digoxin tablets must assay between 92% and 108% of label claim.   *(18c:II–4)*

14. **(E)** Both nitroglycerin and Isordil are available in a sublingual dosage form for use as coronary vasodilators in the treatment or prevention of anginal attacks. Hydergine is claimed to be a mood elevator, perhaps useful for senile dementia.   *(1:844,1040)*

15. **(A)** A chelate is a compound formed by the combination of an electron donor with a metal ion to form a ring structure. The molecule that forms the ring structure with the metal is called a ligand or chelating agent. Metals in chelates are generally multivalent, and the electron donor atoms are limited almost entirely to nitrogen, oxygen, and sulfur.   *(1:166)*

16. **(C)** Edetate calcium disodium (Versenate) is used parenterally (generally intramuscularly) to reduce blood levels and depot stores of lead in acute and chronic lead poisoning and lead encephalopathy. The chelate formed with lead is stable, water-soluble, and readily excreted by the kidneys.   *(1:824; 4:56)*

17. **(E)** All three forms, as well as Purified Water, Sterile Water for Injection, and Sterile Water for Irrigation, are official. Water for Injection is a parenteral solvent, free from pyrogens, that is used in manufacturing. Bacteriostatic Water for Injection is used in reconstitution of powders in small vials. Sterile Water for Inhalation is labeled for inhalation use only, not for parenteral administration. It is sterile and free of bacterial endotoxins. It does not contain an antimicrobial agent except when intended for use in a humidifier.   *(18c:III–281)*

18. **(B)** The hydroxyl group of the alcohols permits hydrogen bonding with water molecules. Water solubility increases as the number of hydroxyl groups is increased and the carbon content is held constant. On the other hand, as the carbon content increases, the molecule becomes more nonpolar and loses water solubility.   *(12:274)*

19. **(B)** Epinephrine, a catecholamine, is very sensitive to oxidation, which results in biologically inactive products. The first indication of oxidation is the development of a pink color that darkens to form a brown precipitate.   *(1:878)*

20. **(A)** Aminophylline consists of theophylline, which has been reacted with ethylenediamine to improve its water solubility. Upon exposure to air, carbon dioxide is absorbed and free theophylline forms. Addition of small amounts of ethylenediamine redissolves these crystals. A note in the monograph for Aminophylline Injection USP states, "Do not use the Injection if crystals have separated."   *(1:867; 18c:III–11)*

21. **(C)**   *(1:1630)*
(A–incorrect) Levigation is the process of reducing the particle size of solids by adding a small amount of a liquid or ointment base to make a paste, which is then rubbed with a spatula on an ointment tile.   *(1:1630)*
(B–incorrect) Sublimation is the conversion of a solid to a vapor without passing through a liquid phase.   *(1:175)*
(D–incorrect) Pulverization by intervention is a process for reducing particle size by using a second agent that can then be readily removed. For example, camphor is reduced by the intervention of alcohol.   *(1:1630)*
(E–incorrect) Maceration is an extraction process in which the ground drug is soaked in the solvent until the cellular structure is penetrated and the soluble constituents have been dissolved.   *(1:1543)*

22. **(B)** Powders that are either directly applied to the skin or are incorporated into topical products should be extremely fine or impalpable. Trituration is often needed to reduce particles to an extremely fine size so that the patient will not discern individual particles when the product is rubbed on the skin. Usually a particle size of 50μ or smaller is desired.   *(30:655)*

23. **(E)** Micromeritics is the study of all aspects of small particles, including particle size, separation of particles, comminution, and behavior of particles in pharmaceutical systems.   *(24:118)*

24. (C) Cafergot is available as tablets (1 mg ergotamine tartrate + 100 mg caffeine) and suppositories (2 mg ergotamine tartrate + 100 mg caffeine). The drug is classified as an antimigraine agent. *(10)*

25. (D) Polymorphs differ in their melting points, x-ray diffractions, infrared spectra, and dissolution rates. For example, riboflavin has three polymorphs, each with significantly different solubilities. Theobroma oil (cocoa butter) can exist in four forms, each differing in melting points. Gentle heating of cocoa butter will favor the formation of the stable beta polymorph. This crystalline form is desired since it melts at 34.5° C, which is close to but lower than body temperature. Metabolic rates of a drug's polymorphs will not vary since once the drug has dissolved the polymorphs no longer exist. *(1:1440–41)*

26. (D) Benzalkonium chloride is a cationic surface active agent. In the presence of anionic agents such as soaps, benzalkonium chloride and similar cationic agents are inactivated because the combination of large cations with large anions of soaps form inactive products. *(1:1164; 6:950)*

27. (C) Hydrogen bonding is an attractive force between hydrogen atoms and electronegative atoms such as oxygen, fluorine, and nitrogen. Although weak, hydrogen bonds can bring about the miscibility of certain solvents or the solubility of certain chemicals. Hydrogen bonding is also responsible for the shrinkage phenomenon that occurs when mixing certain liquids. For example, when equal volumes of Alcohol USP and purified water are mixed, there is approximately 3% shrinkage from the theoretical volume. If one wishes to prepare 100 mL of Diluted Alcohol USP containing 49% V/V ethanol and purified water, equal volumes of each are used. However, one must also remember to use an excess of at least 3% of each to assure obtaining the required volume. *(12:59)*

28. (B) Starch suspension and zinc oxide paste show dilatancy. *(1:314)*
(A–incorrect) A plastic liquid does not flow until a certain minimum shearing stress is applied. After plastic flow begins, the apparent viscosity decreases with increasing rates of shear. *(1:316)*
(C–incorrect) A pseudoplastic liquid does not require a certain minimum shearing stress before it begins to flow. Flow begins as soon as force is applied, and viscosity decreases with increasing rates of shear. *(1:313)*
(D–incorrect) Thixotropy is a property that certain plastic materials exhibit. While standing, the system forms a gel that breaks down to form a liquid sol if agitation is applied. This reversible isothermal gel-sol transformation is known as thixotropy. *(1:318)*
(E–incorrect) Newtonian flow is characterized by constant viscosity at varying rates of shear. *(1:312)*

29. (D) The equation may be expressed as:

$$V = \frac{r^4 \times t \times \Delta P}{8 \times l \times \eta}$$

The volume of liquid (V) passing during a unit of time (t) is directly proportional to the radius of the tube (r) and the pressure differential (ΔP) at each end of the tube and inversely proportional to the length of the tube (l) and the viscosity of the liquid (η). Since the radius is raised to the fourth power, doubling the radius would cause a 16-fold change in the flow provided all other factors remained constant. The capillary can be envisioned as a simple glass tube or a human blood vessel. *(1:313; 12:532)*

30. (C) Potassium chloride is an obvious substitute for sodium chloride since it has a similar salty taste, is crystalline, and is an electrolyte already present in the body. However, the use of these salt substitutes is contraindicated in patients with severe kidney disease or oliguria. Symptoms such as weakness, nausea, and muscle cramps indicate excessive sodium depletion. Increased sodium intake is warranted. *(10)*

31. (B) IV injection of high concentrations of potassium may cause cardiac arrest. Intravenous administration must be by slow infusion to allow dilution of the potassium to occur. When plasma potassium levels are above 2.5 mEq/L, rates up to 10 mEq/h (total of 100 to 200 mEq/day) may be set. In more serious conditions, with plasma levels below 2 mEq/L, rates of 40 mEq/h (total of 400 mEq/day) have been employed. Available injection forms contain 10 to 80 mEq per vial. IV admixtures are prepared by diluting these solutions to 250 to 1000 mL. Oral dosage forms include Kay Ciel elixir, Kaon tablets, K-Lor, and K-Lyte packets. Slow-K tablets have a wax matrix from which the KCl is slowly dissolved in the GI tract. *(1:819)*

32. (B) Topical dosage forms are used. For example, both creams and solutions are available under the tradenames of Efudex and Fluoroplex. In fact, however, fluorouracil is usually administered by intravenous injection. It is not given orally because of irregular absorption from the GI tract. *(3:1951; 6:1229)*

33. (A) Isoclor Liquid (Fisons) is a preparation containing 2 mg of chlorpheniramine maleate and 12.5 mg of pseudoephedrine HCl per teaspoon. It is used for the relief of upper respiratory and bronchial congestion. *(3:769)*

34. (C) Potassium chloride is embedded in a wax matrix core to provide slow release as the salt is leached from the core. Slow release of the potassium in this manner is believed to minimize high local concentration of potassium ion near the GI wall. These preparations have advantages over liquid potassium supplements since they are tasteless and easier to take. It should be pointed out, however, that there have been reports of small-bowel ulceration associated with the use of these slow-release preparations. Although it appears that the incidence of this adverse effect is considerably less than that associated with oral liquid potassium preparations, the clinical significance of these reports remains to be determined.

(9:40.12)

35. (C) Both *Facts and Comparisons* and the *Handbook on Injectable Drugs* present tables comparing the commercial amino acid injections.   *(21:22)*

36. (E) Insulin is usually administered by subcutaneous injection into the arm or thigh. Absorption of the insulin is good, and this route is both convenient and safe for self-administration of the drug.   *(13:113)*

37. (D) Insulin solutions have low viscosities, and only small volumes are injected. Therefore, small-bore needles (25G or 26G) may be used. Short (1/2" to 5/8") needles are adequate for the usual subcutaneous route of insulin administration.   *(13:303)*

38. (D) The winged (scalp-vein, scalp, or butterfly) needle consists of a stainless steel needle with two flexible plastic, wing-like projections. The wings serve two purposes: They ease manipulation of the needle during insertion into the vein and then allow the needle to be anchored with tape to the skin. *(13:303)*

39. (B) Hypodermic needle sizes are expressed by a gauge system based upon the external diameter of the cannula; the larger the number, the smaller the diameter of the needle. For example, the 21-gauge needle is smaller in diameter than the 19-gauge needle. Generally, the length of the cannula is specified also. This measurement, expressed in inches, represents the distance from the needle tip to the junction with the hub.   *(13:302)*

40. (A) The Busher Automatic Injector is a metal device into which the patient places a filled hypodermic syringe and needle. By releasing a spring on the unit, the patient administers the injection automatically. This unit is used mainly by patients using insulin.

(24:275)

(D–incorrect) The Bristol unit is called the Bristoject.
(E–incorrect) Wyeth's cartridge and metal syringe system is known as the Tubex system.

41. (D) The pH of solutions is often adjusted during the manufacturing procedure by the addition of either acid (hydrochloric acid) or alkali (sodium hydroxide). The amount needed may vary from batch to batch. Therefore, the label cannot specify an exact quantity. Also, isotonicity adjustors may be listed by name only with a statement as to their purpose.   *(18c:II–7)*

42. (B) Either 5% or 5.5% dextrose in water is isotonic depending upon whether the anhydrous or hydrous form of dextrose is used.   *(4:770)*

43. (C) The term venoclysis is synonymous with intravenous infusion.   *(13:116; 33:497)*

44. (A) Partially filled glass containers (minibottles) usually consist of 250-mL bottles containing 50, 100, or 150 mL of either D5W or NS. To these bottles, one can easily add drug solutions, taking advantage of the vacuum present in the minibottle. Plastic bags are also employed for preparing parenteral admixtures. The plastic units do not have a vacuum but are flexible enough to accommodate additional liquids.   *(1:1572; 13:140)*

45. (A) Intermittent therapy refers to administration of parenteral drugs at spaced intervals. One of the most convenient methods for administration is to attach a minibottle to the tubing of a large-volume parenteral (LVP) bottle already hanging on the patient. The minibottle is a 250-mL bottle containing 50 to 150 mL of either 0.9% sodium chloride or 5% dextrose solutions plus an active drug such as an antibiotic. The piggyback concept saves the patient from multiple injections and assures high blood levels of the additive drug since the minibottle solution is infused in a short period of time.   *(1:1574,13:143)*

46. (B) While the maximum volume will vary depending upon the condition of the patient, daily volumes greater than 3 to 4 L may cause a fluid overload.

(1:1579; 13:213)

47. (A) There have been reports that diazepam will precipitate even when added to normal saline or 5% dextrose solution.   *(21:289)*

48. (E) While the most widely used syringe size is the 1-mL syringe, Becton Dickinson markets a Lo-Dose 0.5-mL disposable insulin syringe. This size is particularly useful for administering small volumes (0.1 or 0.2 mL) of insulin.

49. (C) Purified Water USP may be prepared by distillation, ion-exchange treatment, reverse osmosis, or other suitable processes, provided that assay requirements are met. Labels must indicate the method of preparation. One possible disadvantage of ion exchange is the higher microbial count, which occurs in deionized water because the resin beds generally become contaminated.   *(18c:VI–36)*

50. (D) Although there is some disagreement concerning the shelf life of ampicillin solutions, it is generally agreed that sodium chloride solutions are more stable (approximately 8 hours at room temperature) than dextrose solutions (less than 4 hours at room temperature).   *(21:66)*

51. (B) While many of the parenteral admixtures are chemically stable for long periods of time, potential contamination of the products during preparation by the pharmacist is of prime concern. Usually no significant microbial growth will occur until after 24 hours. Therefore, an expiration date of 24 hours is safest unless the solution is known to be less stable chemically. Refrigeration also helps to retard microbial growth.   *(13:237)*

52. (A) Folvite Injection contains folic acid as the active ingredient. Actually, the drug is present as the sodium salt, and the aqueous solution has a pH of approximately 9. All of the other drug solutions have pH's less than 7, as they consist of acid salts; (B–incorrect) metoclopramide HCl, (C–incorrect) oxymorphone HCl, (D–incorrect) octreolide acetate, and (E–incorrect) ranitidine HCl.   *(21:403)*

53. (E) A subcutaneous injection will come into contact with a large number of nerve endings and may remain at the injection site for a long period of time. Extreme pain will be felt if the solution is not isotonic. The potential isotonicity effects of hypotonic or hypertonic intravenous solutions are offset by their dilution in the large volume of blood into which they are injected, provided the volume injected is not excessive and the rate of injection is slow.   *(32:244)*

54. (A) The osmotic pressure of the dextrose solution will be approximately one half that of an equimolar sodium chloride solution. The osmotic pressure of a substance in a solution is an example of a colligative property. Equimolar concentrations of nonelectrolytes will have similar osmotic pressures. However, electrolytes ionize to form particles that quantitatively increase the magnitude of the colligative property. Since sodium chloride ionizes into two particles, a 0.1 molar solution has twice the osmotic pressure of a 0.1 molar solution of a nonelectrolyte such as dextrose. Deviations from this simple theory arise from interionic attractions, solvation, and other factors.   *(1:1482)*

55. (E) Osmolarity, expressed as mOsm/L, is included on the labels of many large-volume parenteral bottles. Those injections with a value of approximately 300 mOsm/L will be isoosmotic and presumably isotonic with the blood. For example, 5% dextrose injection has a value of 280 mOsm/L, whereas 0.9% sodium chloride injection has a value of 308 mOsm/L. One calculates the osmolarity of a solution by first determining the millimoles of chemical present, then multiplying by the number of ions formed from one molecule. One liter of 0.9% sodium chloride solution contains 9 g of sodium chloride (MW = 58.4). The millimole concentration will be:

$$\frac{9\,g}{58.4} = 0.154 \text{ mol or } 154 \text{ mmol}$$

The milliosmole (mOsm) concentration will be:
154 mM × 2 (ions present in NaCl) = 308 mOsm

(1:1483; 13:208)

56. (E) Water for Injection (WFI) is pyrogen-free water that is freshly prepared by careful treatment of distilled water. If not used within 24 hours, it is discarded since it may contain microorganisms. The parenteral prepared with WFI must be sterilized near the end of the manufacturing process. Bacterio-static Water for Injection USP and Sterile Water for Injection USP are also used for parenterals.   *(1:1547)*

57. (D) There is the potential danger of blockage of a blood vessel by suspension particles.   *(24:256; 32:243)*

58. (B) Except for the lactate concentration and the absence of sodium bicarbonate, Lactated Ringer's (Hartmann's) solution closely approximates the extracellular fluid. Although the injection has a pH of 6 to 7.5, it has an alkalinizing effect since the lactate is metabolized to bicarbonate.   *(1:806)*

59. (B) Factors affecting the distribution of a drug in the blood after an IV bolus include the blood volume, heart rate, and injection rate. Assuming that even distribution occurs within 4 minutes, drug sampling may be initiated after that time.   *(13:108)*

60. (C) Not only will an intramuscular injection be painful, but it may cause a localized hematoma.   *(21:439)*

61. (B) The Baxter and McGraw systems use a plastic airway tube that extends from the rubber stopper to above the fluid surface when the bottle is inverted for administration. The Abbott system uses a filtered airway that is an integral part of the administration set.   *(1:1572)*

62. (A) There are two main sites of degradation for insulin—the liver and the kidneys. Insulin is filtered through the glomeruli and reabsorbed by the tubules, where some degradation occurs.   *(6:1467)*
(B–incorrect) When injected intravenously, the half-life is estimated to be 5 to 6 minutes.
(C–incorrect) The volume of distribution approximates the volume of extracellular fluid.
(D–incorrect) Approximately 50% of the insulin that reaches the liver through the portal vein is destroyed.

63. (A) Insulins can be classified by their onset of action after subcutaneous injection and by their duration of action. Fast-acting insulins (Insulin Injection and Prompt Insulin Injection) have an onset of less than 1 hour. The intermediate-acting insulins (Isophane Insulin Suspension, Insulin Zinc Suspension, and Globin Zinc Insulin Injection) have onsets of 1 to 2 hours. The onset of action for the long-acting products (Protamine Zinc Insulin Suspension and Extended Insulin Zinc Suspension) is approximately 4 to 6 hours.   *(6:1476)*

64. (A) Gentamicin sulfate (Garamycin) is stable for 2 years at room temperature. Of the five antibiotics listed, it is the only one manufactured in solution form, ready for injection. The others are packaged as powders for reconstitution.   *(21:312)*

65. (A) While vitamin C's main attribute is in the prevention and cure of scurvy, it has been advocated for the prevention and alleviation of symptoms of the "common cold," to facilitate absorption of iron by maintaining iron in the ferrous state, and as an anti-oxidant in both pharmaceuticals and foods. The fat-soluble vitamin E has also been purported to possess antioxidant properties, especially within the body.

(1:1008,1012)

Vitamin D_2 prevents or treats rickets and is used in the management of hypoparathyroidism and hypo-calcemia. *(1:1010)*

Deficiencies of vitamin A may cause night blindness, skin disorders, and abnormalities of both nerve and connective tissue. *(1:1011)*

66. (B) Vitamin K occurs naturally in two forms, vita-min K_1 and K_4. Phytonadione (Mephyton) is a natu-rally occurring vitamin K_1. Menadione (K_4) is an in-active synthetic derivative that is transformed by the liver into active vitamin K_1. *(1:1011)*

67. (B) Water solubility decreases with an increase in the number of carbons in an alkane chain. Therefore, the butanols will be more soluble than the pentanols. Since side chains tend to improve water solubility, tertiary butanol would be more soluble than n-buta-nol. *(1:221)*

(A–incorrect) The absence of hydroxyl groups in bu-tane would indicate poor water solubility.

68. (B) Esters of p-hydroxybenzoic acid are used as pre-servatives to protect against mold and yeast growth in pharmaceuticals. Toxicity, preservative effect, and lipid solubility all increase as the molecular weight increases. Of the four esters–methyl, ethyl, propyl, and butyl–the latter two are more suitable for oils and fats. They are often used in combination with each other. *(1:1172)*

69. (C) Human immune serum is obtained from human blood. It contains specific antibodies reflecting the diseases contracted by the donor. The immunity is passive since the recipient's body does not actively develop either antibodies or sensitized lymphocytes in response to a foreign antigen. Passive immunity does not last long; usually not more than 2 or 3 weeks of protection are achieved. Active immunity implies that the recipient of the biological will de-velop specific immunity due to an active response to the introduction of antigenic substances.

(1:1390; 24:298)

70. (A) A sterile solution of the diluted, standardized toxic products of growth of the diphtheria bacillus (Diphtheria Toxin for Schick Test USP) is injected intradermally (0.1 mL) into the forearm. A positive reaction denotes susceptibility to diphtheria; a reac-tion consists of redness and infiltration, which ap-pear at the injection site in 24 to 36 hours and per-sist for 4 or 5 days. *(1:1394)*

71. (C) The human immune sera, such as immune glob-ulin and hyperimmune sera, offer passive immunity against specific diseases. *(1:1400)*

72. (B) The immune gamma globulin is used to prevent or modify several diseases, including measles, infec-tious hepatitis, German measles, and chickenpox. The immunity is passive, lasting for 1 to 2 months. There are also special forms for individuals exposed to mumps, pertussis, tetanus, vaccinia, and rabies.

(1:1391)

73. (D) Another intradermal test for detecting tubercu-lin sensitivity is the tuberculin tine test, which uses a disposable stainless steel unit with prongs (tines) tipped with old tuberculin. It has been standardized to conform to the Mantoux test. *(1:1404)*

74. (B) The tuberculin skin test is based on skin hyper-sensitivity to a specific bacterial protein antigen. Tu-berculin can be administered intracutaneously (Mantoux test) or by the multiple puncture method (tine test). The intracutaneous method using puri-fied protein derivative (PPD) is more reliable. Gen-erally, the intermediate strength (5 U/0.1 mL) is used. The first strength (1 U) is generally used for individuals suspected of being highly sensitive, and the second strength (250 U) is exclusively for those who did not react to previous injections of either 1 or 5 units. *(1:1404; 9:36:84)*

75. (E) Serum albumin is the protein in plasma that controls blood volume through its water-containing capacity. Normal Human Serum Albumin USP, which is used in the treatment of shock or hemor-rhage, is available in either a 6% or 25% sterile solu-tion. *(1:803)*

76. (B) The labeling on biologicals is required to specify the recommended storage temperature. With few ex-ceptions, biologicals are stored in a refrigerator at 2° to 8° C. *(24:293)*

77. (C) Booster doses of the common toxoids are re-quired to sustain immunity. For example, a 0.5-mL dose of tetanus toxoid should be administered as a routine booster about every 10 years or, as a booster in the management of minor clean wounds, not more frequently than every 6 years. *(1:1398)*

78. (C) The tuberculin syringe is a small but relatively long 1-mL syringe with easy to read 0.1-mL calibra-tions. It is accurate and convenient to use when mea-suring small volumes. *(1:1878)*

79. (E) Typhoid fever is a bacterial infection. *(1:1394)*

80. (C) Rabies is a viral infection. *(1:1397)*

81. (E) For therapeutic effects, antitoxins are usually administered by the SC or IM routes. While the more slowly absorbed subcutaneous injection is gen-erally preferred for prophylactic effects, the intra-muscular route is also used. *(1:1399)*

82. (B) Passive immunizations are usually accom-plished by the administration of purified and concen-trated antibody solutions (antitoxins) derived from humans or animals that have been actively immunized against a live antigen. Active immunizations are usually accomplished by the administration of one of the following: (1) toxoids (eg, choice A–incorrect), (2) inactivated (killed) vaccines (eg, choices C–incorrect and E–incorrect), (3) live attenuated vaccines (eg, choice D–incorrect). *(1:1402; 24:298)*

83. **(C)** Both ipecac syrup and activated charcoal have proved effective in the treatment of many types of drug poisoning. However, they must not be used concurrently, since the charcoal will adsorb the active alkaloids present in ipecac syrup; the desired emetic effect may thus be lost. If both agents are to be administered, it is best to induce vomiting first with the ipecac syrup, then administer the charcoal to adsorb remnants of the poison. *(2:298)*
(E–incorrect) The "universal antidote" is a mixture of activated charcoal, magnesium oxide, and tannic acid. Only the charcoal in this combination is effective, and its activity is probably reduced by the other two ingredients. *(2:300)*

84. **(B)** Chemicals that are not significantly adsorbed by activated charcoal include boric acid, cyanides, DDT, and ferrous sulfate. *(2:105)*

85. **(D)** While Alcohol USP (95% V/V ethanol) is usually used in the production of pharmaceuticals, labels stating alcohol concentration are based upon 100% V/V ethanol (Absolute Alcohol). Proof strengths of products are easily calculated by simply doubling the % V/V ethanol concentration. *(23:291)*

86. **(A)** Sulfamethoxazole inhibits the conversion of paraaminobenzoic acid to dihydrofolic acid, and trimethoprim inhibits the subsequent conversion to tetrahydrofolic acid. *(1:1178)*

87. **(D)** Each dose of Lomotil tablets and liquid contains 2.5 mg of diphenoxylate HCl and 0.025 mg of atropine sulfate. The diphenoxylate HCl exerts a constipating effect. The atropine sulfate is added to minimize the abuse potential of the product. While the dose of atropine sulfate in this formulation is much too low to exert any significant therapeutic effect, an excessive dose of Lomotil will give rise to unpleasant effects of atropine overdosage. *(1:797)*

88. **(C)** Colostomy pouches are available in several sizes based upon the opening that will surround the stoma on the body. These sizes are designated in inches of diameter. Pouches may be designed as either open end, in which the effluent may be drained while the pouch is on the patient, or closed end, which must be removed to be either emptied or discarded. There is no difference between pouches worn by males or females, but there are pediatric pouches with a smaller capacity. *(1:1886; 2:694)*

89. **(C)** Hygroscopicity is the ability of a substance to attract and retain moisture. Because glycerin will absorb water even in low relative humidities, it is used as a humectant to keep creams and other semi-solid formulations from drying out. *(1:1316)*

90. **(A)** Type I glass consists of borosilicate. This is the best material as it is more resistant to water attack. Type II is a specially treated soda-lime glass. Type III is the typical soda-lime glass. NP (nonparenteral) glass is unsuitable as a parenteral container. *(1:1524,1552; 18c:II–22:1224)*

91. **(C)** The term "leaching" is used specifically to designate the release of a container ingredient into the product. For example, zinc and accelerators may be leached from a rubber closure into a parenteral vial solution. *(24:122)*
(A–incorrect) Adsorption would refer to the binding of a substance onto the surface of the container wall.
(B–incorrect) Diffusion is the passage of a substance through a second substance. For example, volatile oil or dye may diffuse from a solution through the walls of a plastic container.
(D–incorrect) Permeation would denote the solution of a substance in the cell wall followed by passage through the wall.
(E–incorrect) Porosity indicates small holes or passages through which a substance could pass.

92. **(C)** Monoclonal antibodies (MAb) are antibodies derived from single hybrid cells. The resulting product has enhanced selectivity, making it invaluable as a specific diagnostic agent or drug. Gene splicing refers to those procedures resulting in alterations of the DNA make-up of a microorganism. Using recombinant DNA technology, specific antibodies useful for medical and agricultural applications can be developed. *(1:1419)*
Lyophilization is an industrial procedure that removes water from products, thereby increasing their stability. The process is also known as freeze-drying or cryodessication. *(1:1565)*

93. **(E)** The thrombolytic agent urokinase is an enzyme isolated from cultures of human kidney tissue. *(9:20:40)*
(A–incorrect) Humulin is Lilly's human insulin.
(D–incorrect) Protropin (Genentech) is a human growth hormone intended for the long-term treatment of children with growth failure due to insufficient endogenous hormone. A similar product is Lilly's Humatrope. *(1:1426)*
(B–incorrect) Interferon is used in numerous diseases, including AIDS-related Kaposi's sarcoma.
(C–incorrect) Erythropoietin is used in dialysis, anemia, and chronic renal failure. *(24:301)*

94. **(D)** The increased sensitivity of both types of tests is due to the use of monoclonal antibodies (MAb), which allow earlier determination of the specific hormones involved. Ovulation prediction tests detect surges in luteinizing hormone (LH), which indicate that ovulation is about to occur. Pregnancy determination tests detect an increased level of human cho-

rionic gonadotropin (hCG) hormone that occurs when the egg is fertilized. The fecal occult blood tests are based upon the colorimetric detection of hemoglobin. Various chemicals such as guaiac, tetramethylbenzidine, etc., are used to elicit a characteristic color. This last test is not very selective or sensitive. *(2:45–49)*

95. **(A)** Uticort Gel contains the steroid betamethasone benzoate, which has anti-inflammatory, antipruritic, and vasoconstrictive activity for the relief of inflammatory dermatosis. All of the other products are available with either 5% or 10% benzoyl peroxide. These products are used in the treatment of acne vulgaris. The mode of action appears to be a drying and desquamation action plus an antiseptic effect against *Propionibacterium acnes* by hydrogen peroxide. *(1:767; 3:2171,2241)*

96. **(D)** The HLB system was originally designed by using combinations of nonionic surfactants in the preparation of a standard emulsion. Although some anionic and cationic emulsifiers have been assigned HLB values, the system's primary use is to classify the hundreds of nonionics that are commercially available. In the HLB system, emulsifiers are given numerical designations between 1 and 20, depending on the relative strength of the hydrophilic and hydrophobic portions of the molecule. Emulsifiers with low HLB values are hydrophobic, whereas emulsifiers with high HLB values are hydrophilic. Generally, an emulsifier with an HLB of less than 9 will produce water in oil (W/O) emulsions, those with values of greater than 11 will produce oil in water (O/W) emulsions, while those with intermediate values (9 to 11) are susceptible to other factors influencing the type of emulsion that is formed. *(1:324)*

97. **(D)** Sorbitan monopalmitate is a sorbitan fatty acid ester, commercially available as Span 40. It is classified as nonionic since the molecules would not have the tendency to migrate to either pole in an electric field. *(1:304,1605)*
(A–incorrect) (C–incorrect) (E–incorrect) These compounds are anionic surfactants. This designation implies that the large, active portion of the surfactant molecule would bear a negative charge, and therefore, would migrate to the anode in an electric field. For example, the stearate portion of triethanolamine stearate is considered the active ion.
(B–incorrect) Cetylpyridinium chloride is a cationic surfactant. The active surfactant portion, cetylpyridinium, has a positive charge and migrates to the cathode.

98. **(C)** Both ophthalmic and nasal preparations should have only mild buffer capacity so that the organ's natural buffer system can overcome any pH differences. Otherwise, irritation might result.
(A–incorrect) Nasal preparations usually have a pH

in the range of 5.6 to 7.5. Often, phosphate buffers are used.
(B–incorrect) Rendering the nasal solution isotonic will decrease potential for damage to the local tissue.
(D–incorrect) The presence of an antimicrobial preservative is important because there may be accidental contamination of the dropper or nasal spray tip. *(20:157)*

99. **(C)** Neoloid is an aqueous emulsion containing 36% castor oil as the active ingredient. *(2:375)*

(A–incorrect) Agoral contains mineral oil and phenolphthalein. *(2:366)*
(B–incorrect) Kondremul contains mineral oil and the bulking agent chondrus. *(2:373)*
(D–incorrect) Haley's M-O is an aqueous emulsion of mineral oil and magnesium hydroxide gel. *(2:373)*
(E–incorrect) Neo-Cultol is a chocolate-flavored, refined mineral oil jelly. *(2:375)*

100. **(E)** The tablets are enteric coated to avoid gastric irritation. They should not be taken within 1 hour of ingestion of milk or antacids since the enteric coating may be dissolved prematurely. *(4:870)*

101. **(D)** InFeD is Iron Dextran Injection USP, a colloidal solution of ferric hydroxide complexed with partially hydrolyzed dextran. It is intended for treatment of confirmed cases of iron-deficiency anemias, particularly among those patients who cannot tolerate or who fail to respond to oral administration of iron. *(1:841; 4:2123)*

102. **(E)** The FDA OTC panel on laxatives, antidiarrheals, antiemetics, and emetics reported that only the opiates and polycarbophil were recognized as safe and effective as antidiarrheal agents. Polycarbophil absorbs large quantities of water, allowing the formation of stools. There does not appear to be any effect on the digestive enzymes or nutrients. The drug itself is not absorbed systemically. Polycarbophil is present in Mitrolan and FiberCon. *(1:796; 2:323)*
(A–incorrect) Activated charcoal possesses good adsorption properties but is seldom used as an antidiarrheal. *(2:300)*
(C–incorrect)(D–incorrect) Kaolin and attapulgite are typical examples of adsorbent clays. Attapulgite is a colloidal hydrated magnesium aluminum silicate clay. Studies have indicated that it is an effective adsorbent for alkaloids, toxins, bacteria, and strains of human enteroviruses. However, attapulgite and kaolin are not selective and will also adsorb nutrients and digestive enzymes. Probably their greatest efficacy will be in the treatment of mild, functional diarrhea. *(2:325)*

103. **(C)** Perdiem consists of granules containing both a stimulant laxative, senna, and a bulking agent, psyllium.
Persons sensitive to phenolphthalein may develop a

polychromatic rash. Phenolphthalein-induced rashes vary greatly in size and color. Usually the rash itches or causes a burning sensation. Among the other commercial products containing phenolphthalein are Ex-Lax, Espotabs, and Feen-A-Mint.

(2:354,375)

104. **(D)** Pepto-Bismol contains bismuth subsalicylate. The subsalicylate salt is the preferred insoluble form since the subnitrate may form the nitrite ion in the gut. Absorption of this ion could cause hypotension and possibly methemoglobinemia. The FDA panel concluded that the bismuth salts are safe when taken orally, but data establishing effectiveness of bismuth in diarrhea are questionable. *(2:325,331)*
(A–incorrect) Bisodol is an antacid product containing calcium carbonate, magnesium oxide, and sodium bicarbonate. *(2:284)*

105. **(E)** Kaopectate tablets contain 750 mg of attapulgite. *(2:330)*
(A–incorrect) Donnagel contains kaolin as the adsorbent clay. Another component is pectin, a purified carbohydrate extracted from citrus fruit rinds. Pectin is classified as an intestinal adsorbent, absorbent, and protective. Several belladonna alkaloids are included for antispasmodic activity, but their effectiveness is questionable because of the low dosage used. *(2:329; 4:971)*
(B–incorrect) Kaopectate suspension contains kaolin and pectin. *(2:329)*
(C–incorrect) Bacid contains the microorganism *Lactobacillus,* intended to restore normal flora in the intestine. *(2:329)*
(D–incorrect) Parepectolin is a suspension containing kaolin, pectin, and paregoric. *(2:331)*

106. **(A)** Iron should not be consumed simultaneously with vitamin E since the iron appears to prevent the absorption of the vitamin. *(2:467)*
(B–incorrect) Large doses of vitamin E have been administered without toxicity. It is interesting to note that the RDA for the adult is only 15 international units (IU), yet vitamin E capsules containing 400 and 1000 IU are marketed. *(2:465)*
(D–incorrect) Deficiencies of vitamin E are rare. The vitamin is readily available in vegetable oils, nuts, cereals, etc. *(2:466)*
(E–incorrect) Because of its antioxidant properties, vitamin E has been suggested for slowing the aging process. This activity has not been proved or disproved. *(2:466)*

107. **(C)** Phenylpropanolamine appears to suppress the appetite center in a manner similar to that of the amphetamines. While phenylpropanolamine appears to have anorexigenic properties, the dose present in most OTC products (25 mg) is too low. However, higher doses increase the incidence of side effects, such as nervousness, insomnia, hypertension, nausea, and tachycardia. *(2:568)*

108. **(E)** Bacid is used in the treatment of diarrhea. It contains the microorganism *Lactobacillus acidophilus,* which aids in the rebalancing of intestinal flora. Usually normal bowel function is established within 24 to 48 hours after the start of therapy. A similar product is Lactinex, which contains both *L acidophilus* and *L bulgaricus.* *(2:326; 4:850)*

109. **(D)** Excedrin contains aspirin, caffeine, salicylamide, and acetaminophen but no buffering agents. All of the other preparations contain aluminum hydroxide, magnesium hydroxide, magnesium carbonate, or some combination of these antacids. *(2:209)*

110. **(B)** Magnesium salicylate is similar to sodium salicylate in its analgesic activity, but there is the danger of systemic magnesium toxicity, especially in the renally impaired patient. *(2:65,81)*

111. **(E)** The usual adult dose is 30 mg every 6 to 8 hours, with a maximum daily dose of 120 mg. Individual doses of 30 mg or higher do not appreciably increase antitussive activity. *(2:154)*

112. **(D)** Emetrol is a phosphorated carbohydrate solution containing levulose, dextrose, and orthophosphoric acid with a pH adjusted to 1.5. Its effectiveness in preventing or treating motion sickness has not been proven. The Emetrol label states that the oral solution should not be diluted with or accompanied by other fluids. *(2:302)*

113. **(B)** Calcium carbonate is a rapid prolonged, potent neutralizer of gastric acid. Some scientists and consumer groups have advocated its use because of its high effectiveness and low cost. However, the listed side effects should warrant curtailment of its use, particularly for chronic therapy. *(2:257)*
(A–incorrect) Some of the insoluble calcium carbonate is converted to soluble calcium chloride, which is absorbed. Significant amounts of calcium may be absorbed after a few days of antacid therapy.
(D–incorrect) Gastric hypersecretion is believed to be caused by the local effect of calcium on the gastrin-producing cells.

114. **(D)** The generic name for Ayerst's Riopan is magaldrate. The product is a chemical rather than a physical combination of aluminum and magnesium hydroxides. While this chemical form has a lower neutralizing capacity, it is still considered to be an effective antacid with a low sodium level and does not cause electrolyte imbalance in the body.

(1:776; 2:260)

115. **(E)** Rolaids contains dihydroxyaluminum sodium carbonate, which combines the antacid properties of aluminum hydroxide and sodium bicarbonate. The approximate sodium level is 53 mg per tablet.

(2:290)

116. **(E)** Since para-aminobenzoic acid (PABA) absorbs UV light, especially in the 260 to 313-nm range, it is

included in several OTC sunscreening products. However, newer agents with a lower incidence of causing contact dermatitis and photosensitivity have replaced PABA. These agents include the padimates, oxybenzones, and cinnamates. *(1:769; 2:915)*

117. **(E)** Picking occurs when the tablet powder sticks to the punch face.
(D–incorrect) Mottling is uneven color distribution, probably due to poor mixing of the tablet granulation. *(20:62)*

118. **(A)** Excessive compression would result in hard tablets that would not stick to the punches and would not be picked. However, excessively hard tablets may not disintegrate in the body fluids. *(20:62)*

119. **(A)** Magnesium stearate (as well as other stearates) is included in tablet formulations as a lubricant. *(1:1323; 20:57)*

120. **(C)** Tablet lubricants are characterized by lubricity, as they are usually water insoluble and difficult to wet. The waterproofing property might retard disintegration and dissolution. *(1:593; 20:56)*

121. **(B)** Ingredients such as potato or corn starch speed the flow of tableting powder into the dies, thereby increasing production rates. These starches also act as disintegrants in the tablet. *(20:58; 33:382)*

122. **(A)** Capping implies that the compressed powder is not cohesive. A tablet lubricant ensures feeding of granules into the dies and prevents sticking of powder to the dies and punches. Excessive lubricant may render the granulation too slippery, preventing cohesiveness, but will not cause capping. *(20:62)*

123. **(A)** Carnauba wax and beeswax combinations are commonly used as a polishing coat for sugar coating, but not for film coating.
(B–incorrect) (C–incorrect) (D–incorrect) (E–incorrect) In film coating, a thin film of coating material is applied or sprayed onto tablets. Alcohol solutions of cellulosic polymers are commonly used. The thin film does not change the shape of the tablet, and designs imprinted on the tablet are easily seen through the coating. *(20:69)*

124. **(B)** Products such as Potassium Chloride Enseals are enteric coated to protect the stomach from irritating substances or to prevent drug decomposition in the stomach. *(10; 24:158)*
(A–incorrect) Endurets are sustained-release tablets. Preludin is an example.
(C–incorrect) Extentabs are prolonged-action tablets (for example, Dimetane Extentabs).
(D–incorrect) Filmtabs are tablets coated with a transparent protective coating (for example, Eutron Filmtabs).

125. **(D)** Mannitol possesses characteristics that make it an almost ideal sweetener for chewable tablets. While not as sweet as sucrose, it leaves a cool taste in the mouth and is nonhygroscopic. Mannitol is also easily compressed by wet granulation. *(24:182)*

126. **(B)** Sterile powders of water-unstable drugs are often prepared by lyophilization (freeze-drying). Mannitol may be included in the formula to build up the dry powder, known as the cake. The larger, more visible cake is helpful in that the pharmacist can more readily ascertain when dissolution is completed. *(33:508)*

127. **(A)** Benzyl alcohol is used in many parenterals, especially in Bacteriostatic Sterile Water for Injection as an antimicrobial agent. While its relative toxicity is low, there are a few reports of hypersensitivity. Also, it is contraindicated for use in premature infants because of incidences of fatal toxic syndrome. *(13:16,379)*

128. **(D)** A pseudoplastic flow is characterized by a greater flow rate after the system has been agitated. Thixotropy refers to a reversible sol-gel system; it is characterized by a gel that forms a flowable sol when shaken. Upon standing, the reformation of the gel will slow particle settling. Caking is undesirable since settling particles form a dense pack in the bottom of the container. It is very difficult to break this cake and to reconstitute the original suspension. *(1:313,316,1538; 20:174)*

129. **(C)** Inhalation aerosol products may be intended for either localized activity (bronchodilators for asthma) or systemic action (ergotamine for migraine). In either situation, the onset of action will be fast. When the drug is absorbed through the alveolar-capillary membrane, the first-pass metabolism in the liver is avoided. Because of the limited capacity of aerosol units, especially in the small chamber metered valves, only a limited amount of drug can be administered. *(1:1694)*

130. **(A)** Epinephrine is the active bronchodilator in such OTC products as Bronkaid Mist and Primatene Mist. Ephedrine is available OTC only in tablet and syrup dosage forms. Metaproterenol aerosol products are by prescription only. *(2:213)*

131. **(C)** Thyrolar (sodium levothyroxine with sodium liothyronine in a ratio of 4:1) is a combination product designed to mimic the natural secretion of the thyroid gland. *(6:1371)*
(A–incorrect) Proloid is thyroglobulin extracted from animal thyroid glands and contains T_4 and T_3 in the ratio of 2:1.
(B–incorrect) (D–incorrect) Synthroid and Levothroid are products containing pure sodium levothyroxine (T_4).
(E–incorrect) Cytomel contains pure sodium liothyronine (T_3)

132. **(A)** Diacetylmorphine is commonly known as heroin. It is a Class I controlled substance; this means that it may be used only for experimental work by special permit. *(1:1101)*

133. (A) The first-degree burn is the mildest injury since only the epidermis is affected.
(C–incorrect) These are characteristics of a second-degree burn, which affects the epidermis and portions of the dermis.
(D–incorrect) A third-degree burn penetrates through the entire skin. Damage may be permanent.
(E–incorrect) These are characteristics of the fourth-degree or char burn. Both the skin and underlying tissues are affected. *(2:891)*

134. (A) Benzocaine is widely used for surface anesthesia of the skin and mucous membranes. It remains on the skin for a long period of time since it has poor water solubility and is poorly absorbed. Systemic toxicity is rare. While the possibility of local sensitization should be considered, the incidence is low considering the frequent use of benzocaine. *(1:1054; 2:898)*
(B–incorrect) Butamben picrate is available only in Butesin Picrate ointment. *(2:904)*
(C–incorrect) Lidocaine is present in Medi-Quik Aerosol, Bactine, and Unguentine Plus. *(2:905)*
(D–incorrect) Although phenol (carbonic acid) possesses both antiseptic and local anesthetic effects, there is the possibility that it may accentuate tissue damage because of its caustic properties. *(1:1323)*
(E–incorrect) Tetracaine is present in Pontocaine Cream and Ointment. *(2:906)*

135. (D) Debrisan is not useful in the treatment of non-secreting wounds. Its action appears to be absorption of fluids and particles that impede tissue repair. The product is available as 0.1- to 0.3-mm spherical beads (4-g packets) that are sprinkled onto secreting wounds. The hydrophilic nature of the beads creates a strong suction force; each gram absorbs about 4 mL of fluid. The beads become grayish yellow when they are saturated with fluid; they should then be washed away by irrigating with sterile water or saline.
(1:773,1900)

136. (E) A topical preparation should contain a minimum of 5% benzocaine. Some studies have indicated that 10% to 20% of the drug is needed. *(2:899; 4:155)*

137. (A) The rectal thermometer bulb has a strong, blunt shape that facilitates insertion into the rectum and retention by sphincter muscles. The oral bulb is cylindrical, elongated, and thin walled for quick registration of temperature. Rectal thermometers can be used orally. The oral bulb is too easily broken and is not suitable for rectal use. The short, sturdy security bulb represents a compromise intermediate shape.
(1:1882; 22:165)

138. (B) Since fertilization can occur within only a few hours (perhaps 24) after ovulation, accurate knowledge of this event could permit timing of intercourse to either increase or decrease the possibility of conception. Basal temperature (the lowest temperature of the body during waking hours) typically passes through a biphasic cycle over the course of the menstrual cycle. From an initially low temperature, a midcycle thermal shift occurs to a high level, where it remains until it again becomes low premenstrually. The temperature rise roughly corresponds with the time of ovulation. *(1:1842)*
(A–incorrect) The thermometer is used orally or rectally once daily, immediately upon awakening in the morning and before getting out of bed.
(D–incorrect) The scale may be either Fahrenheit or Celsius. The temperature rise is only about 0.5° F, which would be difficult to measure on the usual clinical thermometer. The basal thermometer scale ranges only from 96 to 100° F and is graduated to 0.1° F.

139. (C) One French unit equals 1 mm in outside circumference. A catheter with an outside circumference of 20 mm is identified as a 20F or 20Fr size. Sizes range from 10F to 34F. *(1:1888)*
(D–incorrect) Catheters are less commonly sized by the American or English scales.
(E–incorrect) The Foley catheter is a type of self-retaining or indwelling catheter.

140. (D) While the venoms of some insects are potent, the amounts injected are too small to be toxic. The severity of the sting reaction in some individuals is due to hypersensitivity to certain proteins in the venom. This results in the anaphylactic shock. *(2:946)*

141. (D) Persons who experience severe anaphylactic reactions to insect stings or bites should carry emergency kits. These kits usually contain antiseptic pads (to clean and disinfect the area), both an antihistamine and epinephrine injection (to counteract the anaphylactic reaction), and tweezers (to remove the stingers). A tourniquet would be of little value since the amount of venom is very small. *(2:953)*

142. (A) Eucerin consists of equal parts of Aquaphor and water resulting in a W/O emulsion base. *(20:274)*

143. (D) Debrox drops are intended to clean cerumen from ears. The carbamide peroxide will effervesce, thereby softening the waxy material while the glycerin acts as a solvent. *(2:647,652)*

144. (E) Diffusion of a drug from a vehicle into the skin is often related to the solubility of the drug in the vehicle relative to the solubility in the skin, ie, the partition coefficient. Drugs that are very soluble in a vehicle will tend to remain in the vehicle and will penetrate more slowly than drugs with poorer solubility in the vehicle.
(A–incorrect) Covering the area to which a topical drug has been applied will often enhance the rate of absorption. Sweat accumulation at the skin-vehicle interface induces hydration of the skin, a condition that facilitates penetration of drugs.
(B–incorrect) Poorer solubility of the drug in PEG

ointment than in white ointment may lead to faster diffusion. This is the converse of choice E.

(C–incorrect) The thicker epidermis of the palms results in slower drug penetration than that which occurs on the backs of the hands.

(D–incorrect) Higher drug concentrations will increase the rate of diffusion and penetration.

(1:1597–1602; 20:80)

145. **(E)** White ointment is composed of white wax and white petrolatum, both consisting of hydrophobic aliphatic hydrocarbons. This ointment base has a very low "water number." The water number is defined as the largest amount of water that 100 g of an ointment base will hold at 20° C. *(1:1603; 20:274)*

146. **(E)** Polysorb Hydrate contains the lipophilic sorbitan sesquioleate as an emulsifier. Two other W/O emulsion bases are Eucerin and Nivea Cream, both of which contain wool wax alcohols as emulsifiers. *(20:198)*

147. **(E)** Allantoin is included in many topical formulations as a healing agent. Presumably, it stimulates cell proliferation. *(1:773; 3:Sect. 10)*

148. **(B)** The official Cold Cream USP contains a borate/fatty acid surfactant system and mineral oil. Rose Water Ointment NF (cold cream, Galen's cerate) contains a similar surfactant system but with almond oil rather than mineral oil. *(1:1312)*

149. **(D)** The extent of drug release and absorption will vary depending upon the properties of the drug, the suppository base, and the condition of the colon. Oil-soluble drugs will be poorly released from a cocoa butter base because of the high lipid/water solubility. *(24:343)*

(A–incorrect) The rectal fluid pH is essentially neutral and has a low buffer capacity. Therefore, drugs that can be destroyed by the acidity of the stomach may be successfully administered rectally.

(B–incorrect) Drugs that are absorbed through the colon pass into the lower hemorrhoidal veins and into the general systematic circulation. Avoidance of first-pass exposure to the liver may enhance the effect of drugs that the liver inactivates. Drugs that are absorbed from the upper intestinal tract pass directly through the portal vein into the liver, where metabolism to inactive products can occur.

(E–incorrect) The lesser dose frequency and lower propensity for irritation are the reasons certain drugs can be administered rectally but not orally.

150. **(E)** Selected combinations of the polyethylene glycols (PEGs) can be formulated into water-miscible suppositories with a range of consistence. They are easy to insert and do not require refrigeration. *(24:377)*

151. **(A)** Lactose is a readily compressible, water-soluble, inert ingredient. It also encourages the growth of Döderlein's bacilli, a microorganism present in the healthy vagina. *(24:386)*

152. **(C)** The active ingredient in Norforms vaginal suppositories is the quaternary ammonium germicide methylbenzethonium chloride, which decreases odor-producing microorganisms. *(2:416; 10)*

153. **(E)** Mycostatin tablets contain the antibiotic nystatin, which is unstable at elevated temperatures. *(10)*

154. **(D)** The dextrans are plasma extenders that will restore blood volume. Since they have no oxygen-carrying capacity, however, they are not substitutes for blood. Therefore, plasma or blood should be administered as soon as possible after the use of dextrans in emergency situations. Dextran 40 is used to prevent aggregation of erythrocytes during surgery and as a plasma expander during hypovolemic shock. Dextran 75 is mainly used in the treatment of hypovolemic shock, especially for toxemia of pregnancy and for nephrosis. *(1:804)*

155. **(A)** Properties of a solution that depend on the number of particles of the solute and are independent of the chemical nature of the solute are termed colligative properties. The magnitude of vapor pressure and freezing point reduction, boiling point elevation, and osmotic pressure are all related to the number of particles in solution. *(1:228)*

156. **(A)** Solutions with equal osmotic pressure are isoosmotic; they also are isotonic if separated by a membrane permeable to the solvent but impermeable to the solute. Any of the colligative properties can be used to determine tonicity of solutions. Freezing-point depression is most frequently used. The freezing point of a 0.9% aqueous solution of sodium chloride is −0.52° C, the same as that of human blood and tears. Saline solutions of this concentration are isotonic with these body fluids. More concentrated solutions are hypertonic; less concentrated are hypotonic. *(1:1488)*

157. **(C)** An electric current is conducted in an electrolytic solution by the movement of ions. Conductivity (the ability to conduct current) depends upon the number and type of ions present. It is the reciprocal of the resistance of the solution. *(1:228)*

158. **(D)** Solutions with the same osmotic pressure as blood are usually isotonic with blood. Solutions that have a higher osmotic pressure (ie, hypertonic) will cause water to pass out of the red blood cells. Solutions that have a lower osmotic pressure (ie, hypotonic) will allow water to pass into the cells. This causes them to swell and rupture with a release of hemoglobin (hemolysis). *(1:1482; 12:234)*

159. **(B)** Appendix A in *Remington's Pharmaceutical Sciences* lists sodium chloride equivalents, freezing-point depressions, and the hemolytic effects of many

chemicals in aqueous solutions. Even when boric acid, glycerin, propylene glycol, and urea solutions are isoosmotic, hemolysis occurs when red blood cells are added. Glucose does not cause hemolysis. If it did, it could not be used in large-volume parenterals for infusion into the bloodstream. *(1:1491)*

160. **(C)** A hypertonic solution will draw water from within the cell until an equilibrium is reached with equal pressure on each side of the cell membrane. Because of the loss of volume, the cell will shrink and take on a wrinkled appearance (crenation). *(12:234)*

161. **(A)** A sodium chloride equivalent is the weight of sodium chloride that will produce the same osmotic effect as 1 g of the specified chemical. For example, morphine hydrochloride has an E value of 0.15. This indicates that 1 g of morphine hydrochloride produces the same osmotic pressure (and depression of freezing point) in solutions as 0.15 g of sodium chloride. *(1:1490)*

162. **(C)** Any two solutions that have the same freezing points will have the same osmotic pressure and should be isotonic. Since blood freezes at −0.52° C, any solution that freezes at this temperature will be isoosmotic. The use of freezing-point data for isotonicity adjustment for both ophthalmic and parenteral solutions is common in the pharmaceutical industry because freezing points can be easily measured. *(1:1488)*

163. **(D)** Aqueous solutions that freeze at the same temperature as blood have the same osmotic pressure as blood (ie, are isoosmotic with blood and each other). However, to be isotonic a solution must maintain a certain pressure, or "tone," in the red blood cells. If the chemical in a solution passes freely through the red blood cell membrane, equalized pressure on both sides of the membrane is not possible without changes in the cell volume. Tone will not be maintained, and the solution will not be isotonic, though it might be isoosmotic with blood. *(1:1482)*

164. **(E)** Although it is possible to experimentally determine whether a solution is isoosmotic with a 0.9% sodium chloride solution or blood, one cannot assume that the solution is also isotonic. The pharmacist in product development will adjust a solution to the correct isoosmotic pressure, then mix the solution with red blood cells to observe whether hemolysis occurs. *(1:1489)*
(C–incorrect) *Remington's Pharmaceutical Sciences* presents extensive tables of values. *(1:1491)*
(D–incorrect) Other chemicals may be used as tonicity adjustors. Concentrations of chemicals that are isoosmotic are listed in the Remington or can be calculated by simple proportions. *(1:1491)*

165. **(B)** Increasing the contact time between a drug and the cornea will often increase the amount of drug absorption that will occur. *(1:1590)*

166. **(B)** Fluorescein sodium is an ophthalmic diagnostic agent. It is instilled into the eye to delineate scratches and corneal lesions. It would be very dangerous to place a contaminated solution on a damaged cornea through which microorganisms may easily pass. Pharmacists should not extemporaneously prepare fluorescein sodium solutions unless sterility can be guaranteed. Pharmaceutical manufacturers supply fluorescein as unit-dose solutions or individual paper strips. *(1:1282)*

167. **(A)** The combination of benzalkonium chloride and EDTA (0.01% of each) is effective against most common microorganisms, including strains of *Pseudomonas aeruginosa* that are resistant to benzalkonium chloride. *(1:1591; 20:148)*

168. **(D)** Sodium Sulamyd is a brand of sulfacetamide sodium manufactured by Schering. The label specifies storage in a "cool place", which, according to the USP, has a temperature range between 8 and 15° C. However, storage of Sulamyd Ophthalmic Solution in the refrigerator (2 to 8°C) will not damage the product.
(10)
(A–incorrect) Chloroptic is Allergan's brand of chloramphenicol 0.5% solution.
(B–incorrect) Barnes-Hind's Eppy is a borate complex containing the equivalent of 1% l-epinephrine.
(C–incorrect) Parke-Davis markets Ophthochlor, which is a 0.5% solution of chloramphenicol.

169. **(E)** Tetracaine hydrochloride is useful for topical eye anesthesia since it is five to eight times more potent than cocaine. A 0.5% solution produces local anesthesia within 25 seconds and lasts for 15 minutes. *(4:2001; 9:52:16)*

170. **(E)** In spite of its name, veegum is not an organic gum but is an inorganic clay. It is water insoluble and would probably be unsuitable for ophthalmic administration since insoluble particles could be deposited in the ocular areas. *(20:147)*

171. **(D)** Papain is a proteolytic enzyme aiding in the removal of proteinaceous residues that slowly build up on soft lenses. Allergan markets Soflens Enzymatic Contact Lens Cleaner as tablets containing papain. Once weekly, the soft lenses are soaked overnight in a solution prepared from the tablets. *(2:614)*

172. **(C)** Sodium bisulfite and sodium metabisulfite are included in pharmaceutical solutions as antioxidants. For example, the oxidation of epinephrine may be retarded by the presence of sodium bisulfite, which is preferentially oxidized. Unfortunately, some individuals are sensitive to the bisulfites and must avoid products containing them. *(1:1288)*

173. **(A)** One of the first signs of sensitivity to bisulfites is difficulty in breathing. Also, the patient may experience hives, abdominal pain, and wheezing. *(24:104)*

174. **(A)** Investigators have shown that solutions with a

range of sodium chloride concentrations from 0.5 to 2.0% can be instilled into either normal or inflamed eyes without causing pain or detectable tissue change. Purified water will sting because it has such a low tonicity.   *(20:147)*

175. **(E)** The three layers of the cornea are the corneal epithelium (outermost layer), the stroma or substantia propria, and the corneal endothelium (inner layer). Of the three layers, the stroma is the deepest and most hydrophilic. Because of the presence of both lipophilic and hydrophilic layers, drugs that possess biphasic solubility will usually pass through the cornea. Few drugs exhibit both oil and water solubility. Therefore, the ability of the drug to coexist in both the ionized (water-soluble) and the unionized (oil-soluble) forms at a physiologic pH is important.   *(1:1583)*

176. **(A)** The capacity of the cul-de-sac is estimated to be not more than 0.03 mL, with a normal tear volume of approximately 0.007 mL. Probably less than 0.02 mL of an ophthalmic solution can be successfully placed in an eye at one time. This volume is less than the nominal 0.05 mL (1 drop) usually requested in prescription directions. This implies that a portion of the dose is lost through drainage or overflow onto the cheek.   *(1:1583)*

177. **(D)** By definition.   *(1:237; 12:195)*

178. **(C)** The Henderson-Hasselbalch equation, or buffer equation for a weak acid and its salt, is represented by:

$$pH = pKa + \log \frac{salt}{acid}$$

where pKa is the negative log of the dissociation constant for the weak acid and salt/acid is the ratio of the molar concentration of salt and acid in the system.   *(12:223)*

179. **(E)** According to the Henderson-Hasselbalch equation, pH will equal pKa when the expression

$$\log \frac{[salt]}{[acid]} \text{ is equal to zero}$$

This can occur only when the salt/acid ratio equals 1, since the log of 1 is 0. The point where the salt concentration equals the acid concentration is the half-neutralization point.   *(32:65)*

180. **(D)** For many years, the curie (Ci) has been the basic unit for expressing radioisotope decay. Now the becquerel is recognized as the "official" unit. One becquerel equals one decay per second (dps).

$$1 \text{ curie} = 3.7 \times 10^{10} \text{ bq (dps)}$$

The rad is a quantitative measure of radioactivity.   *(1:609; 18c:II–5)*

181. **(D)** Since ^{32}P is metabolized in a manner similar to naturally occurring phosphorus, the isotope is readily distributed to all tissues and is concentrated in those tissues where proliferation is most rapid. A therapeutic dose of ^{32}P (1.5 to 5mCi) will concentrate in bone marrow and partially suppress erythrogenesis.   *(1:649)*

182. **(B)** Although it is desirable to use isotopes with short half-lives to minimize the radiation dose received by the patient, it is evident that the shorter the half-life, the greater the problem of supply. Radioisotope generators, or "cows," have been developed to deal with this problem. A radioisotope generator is an ion-exchange column containing a resin of alumina upon which a long-lived parent nuclide is absorbed. Radioactive decay of the long-lived parent results in the production of a short-lived daughter nuclide that is eluted or "milked" from the column by means of an appropriate solvent such as sterile, pyrogen-free saline.   *(1:613)*

183. **(B)** ^{90m}Tc is available commercially as a technetium generator (various manufacturers) in which molybdenum ^{99}Mo is the parent nuclide. The half-life of technetium (6 hours) is long enough to allow completion of usual diagnostic procedures for which it is used, yet short enough to minimize the radiation dose to the patient. Lack of a beta component in its radiation further decreases the dose delivered to the patient. The gamma energy is weak enough to achieve good collimation, yet strong enough to penetrate tissue sufficiently to permit deep-organ scanning.   *(1:613,640)*

184. **(E)** The number of protons in the nucleus of an atom defines its atomic number. This is equal to the number of orbital electrons. The atomic weight or mass number of an element is equal to the number of protons and neutrons in the nucleus. Isotopes are species of nuclides that possess the same number of protons (ie, atomic number) but a different number of neutrons (hence, a different mass number). Isotopes represent the same chemical element, and therefore have the same chemical properties.   *(1:606)*

185. **(B)** Decay rate is the rate at which atoms undergo radioactive disintegration. The rate of decay (-dn/dt) is proportional to the number of atoms (n) present at any time (t). Mathematically this may be expressed as

$$-dn/dt = \gamma N$$

where gamma (γ) is a proportionality constant (the decay constant). The decay of radioactive atoms is therefore a first-order process.   *(1:608)*

186. **(C)** Gamma radiation, x-rays, and ultraviolet radiation are forms of electromagnetic radiation and are radiated as photons or quanta of energy. These forms of radiation differ only in wave length and are the most penetrating types of radiation. Gamma

rays are the most penetrating of all and can easily penetrate more than a foot of tissue and several inches of lead. *(1:605,621)*

(A–incorrect) Alpha radiation is particulate radiation consisting of two protons and two neutrons. The range of alpha particles is about 5 cm in air and less than 100 μ in tissue.

(B–incorrect) Beta radiation is also particulate radiation, but exists as two types, the negative electron (negatron) and the positive electron (positron). Both may have a range of over 10 feet in air and up to about 1 mm in tissue. *(1:605,621)*

187. **(E)** Natural ergot alkaloids are morbid fungus growths on various plants, including rye, wheat, and barley. The ergots are marketed as acid salts (ergotamine tartrate, ergonovine maleate, etc); therefore, they would be stable in acid media. *(1:403,946)*

188. **(E)** A surfactant has both hydrophilic (water-solubilizing) and lipophilic (fat-solubilizing) properties in a proper balance (ie, not completely in either direction). The HLB (hydrophile-lipophile balance) system is a semi-quantitative classification of surfactants. *(1:266,304; 31:50,838)*

189. **(C)** Most alkaloids have pKa's above 7; therefore, they are weak bases that form salts with acids (eg, pilocarpine hydrochloride, morphine sulfate).
(D–incorrect) Stereoisomerism is common in alkaloidal structures; large differences in therapeutic activity can be expected among isomers. *(1:395)*

190. **(D)** The United States Adopted Names (USAN) Council establishes nonproprietary drug names. The Council is jointly sponsored by the AMA, United States Pharmacopoeial Convention, and the APhA. Since the USAN is not an official governmental agency, the chosen names are not formally recognized until they are published in the *Federal Register*. *(1:412)*

191. **(B)** A "precaution" is intended to advise the physician of possible problems that may occur with the use of a drug. For example, the use of tetracycline may result in overgrowth of nonsusceptible microorganisms. A "warning" signifies a more serious problem with greater potential for harm to a patient. For example, renal impairment may require reduction in the drug dose. A "contraindication" is the most restrictive limitation since it refers to an absolute prohibition against the use of a drug under certain conditions. For example, the use of penicillin derivatives is prohibited in patients known to be sensitive to penicillin. *(24:40)*

192. **(E)** Values for dissociation constants are always less than one and expressed as exponential notations. To provide whole numbers for ease of comparison and calculation, the reciprocal log of the dissociation constant (1/log Ka) or (–log Ka) is used to express acid strength. For example, the Ka of acetic acid is 1.75×10^{-5}. The pKa of acetic acid may be calculated as:

$$pKa = -\log Ka$$
$$= -(\log 1.75 \times 10^{-5})$$
$$= -(\log 1.75 + \log 1 \times 10^{-5})$$
$$= -(0.24 - 5)$$
$$= -(-4.76)$$
$$= 4.76$$

(12:196)

193. **(C)** Hydrochloric acid is classified as a strong acid. Strong acids ionize almost completely into hydronium ions and the corresponding anions. Other strong acids are sulfuric and nitric. These acids do not have pKa values listed since the values would be close to 0. The fact that all of the other acids listed in the question have pKa's indicate that they are weaker acids (with less ionization) than hydrochloric acid. *(12:188)*

194. **(C)** Stronger acids have larger ionization constants than weaker acids. Since the pKa is the reciprocal of the log of the ionization constant, stronger acids have lower pKa's than weaker acids. Of the acids listed, boric acid has the highest pKa, thus, it is the weakest of these acids. Salicylic acid, which has the lowest pKa on the list, is the strongest. *(12:188)*

195. **(D)** A buffer system consists of a weak acid or base and its corresponding strong salt. In preparing a buffer system, one should choose an acid or base with a pKa value close to the desired pH. For example, lactic acid and sodium lactate can be combined to obtain a pH of exactly 4.0. The needed molar concentration of each may be calculated by using the Henderson-Hasselbalch equation. *(1:242; 12:233)*

196. **(B)** For determining the ratio of a weak acid to its salt present at a given pH, the Henderson-Hasselbalch equation is utilized.

$$pH = pKa + \log \frac{[\text{dissociated}]}{[\text{undissociated}]}$$

If the values for pH and pKa are used in this equation, it can be seen that the ratio of the dissociated form of the drug to the undissociated form will be the antilog of 2, which is equal to 100. *(24:54)*

197. **(C)** Sustained release dosage forms are intended to reduce dosing frequency while maintaining relatively consistent blood levels of the drug. The duration of activity of drugs with half-lives between 2 and 8 hours can be extended to obtain convenient once- or twice-daily dosing. While it would be desirable to increase the therapeutic duration of drugs with half-lives of less than 2 hours, the necessary high drug release rates and high drug concentration in the dosage form reservoir usually preclude sustained release dosage formulation. Also, individual biological variation could result in either sub- or hypertherapeutic blood levels. Drugs with half-lives

greater than 8 hours usually have long intervals between dosing, making sustained release formulations unnecessary.   *(1:1682)*

198. **(A)** Besides the other listed strengths, Inderal is available as 60-mg tablets, long-acting capsules (Inderal LA at 80, 120, or 160 mg), and an injection (1-mL ampules containing 1 mg of drug).   *(25)*

199. **(D)** Coumadin is DuPont's brand of warfarin sodium and is available in several strengths for convenient dosage adjustments. Tablets containing 2, 2.5, 5, 7.5, and 10 mg are marketed.   *(25)*

200. **(C)**   *(25)*

201. **(D)** Valium tablets are available in strengths of 2, 5, and 10 mg. The injection solution is supplied as 2-mL ampules and 10-mL vials both containing 5 mg/mL of drug. Because of limited water solubility, the injection solution has a mixed solvent system of 40% propylene glycol, 10% ethanol, and water.   *(25)*

202. **(B)**   *(25:1–40)*

203. **(C)**   *(25:1–40)*

204. **(A)**   *(25:1–40)*

205. **(E)**   *(25:1–40)*

206. **(C)**   *(25:1–40)*

207. **(D)**   *(25:1–40)*

208. **(A)**   *(25:1–40)*

209. **(B)**   *(25:1–40)*

210. **(D)**   *(25:1–40)*

211. **(E)**   *(25:1–40)*

212. **(A)**   *(25:1–40)*

213. **(C)**   *(25:1–40)*

214. **(B)**   *(25:1–40)*

215. **(E)**   *(25:1–40)*

216. **(A)**   *(25:1–40)*

217. **(D)**   *(25:1–40)*

218. **(C)**   *(10)*

219. **(A)**   *(10)*

220. **(D)**   *(10)*

221. **(E)**   *(10)*

222. **(B)**   *(10)*

223. **(E)**   *(10)*

224. **(C)**   *(10)*

225. **(B)**   *(10)*

226. **(A)**   *(10)*

227. **(D)**   *(10)*

228. **(D)**   *(10)*

229. **(A)**   *(10)*

230. **(E)**   *(10)*

231. **(B)**   *(10)*

232. **(C)**   *(10)*

233. **(B)**   *(10)*

234. **(A)**   *(10)*

235. **(D)**   *(10)*

236. **(E)**   *(10)*

237. **(C)**   *(10)*

238. **(C)**   *(10)*

239. **(A)**   *(10)*

240. **(E)**   *(10)*

241. **(D)**   *(10)*

242. **(B)**   *(10)*

243. **(A)** Procainamide   *(10)*

244. **(C)** Hydrochlorothiazide   *(10)*

245. **(D)** Isosorbide dinitrate   *(10)*

246. **(E)** Albuterol   *(10)*

247. **(B)** Verapamil   *(10)*

248. **(D)** Erythromycin ethylsuccinate   *(10)*

249. **(E)** Lithium carbonate   *(10)*

250. **(A)** Erythromycin   *(10)*

251. **(B)** Nystatin   *(10)*

252. **(C)**   *(2:199)*

253. **(D)**   *(2:194)*

254. **(A)**   *(2:198)*

255. **(B)**   *(2:200)*

256. **(E)**   *(2:200)*

257. **(C)**   *(4:1972)*

258. **(A)** Demecarium is a long-acting anticholinesterase.   *(4:1972)*

259. **(B)** Echothiophate iodide is a potent long-acting anticholinesterase marketed as a lyophilized powder for reconstitution.   *(4:1972)*

260. **(D)**   *(6:320)*

261. **(E)**   *(6:321)*

262. **(A)**   *(6:320)*

263. **(C)**   *(6:321)*

264. (A) Despite its slow onset of action and low neutralizing capacity, aluminum hydroxide is a commonly used antacid because of its nonabsorbability, demulcent activity, and ability to adsorb pepsin.

(2:258,284)

265. (C) Magnesium trisilicate appears to be longer acting than aluminum hydroxide. Also, magnesium trisilicate reacts with hydrochloric acid to form hydrated silicon dioxide, which may coat ulcers, thereby providing symptomatic relief. Gaviscon also contains alginic acid, which forms a viscous solution, thereby prolonging contact time. The product is claimed to be effective in the relief of gastro-esophageal reflux.

(2:286)

266. (B) Magnesium hydroxide has been mixed with aluminum hydroxide in an attempt to reduce the incidence of constipation attributed to the aluminum ion.

(2:259,289)

267. (D) Calcium carbonate is often considered the antacid of choice because of its rapid onset of action, high neutralizing capacity, and relatively prolonged action. Side effects include constipation, which may be prevented by combining calcium carbonate with either magnesium carbonate or magnesium oxide. Prolonged use of calcium carbonate may result in the formation of urinary calculi. Also, increased blood levels of calcium have been reported.

(2:257,291)

268. (D)   *(2:288)*

269. (C)   *(13:272)*

270. (E)   *(13:272)*

271. (D)   *(13:272)*

272. (A)   *(13:272)*

273. (D)   *(1:1572)*

274. (A)   *(1:1572)*

275. (B)   *(1:1572)*

276. (C)   *(1:1019)*

277. (D)   *(1:1018)*

278. (B)   *(1:1017)*

279. (A)   *(1:1022)*

280. (D) Alcohol USP, sometimes known as grain alcohol, contains 94.9% V/V or 92.3% W/W of C_2H_5OH. The remaining portion is water.

(1:1314)

281. (A) Diluted alcohol is prepared by mixing equal volumes of Alcohol USP and purified water. Because of some volume shrinkage (about 3%), the final strength is somewhat higher than that calculated by simple alligation.

(1:1315)

282. (B) Rubbing alcohol is a form of denatured alcohol containing approximately 70% V/V of absolute alcohol. This product is used as a germicide and an external rubefacient.

(1:1164)

283. (C) The needle hub can be made of plastic or metal. It is fitted into the syringe body by either a locking system such as the Luer-Lok or by a simple friction fit.

(13:301; 20:197)

284. (A) The bevel is ground to sharpness, but the back portion (heel) of the bevel is left dull. A dull heel has been shown to decrease the incidence of coring of the rubber closure and the skin.

(13:302)

285. (B) Needle cannulae are made of various grades of steel. Both strength and flexibility are needed.

(13:301)

286. (E)   *(13:301)*

287. (D)   *(1:764; 2:647)*

288. (A)   *(1:762)*

289. (E)   *(1:1247)*

290. (C)   *(1:764)*

291. (E) The normal pH range for the blood is 7.36 to 7.40 for venous samples and 7.38 to 7.42 for arterial samples. It is essential that the blood pH remains within the range of 7.35 to 7.45. Normal acid-base balance is generally maintained by three homeostatic mechanisms using chemical buffers (eg, bicarbonate and carbonic acid), respiratory control, and renal function. An impairment in any of these mechanisms can result in either acidosis or alkalosis.

(1:514)

292. (E) The pH of the lacrimal fluid is approximately 7.4 but varies with certain ailments. The eye can tolerate a pH from 6 to 8 with a minimum of discomfort. The buffering system of the lacrimal fluid is efficient enough to adjust the pH of most ophthalmic solutions. However, some solutions, particularly those containing strongly acidic drugs, will cause discomfort.

(1:1589)

293. (B) The pH of the skin is usually based upon measurements of the lipid film that covers the epidermis. Although the value varies greatly between individuals and in various areas of the body, the average value is reported to be 5.5, with a range of 4.0 to 6.5.

(1:1596)

294. (A) The acidic pH (3.5 to 4.2) of the vagina discourages the growth of pathogenic microorganisms while providing a suitable environment for the growth of acid-producing bacilli.

(2:398)

295. (C)   *(4:157)*

296. (E)   *(4:160)*

297. (B)   *(4:161)*

298. (B) One major use of bupivacaine (Marcaine, Sensorcaine) is for epidural anesthesia during labor because of its relative long duration of action (2 to 3 hours).   *(4:155)*

299. (A) Because of its rapid onset when injected intramuscularly, ketamine (Ketalar) is used for repeat anesthesia in burn patients and sedation of uncontrollable patients.   *(4:176)*

300. (D) Tetracaine is often used for spinal anesthesia.   *(4:162)*

301. (C) Triaminic tablets are designed to release an initial dose, followed by a second dose at a later time. This type of product reduces the number of doses the patient must take during the day. Similarly designed products include Schering's Repetabs (Chlor-Trimeton, Polaramine, and Demazin).   *(20:55; 34:200)*

302. (E) This type of product is formulated by mixing the drug with an insoluble material and compressing it into a tablet. The tablet does not disintegrate; instead, it maintains its geometric shape and releases drug as erosion takes place at the surface of the tablet. Other examples of this principle include Disophrol Chronotabs and Dimetane Extentabs.   *(1:1685; 20:55; 34:200)*

303. (B) This dosage form is prepared by compressing medicated pellets into tablets. Release can be designed for one or more time spans. Product examples include Bellergal-S tablets and Theo-Dur.   *(34:201)*

304. (A) The Durabond principle consists of complexing amine drugs with tannic acid to form the corresponding tannates. These relatively insoluble drug forms are slowly released over a 12-hour period.   *(34:201)*

305. (D) For this type of drug, an initial dose is not as important as a prolonged blood level. Therefore, the equivalent of three normal doses is formulated into a core that slowly releases the drug by surface erosion. Unlike Extentabs, no initial dose is released. Another example of a slow erosion core is Tepanil Ten-Tab.   *(34:200)*

306. (B) The active drug (phentermine) in Ionamin capsules is combined with a polystyrene sulfonic acid resin. As the capsule passes through the GI tract, the resin exchanges active drug for ions such as sodium and potassium. Biphetamine capsules are similarly formulated.   *(1:1685)*

307. (D) Drug particles can be coated by encapsulation with a thin film that acts as a dialysis membrane. GI fluids slowly diffuse into the coated powder and dissolve the drug, which then diffuses out of the microcapsule.   *(1:1684; 34:206)*

308. (A) SKB's spansule formulation consists of medicated pellets in a capsule dosage form. Some pellets are uncoated to give almost immediate release; other pellets have lipid coatings of various thicknesses. Thus, the initial dose is reinforced with additional drug release over a period of time. Another group of products based upon medicated pellets are Lederle's Sequels (eg, Diamox Sequels).   *(1:1685)*

309. (C) Abbott's Gradumets consist of an insoluble plastic matrix containing active drug. As the tablet passes through the body, drug leaches from the matrix.   *(1:1684; 34:204)*

CHAPTER 4

Pharmaceutical Compounding

Compounding is considered an intrinsic skill of the pharmacist. Although the number of extemporaneously compounded prescriptions is steadily declining, there is a growing demand for hospital pharmacists to prepare parenteral admixtures. The emerging field of home health care has called upon both community and institutional pharmacists to prepare sterile chemotherapeutic, analgesic, and nutritional formulations.

This chapter reviews some of the compounding techniques, ingredients, and calculations that the practicing pharmacist may need to use.

Questions

Questions 1 through 5

Questions 1 through 5 relate to the following parenteral admixture order as received in a hospital pharmacy:

Patient: Clinton Reynolds	Age: 54	Room No. 234
Aminophylline *alkaline*		400 mg
Pot. Chloride *pH neutral 5-7*		20 mEq
D5W		500 mL

Infuse over 4 h at 1000, 1600, 2200 for 3 days.

39.1
× 60
234

1. How many ampules of 20 mL Aminophylline Injection (25 mg/mL) are needed daily for this order?

   (A) 1
   (B) 2
   (C) 3
   (D) 4
   (E) 5

   20 × 25 = 500 mg /amp
   400 × 3 = 1200

2. When reviewing this order, the pharmacist should

   (A) inform the prescriber that an incompatibility exists between aminophylline and potassium chloride
   (B) inform the prescriber that the dose of aminophylline is too high
   (C) inform the nursing staff to protect the mixture from sunlight
   (D) inform the prescriber that aminophylline will precipitate when added to D5W
   (E) fill the order as written

   pH 8-9

3. Correct method(s) for preparing the above admixture include

   I. add the potassium chloride solution to the D5W, followed by the aminophylline solution
   II. add the aminophylline solution to the D5W first then add the potassium chloride solution
   III. mix the aminophylline solution and the potassium chloride solution then add this mixture to the D5W

   (A) I only
   (B) III only
   (C) I and II only
   (D) II and III only
   (E) I, II, and III

4. The total amount (mg) of potassium administered daily in the admixture (K = 39.1; Cl = 35.5) is

   (A) 780
   (B) 1180
   (C) 2340
   (D) 4480
   (E) 2240

   20 × 3 = 60
   60 mEq = 10 mEq
   × mg = 750
   4500

5. Which of the following commercial parenteral solutions would be incompatible with the original admixture?

   I. dobutamine
   II. morphine *HCl*
   III. sodium bicarbonate

   (A) I only
   (B) III only
   (C) I and II only
   (D) II and III only
   (E) I, II, and III

   acidic

Answer questions 6 and 7 in reference to the following medication order:

Pot. Pen G	2 million units in 100 mL minibt q6h

Note: The pharmacy has vials containing 5 million units of potassium penicillin G which, when reconstituted with diluent, will contain 750,000 units/mL. The label on the vial states that the powder contains a citrate buffer to maintain a pH of 6 to 6.5.

6. Which of the following vehicles is(are) suitable for the above order?
   - I. D5W (pH = 4.5)
   - II. N/S (pH = 6.0)
   - III. D2.5W/.45NS (pH = 5.0)

   (A) I only
   (B) III only
   (C) I and II only
   (D) II and III only
   (E) I, II, and III

7. Which of the following procedures should the pharmacist use in preparing the minibottles?

   (A) Remove 2.7 mL of vehicle from the minibottle, then inject 2.7 mL of penicillin solution.
   (B) Inject 2.7 mL of penicillin solution directly into the minibottle.
   (C) Remove 6.7 mL of vehicle from the minibottle, then inject 6.7 mL of penicillin solution.
   (D) Inject 6.7 mL of penicillin solution directly into the minibottle.
   (E) Inject 4 mL of penicillin solution directly into the minibottle.

Questions 8 through 13

Answer the following series of questions based upon the following hospital medication order:

Patient: Margaret Kelly	Room No. 604-3
Potassium Chloride	40 mEq
Sodium Chloride	20 mEq
Potassium Phosphate	40 mEq
MVI	1 vial
Zinc Chloride	1 mg
Insulin	20 units
Calcium Gluconate	10 mL
Liposyn 10%	200 mL
FreAmine III	400 mL
D50W	400 mL

8. The TPN formula is best prepared by

   (A) adding the D50W to the FreAmine bottle
   (B) adding the FreAmine to the D50W bottle
   (C) transferring both the FreAmine and the D50W to a sterile, evacuated 1-L bottle
   (D) hanging the FreAmine and the D50W solutions separately on the patient
   (E) piggybacking the D50W into the Y-tubing of the FreAmine administration set

9. A potential problem is the incompatibility between

   (A) potassium chloride and calcium gluconate
   (B) potassium chloride and insulin
   (C) potassium phosphate and calcium gluconate
   (D) potassium phosphate and zinc chloride
   (E) insulin and zinc chloride

10. A second method to reduce the chance of precipitation when mixing calcium salts with phosphates is to

    (A) follow a specific order of mixing
    (B) use sodium rather than potassium phosphate
    (C) use calcium chloride rather than calcium gluconate
    (D) adjust the pH with hydrochloric acid
    (E) adjust the pH with sodium bicarbonate

11. Potassium phosphate has been included in the formula as a(n)

    (A) source of phosphorous
    (B) source of potassium
    (C) buffer
    (D) antioxidant
    (E) stabilizer

12. The prescribing physician should be encouraged to order the potassium phosphate using concentration expressions of

    (A) milliequivalents
    (B) milligrams
    (C) milliliters
    (D) millimoles
    (E) milliosmoles

13. The physician should also be aware that

    (A) approximately half the insulin will be adsorbed onto the glass container walls
    (B) he or she must specify which strength insulin–U-40 or U-100–is desired
    (C) he or she did not indicate whether insulin solution or suspension was desired
    (D) the MVI will cause a precipitate of the insulin
    (E) the inclusion of insulin in TPNs is contraindicated

14. Which of the following laminar flow hoods is(are) considered a suitable working area for preparing parenteral admixtures?
    I.   horizontal
    II. vertical Class I
    III. vertical Class II

    (A) I only
    (B) III only
    (C) I and II only
    (D) II and III only
    (E) I, II, and III

15. When preparing a parenteral admixture in a horizontal laminar flow hood, the pharmacist will work
    I.   with the hood motor turned off
    II. in an area within 6 inches of the HEPA filter
    III. in an area at least 6 inches from the edge of the benchtop

    (A) I only
    (B) III only
    (C) I and II only
    (D) II and III only
    (E) I, II, and III

16. Which one of the following steps is INCORRECT when one is removing 5 mL of solution from a 30 mL multidose vial?

    (A) draw up 5 mL of air into the syringe
    (B) place point of syringe needle onto the vial's rubber closure at a 45-degree angle
    (C) rotate needle so that the bevel opening is facing upwards
    (D) raise the needle angle to 90 degrees and insert needle through the rubber closure
    (E) after injecting the air, remove 6 mL of solution and aspirate excess solution into an alcohol swab

17. When obtaining a 3 mL dose from a 5 mL ampule, which one of the following steps is INCORRECT?

    (A) Draw up 3 mL of air into the syringe.
    (B) Disinfect the neck of the ampule using an alcohol swab.
    (C) Break ampule neck by snapping neck toward the side of the laminar flow hood.
    (D) Place needle tip into solution while holding the ampule almost horizontally.
    (E) After drawing up approximately 4 mL of solution, aspirate excess into alcohol swab.

18. After removing solution from an ampule, the pharmacist should pass the solution through a device such as a filter needle. The filter needle will remove
    I.   particulate matter
    II. microorganisms
    III. pyrogens

    (A) I only
    (B) III only
    (C) I and II only
    (D) II and III only
    (E) I, II, and III

19. A filtering device similar to the filter needle is the filter transfer tube or straw. This device is suitable when the pharmacist wants to
    I.   transfer the complete contents of an ampule
    II. transfer a portion of the contents of an ampule
    III. transfer the contents of a vial

    (A) I only
    (B) III only
    (C) I and II only
    (D) II and III only
    (E) I, II, and III

20. The pharmacist will NOT be able to use the filter straw with which of the following parenteral systems?
    I.   Abbott's Lifecare
    II. McGaw's Accumed
    III. Travenol's Viaflex

    (A) I only
    (B) III only
    (C) I and II only
    (D) II and III only
    (E) I, II, and III

21. Plastic parenteral bottles and bags differ from glass units in that the plastic units have
    I.   an air tube in the unit
    II. a vacuum
    III. two entry ports

    (A) I only
    (B) III only
    (C) I and II only
    (D) II and III only
    (E) I, II, and III

22. Which one of the following IV fluids used as vehicles for parenteral admixtures has the lowest pH value?

    (A) Dextrose 5% Injection (D5W)
    (B) Lactated Ringer's Injection
    (C) Ringer's Injection
    (D) 0.9% Sodium Chloride Injection
    (E) 0.45% Sodium Chloride Injection

Questions 23 through 26 relate to the following prescription:

For: James Brady	Age: 3
Rx	
Sodium Fluoride	500 µg
M & Ft cap. DTD # LX	
Sig: 1 qd	#60

23. How many mg of sodium fluoride are required to prepare this prescription?

.5 × 60 = 30

    (A) 0.5
    (B) 30
    (C) 50
    (D) 300
    (E) 500

24. Problem(s) that the pharmacist should anticipate in preparing this prescription include
    I. caustic nature of sodium fluoride
    II. poor water solubility of sodium fluoride
    III. difficulty in weighing small quantity of powder

    (A) I only
    (B) III only
    (C) I and II only
    (D) II and III only
    (E) I, II, and III

25. The best choice of a diluent for stock powders, especially when preparing capsules, is

    (A) ascorbic acid
    (B) lactose
    (C) sodium chloride
    (D) starch
    (E) talc

26. When filling the first capsule, the pharmacist discovers that the net weight of the powder in a #2 gelatin capsule is 40 mg too light. The pharmacist may elect to

    (A) use a #00 capsule
    (B) use a #1 capsule
    (C) use a #3 capsule
    (D) use a #4 capsule
    (E) place additional powder into the head of the capsule

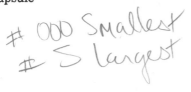
000 Smallest
5 largest

Questions 27 and 28

Questions 27 and 28 refer to the following prescription:

For: Carolyn Pfifler	Age: 10
Rx	.12 .84
Codeine Phosphate	210 mg
Dimenhydrinate	1000 mg
Acetaminophen	3000 mg
M & Ft Cap # xx	20 3y
Sig: i q.i.d. p.r.n. pain	4 12

NOTE: The pharmacist has 50-mg dimenhydrinate tablets, each weighing 200 mg, and 1/2 grain codeine phosphate tablets, each weighing 100 mg. Acetaminophen is available as a powder.

27. Which of the following statements concerning the prescription is (are) true?
    I. The amount of codeine being consumed per day is an overdose. 360/day
    II. There is a chemical incompatibility between dimenhydrinate and codeine.
    III. The patient should be cautioned about the possibility of drowsiness from the capsules.

    (A) I only
    (B) III only
    (C) I and II only
    (D) II and III only
    (E) I, II, and III

28. The final weight of each capsule will be approximately

    (A) 150 mg
    (B) 210 mg   7 × 200mg = 1400
    (C) 235 mg   × 100
    (D) 360 mg
    (E) 385 mg

Questions 29 through 31

Answer questions 29 through 31 based upon the following prescription written by a physician's assistant:

For: Rebecca Collins	Age: 6
Rx	
Codeine Salt	5 mg/tsp
Dextromethorphan	10 mg/tsp
Potassium Chloride	1 g
Flavored Syrup Vehicle	qs ad 4 f oz
Sig: 3 i q.i.d. for cough and phlegm	

29. The prescriber should be consulted concerning which of the following?
    I. the combined use of codeine and dextromethorphan
    II. the purpose of the potassium chloride
    III. the acid-base reaction between codeine and potassium chloride

    (A) I only
    (B) III only
    (C) I and II only
    (D) II and III only
    (E) I, II, and III

30. Which of the following ingredients should be included in this preparation?

    I.   alcohol
    II. codeine base
    III. codeine phosphate

    (A) I only
    (B) III only
    (C) I and II only
    (D) II and III only
    (E) I, II, and III

31. The amount of dextromethorphan required for this prescription is

    (A) 40 mg
    (B) 120 mg
    (C) 200 mg
    (D) 240 mg
    (E) 320 mg

32. When selecting a liquid oral dosage form, elixirs may be preferred over syrups because elixirs have better solvent properties for
    I.   weak organic acids
    II. weak organic bases
    III. flavoring oils

    (A) I only
    (B) III only
    (C) I and II only
    (D) II and III only
    (E) I, II, and III

33. Which of the following is NOT suitable for inclusion in an elixir or syrup formula as a sweetening agent?

    (A) aspartame
    (B) glycerin
    (C) lactose
    (D) saccharin
    (E) sorbitol

    low sweetness ability

Questions 34 through 36

Questions 34 through 36 relate to the following prescription:

Rx	
Burow's Solution	15 mL
White Petrolatum	45 g
Sig: Apply b.i.d. AM and hs	

34. The active ingredient in Burow's solution is

    (A) acetic acid
    (B) aluminum acetate
    (C) aluminum chloride
    (D) alum
    (E) hydrogen peroxide

35. When preparing this prescription, the pharmacist may wish to include

    (A) alcohol
    (B) Aquaphor
    (C) glacial acetic acid
    (D) Tween 80
    (E) potassium iodide

36. The concentration (% W/W) of Burow's solution in the final preparation will be

    (A) 15
    (B) 16.7
    (C) 20
    (D) 22.5
    (E) 25

    $15 \div 60 = 25\%$

37. The process of wetting and smoothing zinc oxide with mineral oil in preparation for incorporation into an ointment base is

    (A) attrition
    (B) levigation
    (C) milling
    (D) pulverization by intervention
    (E) trituration

38. Which form of sulfur should a pharmacist use when extemporaneously preparing an ointment?

    (A) cake of sulfur
    (B) flowers of sulfur
    (C) precipitated sulfur
    (D) sublimed sulfur
    (E) washed sulfur

Questions 39 through 42

Questions 39 through 42 are based upon the following order received from a hospital outpatient clinic:

For: Happy Hospital EENT Clinic	
Tetracaine	1.0%
Boric Acid	0.5%
Pur. Water	qs 60.0 mL

Please make isotonic and sterilize. Label as "Tetracaine Anesthetic Ophthalmic Solution."

39. Which of the following characteristics concerning tetracaine in the above formula is (are) true?
  I. poor water solubility
  II. chemically incompatible with boric acid *NO*
  III. not effective as a local anesthetic *NO*

  (A) I only
  (B) III only
  (C) I and II only
  (D) II and III only
  (E) I, II, and III

40. Boric acid is present in the formula as a (an)
  I. antioxidant
  II. antimicrobial preservative
  III. buffering agent

  (A) I only
  (B) III only
  (C) I and II only
  (D) II and III only
  (E) I, II, and III

  weak antimicrobial

41. How many mg of sodium chloride are needed to adjust the tonicity of the formula? The following "E" values are available: tetracaine HCl = 0.18; boric acid = 0.50; sodium borate = 0.42.

  (A) 260
  (B) 280
  (C) 440
  (D) 540
  (E) 640

42. The most practical method for sterilizing the ophthalmic solution is

  (A) autoclaving for 15 minutes
  (B) autoclaving for 30 minutes
  (C) membrane filtration through 0.2 micron filter
  (D) membrane filtration through 5 micron filter
  (E) the use of ethylene oxide gas

Questions 43 through 45

Questions 43 through 45 refer to the following prescription:

Rx	
Retinoic acid	0.05%
Ac. Sal.	2%
Emulsion Base qs	60 g

Sig: Apply small amount onto spot hs

43. Which of the following statements concerning this prescription is (are) true?
  I. Another name for retinoic acid is tretinoin.
  II. The amount of aspirin needed is 1.2 g.
  III. The term, emulsion base, refers to a brand of ointment base.

  (A) I only
  (B) III only
  (C) I and II only
  (D) II and III only
  (E) I, II, and III

44. Which one of the following ointment bases would result in a chemical incompatibility if used in preparing this prescription?

  (A) cold cream
  (B) hydrophilic ointment
  (C) Eucerin
  (D) Polysorb
  (E) Lubriderm

45. Which of the following should the pharmacist use when compounding this prescription?
  I. pill tile
  II. stainless steel spatulas
  III. alcohol

  (A) I only
  (B) III only
  (C) I and II only
  (D) II and III only
  (E) I, II, and III

  NO b/c Sal Ac.

46. A physician requests a 0.1% strength of a steroidal cream that is commercially available as a 0.25% strength in a "vanishing cream" base. Which one of the following ointment bases is the best choice as a diluent for this order?

(A) cold cream
(B) hydrophilic ointment
(C) lanolin
(D) Vaseline
(E) PEG ointment

47. When preparing the ointment in question 46, the amount of diluent that should be added to 30 g of the 0.25% strength product is

(A) 6.5 g
(B) 12 g
(C) 30 g
(D) 45 g
(E) 75 g

48. The following prescription is received:

> **Rx**
>
> Vitamin E   6000 IU
> O/W Lotion Base   qs   30 mL
>
> Sig: Apply small dab to incision t.i.d.

Which one of the following lotion bases would be the LEAST suitable vehicle?

(A) Allercreme skin lotion
(B) Cetaphil
(C) Keri lotion
(D) Lubriderm
(E) Nivea cream

Questions 49 through 52

Questions 49 through 52 refer to the following prescription:

> **Rx**
>
> Resorcinol   2 g
> Calamine
> Zinc Oxide   aa qs   15 g
> Glycerin   10 mL
> Witch Hazel
> Pur. Water   aa 90 mL
>
> Sig: Use t.i.d. ut dict

49. The final dosage form of this prescription will be a(an)

(A) colloidal solution
(B) elixir
(C) O/W emulsion

(D) W/O emulsion
(E) suspension

50. Calamine powder is a mixture of zinc oxide and

(A) aluminum oxide
(B) amaranth
(C) caramel
(D) cochineal
(E) ferric oxide

51. When preparing the prescription, the pharmacist will
  I. use 7.5 g of calamine
  II. mix the resorcinol, calamine, and zinc oxide together and wet with glycerin
  III. place the final product into a 4-oz amber glass bottle

(A) I only
(B) III only
(C) I and II only
(D) II and III only
(E) I, II, and III

52. Which of the following auxiliary labels should be attached to the container in which the above product is dispensed?
  I. For External Use Only
  II. Shake Well
  III. Keep in a Cool Place

(A) I only
(B) III only
(C) I and II only
(D) II and III only
(E) I, II, and III

53. The following prescription is received:

> **Rx**
>
> Tetracycline HCl   1.5%
> Propylene Glycol   10 mL
> MC 1500   1.5%
> Pur. Water   qs   60 mL
>
> Sig: Apply to inflamed area b.i.d.

When preparing this prescription, the pharmacist should
  I. disperse 900 mg of methylcellulose 1500 in hot water
  II. empty the contents from four 250 mg tetracycline capsules and weigh out 900 mg of the powder
  III. dissolve the tetracycline HCl powder and the methylcellulose 1500 in the propylene glycol

(A) I only
(B) III only
(C) I and II only
(D) II and III only
(E) I, II, and III

54. A prescription calls for 10% urea in Aquaphor base. Which of the following is the best technique to make a pharmaceutically elegant product?

   (A) Dissolve urea in water then incorporate into the Aquaphor.
   (B) Dissolve urea in alcohol then incorporate into the Aquaphor.
   (C) Finely powder the urea and incorporate directly into the Aquaphor.
   (D) Dissolve urea in small amount of mineral oil and incorporate into the Aquaphor.
   (E) Melt the Aquaphor and dissolve the urea in the hot liquid.

55. Which of the following statements is(are) true with respect to the following prescription?

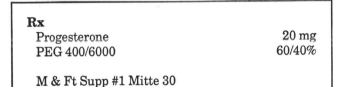

Rx
Progesterone   20 mg
PEG 400/6000   60/40%

M & Ft Supp #1 Mitte 30

   I. The weight of the individual suppository must be determined experimentally.
   II. The volume density of the progesterone must be calculated.
   III. The prescriber should be informed that progesterone is not readily absorbed from the rectum.

   (A) I only
   (B) III only
   (C) I and II only
   (D) II and III only
   (E) I, II, and III

56. Which of the following suppository bases melt rather than dissolve when inserted into the rectum?
   I. cocoa butter
   II. Witepsols
   III. PEGs

   (A) I only
   (B) III only
   (C) I and II only
   (D) II and III only
   (E) I, II, and III only

Questions 57 and 58

Questions 57 and 58 relate to the following prescription:

Rx
Clindamycin   900 mg
Propylene Glycol   15 mL
Diluted Alcohol   ad   60 mL

Sig: Apply small amount ut dict

57. The concentration of ethanol in Diluted Alcohol is

   (A) 20%
   (B) 50%
   (C) 70%
   (D) 92%
   (E) 95%

58. Which of the following are possible sources for the clindamycin?
   I. Cleocin Capsules 150 mg
   II. Cleocin Injection (150 mg/mL)
   III. Cleocin Tablets 75 mg

   (A) I only
   (B) III only
   (C) I and II only
   (D) II and III only
   (E) I, II, and III

59. A lotion formula calls for Coal Tar Solution. Which of the following statements concerning Coal Tar Solution is NOT true?

   (A) Alcohol is used as the solvent.
   (B) L.C.D. is another name for the solution.
   (C) The solution is for external use only.
   (D) Solution is usually diluted 1:9 with water or ointment base.
   (E) The solution contains only coal tar and a volatile solvent.

Questions 60 through 63

Answer questions 60 through 63 based upon the following prescription:

Rx
Ephedrine Sulfate   2%
Menthol   0.5%
Camphor
Methyl Salicylate   aa 0.2%
Mineral Oil   qs   30 mL

Sig: gtt ii both sides t.i.d.

60. Which is NOT true for camphor?

    (A) forms a eutectic mixture with phenol
    (B) can be powdered by rubbing with a small amount of alcohol or ether
    (C) is a ketone
    (D) dissolves readily in water
    (E) is one of the ingredients of Flexible Collodion USP

61. Which of the following ingredients will NOT dissolve in the prescribed solvent?
    I. ephedrine sulfate
    II. menthol
    III. methyl salicylate

    (A) I only
    (B) III only
    (C) I and II only
    (D) II and III only
    (E) I, II, and III

62. This prescription is intended to be placed in the

    (A) eyes
    (B) ears
    (C) nostrils
    (D) lungs
    (E) buccal cavity

63. Methyl salicylate is also known as

    (A) camphorated oil
    (B) peppermint oil
    (C) salicylamide
    (D) oil of wintergreen
    (E) sweet oil

64. Salicylic acid is employed in topical products as a(n)

    (A) antioxidant
    (B) chelating agent
    (C) buffer
    (D) keratolytic
    (E) emollient

65. Which one of the following diluents is LEAST suitable for reconstituting single-dose vials?

    (A) Bacteriostatic Sterile Water for Injection (BSWFI)
    (B) D5W Injection
    (C) N/S Injection
    (D) 1/2 N/S Injection
    (E) Sterile Water for Injection (SWFI)

DIRECTIONS (Questions 66 through 83): Each group of items in this section consists of lettered headings followed by a set of numbered words or phrases. For each numbered word or phrase, select the ONE lettered heading that is most closely associated with it. Each lettered heading may be selected once, more than once, or not at all.

Questions 66 through 77

    (A) oleaginous
    (B) absorption (anhydrous)
    (C) emulsion (W/O type)
    (D) emulsion (O/W type)
    (E) water-soluble

66. cold cream

67. hydrophilic petrolatum

68. Cetaphil

69. lanolin

70. petrolatum

71. polyethylene glycol

72. white ointment

73. wool fat

74. hydrophilic ointment

75. Lubriderm

76. Eucerin

77. Aquaphor

Questions 78 through 83

    (A) cold cream
    (B) hydrophilic ointment
    (C) hydrophilic petrolatum
    (D) PEG ointment
    (E) white petrolatum

78. for an ophthalmic drug

79. for an antibiotic with limited stability

80. for application to a seeping infection

81. for absorbing a large quantity of water

82. to aid in hydrating the skin

83. to clean the skin and impart emolliency

Answers and Explanations

1. **(C)** Each 20 mL ampule contains 500 mg of aminophylline. The pharmacist will have to open an ampule and remove 16 mL of solution every time he or she fills the order. Even assuming that all three admixtures are prepared at the same time (400 mg × 3 = 1200 mg of aminophylline), the equivalent of 48 mL of solution is needed. *(13:345–48; 23:202)*

2. **(E)** Aminophylline injection has a pH range of 8.6 to 9 while potassium chloride concentrated injections have a practically neutral pH (5.0 to 7.0). Therefore, a mixture of these two solutions will result in an alkaline pH without any likelihood of a precipitate. Aminophylline solutions are not sensitive to light nor is the dose requested unrealistic. Adult maintenance doses of 1 mg/kg/h are used. *(13:240; 21:47)*

3. **(C)** Either of the two additives could be added first to the D5W, followed by the other. It is not practical to mix them in syringe before addition to the D5W since the volume measurements may be subject to visual errors. For example, if 9 mL of KCl solution was drawn up instead of the correct 10 mL, 17 rather then 16 mL of aminophylline solution would be used to make 26 mL. *(13:345–48)*

4. **(C)** Total daily infusion of potassium chloride will be 20 mEq × 3 = 60 mEq of potassium chloride or potassium. Since the question asks for mg of potassium only·

$$mg\ (potassium) = \frac{(60\ mEq)\ (39.1)}{1}$$

[where 39.1 = atomic wt of potassium and
1 = valence of potassium]
mg potassium = 2340

(23:204)

5. **(C)** Since the pH of the original admixture will be greatly affected by the alkaline aminophylline solution (pH 8.6 to 9.0), it is likely that the final pH will be above 7.0. Therefore, the addition of either morphine sulfate injection (pH 2.5 to 6.0) or dobutamine HCl injection (pH 2.5 to 5.5) will cause a chemical reaction and probably a precipitate. While one would not be expected to know the exact pH of most phar-

maceuticals, organic bases such as morphine are combined with strong acids such as sulfuric acid or HCl to form salts that are water soluble. Naturally aqueous solutions of a salt combination of a strong acid and weak base will have an acidic pH. Sodium bicarbonate injection has an alkaline pH (7.0 to 8.5) and is not likely to precipitate if mixed with the aminophylline solution. *(21:309,630,832)*

6. **(E)** The citrate buffer system will readily adjust the pH of each listed vehicle to a stable range. Some hospitals prefer to use dextrose solutions for most admixtures to limit sodium intake by the patients. Other hospitals use normal saline injections to avoid supplying the calories present in dextrose solutions. *(1:1190)*

7. **(B)** There is no need to remove vehicle solution when adding small volumes of drug additives. The final volume will always vary since the manufacturer places some excess of solution into each unit. To calculate the mL of penicillin solution required:

$$\frac{750,000\ units}{1\ mL} = \frac{2,000,000\ units}{x\ mL}$$
$$x = 2.7\ mL$$

8. **(C)** FreAmine III is commercially available as 500 mL in a 500 mL bottle. The 50% Dextrose Injection is similarly supplied. Therefore, the transfer into an evacuated 1-L bottle is indicated. *(10)*

9. **(C)** Many calcium salts, such as the phosphate and carbonate, have limited water solubility. Precipitates may occur in parenteral admixtures when certain concentrations of the additives are exceeded. Lowering the concentrations of both the potassium phosphate and the calcium gluconate to 20 mEq each will probably prevent precipitation of calcium phosphate. *(21:131)*

10. **(A)** It is often possible to reduce the incidence of precipitation if the potassium phosphate is dissolved or mixed with the vehicle first; the calcium solution is then added slowly while stirring. *(21:131)*

11. **(A)** Phosphorus is an essential mineral for the body

and is readily available as the phosphate. If a source of potassium is needed, the chloride or acetate salts are usually used.   *(13:222)*

12. **(D)** The commercially available potassium phosphate injections are a mixture of monobasic (potassium) and dibasic (dipotassium) phosphates. Since body phosphate requirements are usually expressed in terms of millimoles (mmol) per kg per day, and the commercial solutions are mixtures, it is more convenient to express the potassium phosphate additive in mmol/L rather than mEq/L, which would be based upon potassium. The average adult needs 10 to 15 mmol phosphorus per day.   *(13:206)*

13. **(A)** When low concentrations of insulin are included in LVPs, the percentage of insulin adsorbed to the walls of the containers and also to the administration sets is significant. One can expect at least 50% insulin loss when only 20 units are added to the container.   *(13:250)*
(B—incorrect) Since the insulin dosage is expressed in units, either U-40 or U-100 can be used.
(C—incorrect) Insulin Injection USP would be used; a suspension would not be used intravenously.

14. **(E)** Air in the horizontal hood flows directly toward the operator, thereby preventing contaminants from entering the admixtures being prepared. This hood provides maximum protection to the parenteral admixture. Vertical hoods have downward air flow, which increases the risk of product contamination but protects the operator. Vertical hoods should therefore be used only for products that pose a significant risk to the operator; for example, when handling chemotherapeutic drugs. The Class I vs II designation refers to the exhaust systems present in vertical hoods.   *(13:55)*

15. **(B)** As the air passing through the HEPA filter nears the edge of the benchtop, it becomes more turbulent, thus defeating the purpose of the laminar flow hood. For this reason, many horizontal laminar flow hoods have a line drawn 6 inches from the edge as a reminder to work further inside the hood. A hood should generally be left running 24 hours a day or should be turned on and left running throughout the workday. Work should not commence until the hood has been running for at least 15 to 30 minutes. It is inadvisable to work within 6 inches of the HEPA filter since this may partially block the laminar air flow.   *(1:1576)*

16. **(E)** It is preferable to aspirate excessive solution and air bubbles while the needle is still in the vial. This prevents accidental contamination of the hood and personnel. Also, there is no point in wasting 1 mL of drug solution that could be used in preparing another admixture. It is necessary to inject a volume of air equal to the volume of solution being removed. Otherwise, a vacuum would occur in the vial, making it difficult to remove solution.   *(13:79,348)*

17. **(A)** There is no reason to inject air into the opened ampule since no vacuum will form when the solution is removed. All ampules are intended as single-dose units and should be discarded after opening.   *(13:79,347)*

18. **(A)** The pore size of the filter is usually 5 microns, which is too coarse to remove either pyrogens or microorganisms. Instead, the filter needle is intended to remove larger particulate matter such as glass fragments that may have fallen into the ampule during the neck-breaking procedure.   *(13:79)*

19. **(A)** The filter straw consists of a plastic tube attached to a needle containing a 5-micron filter. The tube end is placed into an opened ampule, and the needle is inserted into a glass parenteral bottle. The vacuum inside the glass bottle will pull over the entire contents of the ampule. It is impossible to obtain an accurate partial dose, and it is essential that the receiving container have a vacuum.   *(10)*

20. **(E)** None of the listed parenteral systems of large-volume containers have vacuums present.   *(1:1572; 13:133)*

21. **(B)** Parenteral plastic bottles and bags are characterized by the presence of two entry ports or sleeves. One port is covered with a latex-type cap through which the pharmacist or nurse can inject solutions into the unit. When the unit is to be administered to a patient, the spike of the administration set is inserted into the second port. This second port does not have a latex cap. Advantages of the plastic units include their lighter weight and resistance to breakage as compared to glass and their ability to collapse as solution flows out, thus precluding the need for a method to add air as the solution exits. Glass bottles require either an air tube or air filter.   *(13:131)*

22. **(A)** The pH ranges for each are as follows: D5W, 3.5 to 6.5; Lactated Ringer's, 6.0 to 7.5; Ringer's, 5.0 to 7.5; and both Sodium Chloride Injection solutions, 4.5 to 7.0. Despite the apparent acidic pH of some dextrose solutions, one must realize that the solutions have very little buffer capacity. The addition of small volumes of alkaline drug solutions to a liter of D5W will immediately raise the pH to the alkaline range.   *(1:1571)*

23. **(B)** 500 µg is equivalent to 0.5 mg. Since 60 capsules were requested, 0.5 mg × 60 = 30 mg.   *(20:47)*

24. **(B)** The minimum quantity that can be accurately weighed on a Class A prescription balance with an error of not more than 5% is 120 mg. In order to weigh the required 30 mg of sodium fluoride, a stock powder of NaF is needed. In this problem, mixing 120 mg of NaF with 360 mg of diluent and using 120 mg of this stock powder will deliver the required 30 mg of sodium fluoride.
Because of its strong ionic bonds, sodium fluoride is not caustic. A stainless steel spatula can be used for

the weighing procedure. Sodium fluoride has good water solubility.   *(1:78; 23:35)*

25. **(B)** Lactose is a relatively inert, water-soluble substance that also packs well into capsules. An alternative would be the use of starch. For the sodium fluoride prescription, the pharmacist will have to include additional lactose to raise the content of each capsule to a quantity that is weighable and convenient to pack into capsules. For example, a net weight of 300 mg may be arbitrarily selected. *(20:47)*

26. **(B)** Empty capsules are sized by a numbering system, the largest being a #000 and the smallest a #5. If the #2 capsule is too small, the pharmacist should try the next largest, the #1. The correct capsule-filling procedure is to place powder only into the body or base of the empty capsule. It is not good technique to place powder into the head or cap since the fit of the head onto the body may not be tight.

(1:1658; 20:47)

27. **(B)** Both codeine and dimenhydrinate have a tendency to produce drowsiness as a side effect. Codeine is a weak organic base while dimenhydrinate is a combination of diphenhydramine and 8-chlorotheophylline. No chemical reaction between the two drugs would be expected. The amount of codeine consumed per dose is approximately 10 mg or 40 mg daily. This is within the therapeutic dosage range for a 10-year-old child.   *(1:792,1100)*

28. **(E)** The total amount can be calculated as follows:

Drug	Total Weight of Powder
Codeine	7 tabs each weighing 100 mg = 700 mg
Dimenhydrinate	20 tabs each weighing 100 mg = 4000 mg
Acetaminophen (APAP)	powder weighing 3000 mg
	total = 7700 mg

7700 mg divided into 20 caps = 385 mg

(20:47,266)

29. **(D)** There appears to be no synergistic antitussive activity between codeine and dextromethorphan; therefore, the prescriber should be questioned as to why the combination was requested. Potassium chloride is intended to supply potassium ions to the body. If an expectorant action is desired, potassium iodide or ammonium chloride could be used. The potassium chloride will have a neutral pH in an aqueous solution and will not exhibit an acid-base reaction with codeine sulfate.   *(1:834; 2:153–55; 4:441)*

30. **(B)** Codeine phosphate has greater water solubility than codeine base (1 g in 2.5 mL vs 1 g in 120 mL). While the inclusion of alcohol will improve the solubility of dextromethorphan (freely soluble vs 1 g in 65 mL of water), alcohol should not be added to any oral product without the permission of the prescriber. Also, alcohol would increase the degree of drowsiness caused by the product.   *(1:865,1100)*

31. **(D)** Each teaspoonful (5 mL) of prescription is to contain 10 mg of dextromethorphan. Since the prescription calls for 120 mL with a direction of a 5 mL dose, there are 120 mL divided by 5 mL or 24 doses. 10 mg × 24 doses = 240 mg.   *(23:81)*

32. **(E)** Elixirs that are used as vehicles usually contain about 20% ethyl alcohol. Ethanol is a good solvent for most weak organic acids and bases. The water in the elixir will serve as the solvent for the salts of weak organic acids and bases. Therefore, if the pH of the solution changes, the alcohol will keep the un-ionized form of the drug in solution while the ionized portion will remain in solution due to the presence of water molecules. There are limits to the solubility of drugs in an elixir vehicle based upon amount of drug present and competition between the drug and other ingredients in the elixir for solvent molecules. For example, sucrose molecules will compete with ionized drugs for water-solvent molecules. Flavoring oils, which are usually mixtures of terpenes, possess good alcohol solubility.   *(20:128,262; 24:218)*

33. **(C)** Lactose (milk sugar) has only a slight degree of sweetness. The amount needed to sweeten a solution is too great. Saccharin is used because of its high intensity of sweetness (approximately 300 times that of sucrose), but there is some question concerning its potential carcinogenic properties. On the other hand, the amount required is so small that it is unlikely to present a health hazard in pharmaceuticals. Aspartame is a synthetic sweetener that is a dipeptide of L-aspartic acid and L-phenylalanine. When heated, aspartame breaks down into its respective amino acids, with a corresponding decrease in sweetness.   *(1:1322; 2:572)*

34. **(B)** Burow's solution is officially known as Aluminum Acetate Topical Solution. It is classified as a topical astringent dressing.   *(1:761)*

35. **(B)** Aqueous solutions such as Burow's solution cannot be directly incorporated into oleaginous bases such as petrolatum or white petrolatum. Aquaphor will absorb aqueous solutions and will also mix well with petrolatum. While smaller amounts could be used, 15 g of Aquaphor will readily pick up the required amount of Burow's solution. The amount of white petrolatum must be decreased by 15 g to assure the correct concentration of Burow's solution in the final preparation.   *(20:77)*

36. **(E)** The prescription requires 15 mL of Burow's solution plus 45 g of white petrolatum (of which the pharmacist replaced 15 g with Aquaphor). Since Burow's solution is essentially an aqueous solution, one may assume its specific gravity is close to that of water (ie, 1.0). Thus, the total weight of the final ointment will be 60 g, and 15 g divided by 60 g equals 25% W/W.   *(1:95)*

37. **(B)** Incorporating powders into ointment bases may be aided by first wetting the powders with a small

amount of a nonsolvent liquid, then rubbing the paste that forms on an ointment slab with a spatula. Usually mineral oil is employed when the vehicle is oleaginous. Glycerin may be used for more hydrophilic vehicles. *(1:1630,1606; 20:31)*

38. **(C)** Precipitated sulfur has a finer particle size and greater surface area than the other listed forms. A smoother ointment will be formed. *(1:345)* (A–incorrect, B–incorrect, D–incorrect) These are all forms of sulfur purified by sublimation.

39. **(A)** Tetracaine is a weak organic base with poor water solubility (1 g in 1 L of water). The hydrochloride salt, which is very soluble (1 g needs less than 1 mL of water), should be used. Boric acid, which is a very weak acid, is chemically compatible with both tetracaine base and tetracaine HCl. Commercial tetracaine solutions are available under the trade name of Pontocaine. Tetracaine and cocaine are occasionally requested for their local anesthetic activity. Many other local anesthetic agents such as procaine are effective only by injection. *(1:1053; 20:149)*

40. **(D)** Boric acid is an effective buffer in ophthalmic solutions since it will maintain a slightly acidic pH. When placed in the eye, it is quickly neutralized by the buffers in the lacrimal fluid. Boric acid has weak antimicrobial activity. *1:1318,1589; 20:149)*

41. **(B)**

Drug Wt.	"E" values NaCl	Equivalent NaCl
tetracaine HCl	600 mg × 0.18	= 108 mg
boric acid	300 mg × 0.50	= 150 mg
	total =	258 mg

60 mL of solution × 0.9% sodium chloride = 540 mg NaCl
540 mg NaCl – 258 equiv. of NaCl = 282 mg NaCl needed to adjust for tonicity

(1:1490)

42. **(C)** Passing the solution through a 0.2-micron filter using one of the commercially available sterile filter units such as Millipore's Millex is the most convenient sterilization technique available for handling small volumes. Autoclaving may cause some decomposition of the drug. Ethylene oxide gas is not practical for solutions in closed systems. *(20:1447–48)*

43. **(A)** Tretinoin is the official name for retinoic acid. The drug is commercially available under the tradename of Retin-A. The designation of Ac. Sal. refers to salicylic acid, not aspirin (acetylsalicylic acid). The term emulsion base is nondescript. It could refer to a number of ointment bases, including those with either W/O or O/W characteristics. Clarification of the type of ointment base desired should be made. Before compounding this prescription, the pharmacist should contact the prescriber concerning the inclusion of a keratolytic agent such as salicylic acid in a topical preparation containing tretinoin, a compound that exhibits keratolytic activity as a side effect. *(1:768,771)*

44. **(A)** Cold cream is a W/O emulsion base with a borate emulsification system. Acids such as salicylic acid may break the emulsion. *(20:77,274)*

45. **(A)** Incorporating powders or liquids into relatively small amounts of ointment base is best accomplished on a pill tile (also known as an ointment tile). Because of the caustic nature of salicylic acid, rubber spatulas should be used rather than stainless steel, which would discolor. *(1:1606)*

46. **(B)** Hydrophilic ointment is an O/W emulsion base containing sodium lauryl sulfate, petrolatum, and stearyl alcohol. Of the listed bases, it is closest to a vanishing cream base since such a system is characterized by the presence of an O/W stearate emulsion. *(20:77)*

47. **(D)** Let Q_1 and C_1 represent the quantity and concentration desired and Q_2 and C_2 represent the original quantity and strength:

$$[Q_1][C_1] = [Q_2][C_2]$$
$$[x \text{ g}][0.1\%] = [30 \text{ g}][0.25\%]$$
$$x = 75 \text{ g (total amount of ointment that}$$
$$\text{can be prepared)}$$
$$75 \text{ g} - 30 \text{ g (original amount of 0.25\% ointment)} =$$
$$45 \text{ g (amount of diluent to add)}$$

(1:98)

48. **(E)** Nivea cream is a W/O emulsion lotion while all of the other choices are O/W emulsions. The viscosities of each lotion may vary, but the pharmacist can readily adjust each of the O/W vehicles to a pourable consistency by adding purified water after the vitamin E has been incorporated into the formula. *(1:1604; 20:116)*

49. **(E)** The vehicle system for this prescription is the hydroalcoholic Witch Hazel and purified water. A suspension must be prepared since there are water-insoluble powders present. An emulsion is not possible since there is no oil indicated in the formula. *(20:130)*

50. **(E)** Calamine consists of 99% zinc oxide and 1% ferric oxide. The ferric oxide imparts a pink color to the mixture, which is more cosmetically acceptable than the white zinc oxide. *(1:762)*

51. **(A)** The designation "aa qs" translates as "of each enough to make 15 g." Therefore, 7.5 g of calamine and 7.5 g of zinc oxide are needed. These two water-insoluble powders should be mixed together in a mortar and wetted with glycerin. To this mixture, 90 mL of Witch Hazel, in which the resorcinol has been dissolved, should be added slowly. Finally, the 90 mL of purified water can be added. Note that the final volume will be greater than 120 mL. *(20:130)*

52. (C) Most of the ingredients in this preparation are intended for topical use only. While the suspension may not separate or settle immediately, it may do so after a few days. It is standard procedure to place "Shake Well" labels on all suspension formulas. None of the ingredients decompose in the presence of moderate heat; therefore, a "Cool Place" label is not required. *(20:130)*

53. (A) The easiest way to hydrate methylcellulose is to add the powder to hot water and allow the powder to hydrate for 10 to 15 minutes before adding cold water. The thickened solution can then be added to the tetracycline powder that has been wetted with propylene glycol. When emptying the tetracycline capsules, one must weigh the powder since there may be excipients or diluents in the capsule formula. A proportional weight of the powder equivalent to 900 mg of active drug must be used. *(20:120,130–31)*

54. (A) Urea has good solubility in water. The resulting solution can readily be incorporated into the Aquaphor. *(20:277)*

55. (A) Since the exact density of the PEG 400/6000 mixture is not known, the pharmacist must prepare a trial batch to determine the weight of an individual suppository. In this prescription, since the volume occupied by 20 mg of progesterone is insignificant, it is not necessary to determine its volume density. However, one must realize that drugs in larger quantities will contribute to the bulk volume of the suppository. In these situations, one must prepare a trial suppository that includes the active drug to calculate its bulk density. Progesterone has been extemporaneously incorporated into suppositories intended for vaginal administration in the maintenance of pregnancy in luteal phase dysfunction. The usual dose has been 25 mg. *(4:1039; 20:92)*

56. (C) Cocoa butter, a mixture of triglycerides, has been used for over 100 years as a suppository base. A disadvantage of cocoa butter is its inability to absorb aqueous solutions. It melts at slightly below body temperature, and its melting point might be affected by drugs. The Witepsol series of bases consists of natural triglycerides of saturated fatty acids with carbon chains between 12 and 18. Another series of suppository bases that melt is the Wecobees, triglycerides of coconut oil. While cocoa butter suppositories can be hand rolled or prepared by fusion in molds, the other two bases are intended for mold use. Different molecular weight polyethylene glycols (PEGs) can be blended and formed into suppositories by fusion using molds. PEG suppositories do not melt in the body; instead, they slowly dissolve in the limited amount of water in the colon. *(20:92)*

57. (B) Diluted Alcohol is an official product prepared by mixing equal volumes of Alcohol USP and Purified Water. Because of shrinkage due to hydrogen bonding and the use of 95% ethanol, the final strength of Diluted Alcohol is 49% V/V. *(1:1315)*

58. (C) Both 150-mg capsules and a parenteral solution are commercially available. The capsule contains clindamycin HCl while the injectable product contains clindamycin phosphate. However, in both products, the drug concentration is expressed in equivalent weights of clindamycin base. The injectable uses the phosphate form, which is said to cause less gastrointestinal upset. If the capsules were to be used, the pharmacist would empty out the contents of six capsules, mix with 15 mL propylene glycol, and dilute with Diluted Alcohol to make 60 mL. *(20:74)*

59. (E) The solution also contains Polysorbate 80. This nonionic surfactant is included to disperse the water-insoluble components of coal tar, which will precipitate when the highly alcoholic solution is mixed with an aqueous preparation.
(B–incorrect) The Latin name of coal tar solution is Liquor Carbonis Detergens (L.C.D.). *(24:337)*

60. (D) Camphor is soluble in alcohol or organic solvents but is only slightly soluble (1 g in 800 mL) of water. *(1:764,1530)*

61. (A) Ephedrine sulfate is water soluble. It is best to receive the prescriber's permission to use ephedrine base, which is soluble in nonpolar solvents such as mineral oil. *(1:878)*

62. (C) Ephedrine is used as a topical decongestant when administered by the intranasal route. *(1:878)*

63. (D) Methyl salicylate can be used in small quantities as a flavoring or perfuming agent. It is also included in many topical products, such as rubbing alcohols, gels, and liniments, as a counterirritant.
(1:1295; 2:876)

64. (D) Salicylic acid is a keratolytic, which means that it helps to dissolve and loosen keratin. This is a useful property in the treatment of conditions such as psoriasis where the skin becomes hyperkeratotic, ie, the keratin layer thickens. *(1:768)*

65. (A) Product inserts are the best sources of information concerning appropriate diluents for a given drug powder. However, Bacteriostatic Water for Injection should not be used for reconstituting single-dose units since the preservative present would serve no useful purpose, and large amounts of the preservative could increase the incidence or severity of toxicity. The use of BSWFI may be appropriate if a powder in a multidose vial is being reconstituted.
(13:379)

66. (C) *(1:1603)*

67. (B) *(1:1311)*

68. (E) *(20:274)*

69. (C) *(1:1311)*

70. (A)   *(1:1603)*

71. (E)   *(1:1603)*

72. (A)   *(1:1309)*

73. (B)   *(1:1603)*

74. (D)   *(1:1603)*

75. (D)   *(20:274)*

76. (C)   *(20:274)*

77. (B)   *(1:1604)*

78. (E) White petrolatum is a bland base with a very low incidence of irritation to the eye. Also, because of the absence of water, it has low susceptibility to microbial growth.   *(1:1585)*

79. (E) The decomposition of most antibiotics is enhanced by water. White petrolatum is anhydrous and contains few chemically reactive ingredients.   *(1:1603)*

80. (B) Hydrophilic ointment is capable of absorbing serous fluid quite readily. Bases such as petrolatum and hydrophilic petrolatum, which will form a hydrophobic film, should be avoided; they might prevent the desired seepage.   *(1:1604)*

81. (C) Of all the bases listed, hydrophilic petrolatum will absorb the greatest quantity of water.   *(1:1311)*

82. (E) The occlusive characteristic of petrolatum will prevent further water loss through the stratum corneum. Thus, the skin will remain more hydrated.   *(1:1309,1603)*

83. (A) Cold cream will cleanse the skin by removing make-up. It also serves as an emollient.   *(1:1312)*

CHAPTER 5

Biopharmaceutics and Pharmacokinetics

Biopharmaceutics is a scientific discipline concerned with the relationship between the physicochemical properties of a drug in a dosage form and the biologic response observed after its administration. The development of pharmacokinetics, or the study of the absorption, distribution, metabolism, and elimination of drugs as it relates to their therapeutic and toxicologic effects, has led to a better understanding of quantitative aspects of biopharmaceutics.[29] This chapter tests the reader's knowledge of the principles of biopharmaceutics and pharmacokinetics, which is fundamental to the rational selection of quality drug products, the determination of appropriate dose and dosing schedules, and the monitoring of therapy.

Questions

DIRECTIONS (Questions 1 through 70): Each of the numbered items or incomplete statements in this section is followed by answers or by completions of the statement. Select the ONE lettered answer or completion that is BEST in each case.

1. The term biological availability or bioavailability refers to the relative amount of drug that reaches the

   (A) small intestine
   (B) stomach
   (C) systemic circulation
   (D) liver
   (E) kidneys

2. To produce its characteristic pharmacologic action(s), a drug must always

   (A) reach high blood levels
   (B) be absorbed from the gastrointestinal tract
   (C) achieve adequate concentration at its site(s) of action
   (D) be excreted unchanged in the urine
   (E) be formulated into a dosage form that produces the most rapid onset and duration of action

3. Which of the following is the first process that must occur before a drug can become available for absorption from a tablet dosage form?

   (A) dissolution of the drug in the GI fluids
   (B) dissolution of the drug in the GI epithelium
   (C) ionization of the drug
   (D) dissolution of the drug in the blood
   (E) disintegration of the tablet

4. Differences in bioavailability are most frequently observed with drugs administered by which of the following routes?

   (A) subcutaneous
   (B) intravenous
   (C) oral
   (D) sublingual
   (E) intramuscular

5. The relative bioavailability of a drug product can be determined by comparing which of the following values to similar control drug values?
   I. AUCs
   II. total drug urinary excretion
   III. peak blood drug concentrations

   (A) I only
   (B) III only
   (C) I and II only
   (D) II and III only
   (E) I, II, and III

6. The area under the curve (AUC) can be described as being
   I. a theoretical value
   II. a measure of drug concentration–time curve
   III. a value with units of weight and time/volume

   (A) I only
   (B) III only
   (C) I and II only
   (D) II and III only
   (E) I, II, and III

7. The "F" value for a drug product is most closely related to its

   (A) absolute bioavailability
   (B) dosing rate
   (C) clearance rate
   (D) relative bioavailability
   (E) route of administration

8. Determine the F value for a drug available as a 100-mg capsule with a calculated AUC of 20 mg/dL/h when a 100-mg IV bolus of the same drug exhibits an AUC of 25 mg/dL/h.

   (A) 0.2
   (B) 0.4
   (C) 0.8
   (D) 1.25
   (E) 20

9. What is the F value for an experimental drug tablet based upon the following data?

DRUG DOSAGE

Form	Dose	AUC µg/mL/h
Tablet	100 mg PO	20
Solution (control)	100 mg PO	30
Injection (control)	50 mg IV push	40

   (A) 0.25
   (B) 0.38
   (C) 0.50
   (D) 0.66
   (E) 0.90

10. Drug products can also be evaluated by comparing curves of serum concentration vs time (ie, blood level curves). The most important parameters for comparison that can be obtained from such curves are

   (A) peak concentration, biologic half-life, elimination rate constant
   (B) biologic half-life, time of peak concentration, absorption rate constant
   (C) peak concentration, time of peak concentration, total AUC (area under the curve)
   (D) average serum concentration, AUC, biologic half-life
   (E) absorption rate constant, AUC, elimination rate constant

11. The peak of the serum concentration vs time curve approximates the

   (A) point in time when the maximum pharmacologic effect occurs
   (B) point in time when absorption and elimination of the drug have equalized
   (C) maximum concentration of free drug in the urine
   (D) time required for essentially all of the drug to be absorbed from the GI tract
   (E) point in time when the drug begins to be metabolized

12. The time of the peak serum concentration gives some indication of the relative rate of

   (A) absorption
   (B) distribution
   (C) metabolism
   (D) elimination
   (E) biotransformation

13. The area under the serum concentration-time curve represents the

   (A) biologic half-life of the drug
   (B) amount of drug that is cleared by the kidneys
   (C) amount of drug in the original dosage form

   (D) amount of drug absorbed
   (E) amount of drug excreted in the urine

14. Two different oral formulations of the same drug having equal areas under their respective serum concentration-time curves

   (A) deliver the same total amount of drug to the body and are, therefore, bioequivalent
   (B) deliver the same total amount of drug to the body but are not necessarily bioequivalent
   (C) are bioequivalent by definition
   (D) are bioequivalent if they both meet USP disintegration standards
   (E) are bioequivalent if they both meet USP dissolution standards

15. If an oral capsule formulation of the drug A produces a serum concentration-time curve having the same area under the curve as that produced by an equivalent dose of drug A given IV, it can generally be concluded that

   (A) the IV route is preferred to the oral route
   (B) the capsule formulation is essentially completely absorbed
   (C) the drug is very rapidly absorbed
   (D) all oral dosage forms of drug A will be bioequivalent
   (E) there is no advantage to the IV route

16. Differences in bioavailability are especially significant when

   (A) the drug is extensively metabolized
   (B) the therapeutic index is high
   (C) rather specific blood levels of the drug are required
   (D) the drug is given IV
   (E) the drug is rapidly absorbed from the GI tract

17. In vitro dissolution rate studies on drug products are useful in bioavailability evaluations only if they can be correlated with

   (A) disintegration rates
   (B) in vivo studies in humans
   (C) in vivo studies in at least three species of animals
   (D) the chemical stability of the drug
   (E) USP disintegration limits

18. According to pH partition theory, a weakly acidic drug will most likely be absorbed from the stomach because

   (A) the drug will exist primarily in the unionized, more lipid-soluble form
   (B) the drug will exist primarily in the ionized, more water-soluble form
   (C) weak acids are more soluble in acid media
   (D) the ionic form of the drug facilitates dissolution
   (E) weak acids will further depress pH

19. An absorption process is NOT involved when a drug is given by which one of the following routes of administration?
    I. oral
    II. intramuscular
    III. intravenous

    (A) I only
    (B) III only
    (C) I and II only
    (D) II and III only
    (E) I, II, and III

20. In general, the various oral dosage forms can be ranked in which of the following expected orders of availability (fastest to slowest)?

    (A) aqueous solution, capsule, tablet, powder, coated tablet, suspension
    (B) capsule, tablet, coated tablet, powder, suspension, aqueous solution
    (C) aqueous solution, suspension, powder, capsule, tablet, coated tablet
    (D) suspension, aqueous solution, powder, capsule, coated tablet, tablet
    (E) aqueous solution, suspension, capsule, powder, coated tablet, tablet

21. The value of particle size reduction to enhance drug absorption is limited to those situations in which the

    (A) absorption process occurs by active transport
    (B) absorption process is rate-limited by the dissolution of drug in GI fluids
    (C) drug is very soluble
    (D) drug is very potent
    (E) drug is irritating to the GI tract

22. Whenever a drug is more rapidly and/or more completely absorbed from a solution than from a solid dosage form

    (A) it is due to the fact that the solid dosage form did not disintegrate
    (B) a solution is the only practical oral formulation
    (C) it indicates that the solid dosage form is poorly formulated
    (D) it is likely that absorption is rate-limited by the dissolution process
    (E) none of the above

23. Drugs that are absorbed from the GI tract are generally

    (A) absorbed into the portal circulation and pass through the liver before entering the general circulation
    (B) filtered from the blood by the kidney, then reabsorbed into the general circulation
    (C) absorbed into the portal circulation and are distributed by an enterohepatic cycle
    (D) not affected by liver enzymes
    (E) stored in the liver

24. All of the following drugs are believed to undergo significant first-pass hepatic biotransformation EXCEPT

    (A) acetylsalicylic acid
    (B) nortriptyline (Aventyl)
    (C) lidocaine
    (D) morphine
    (E) propranolol (Inderal)

25. Gastric emptying is slowed by all of the following EXCEPT

    (A) vigorous exercise
    (B) fatty foods
    (C) hot meals
    (D) hunger
    (E) emotional stress

26. For many drugs, bioavailability can be evaluated using urinary excretion data. This is based on the assumption that

    (A) bioavailability studies can be done only on drugs that are completely excreted unchanged by the kidneys
    (B) drug levels can be measured more accurately in urine than in blood
    (C) a drug must first be absorbed into the systemic circulation before it can appear in the urine
    (D) all of the administered dose can be recovered from the urine
    (E) only drug metabolites are excreted in the urine

27. Estimating bioavailability from urinary excretion data is less satisfactory than estimates based on blood level data because accurate urinary excretion studies require
    I. complete urine collection
    II. normal or near-normal renal function
    III. that the drug be completely excreted unchanged by the kidney

    (A) I only
    (B) III only
    (C) I and II only
    (D) II and III only
    (E) I, II, and III

28. The excretion of a weakly acidic drug (eg, pKa of 3.5) will be more rapid in alkaline urine than in acidic urine because

    (A) all drugs are excreted more rapidly in alkaline urine
    (B) the drug will exist primarily in the unionized form, which cannot easily be reabsorbed
    (C) the drug will exist primarily in the ionized form, which cannot be easily reabsorbed
    (D) weak acids cannot be reabsorbed from the kidney tubules
    (E) active transport mechanisms function better in alkaline urine

29. If a fixed dose of a drug that is eliminated by first-order kinetics is administered at regular intervals, the time required to achieve a steady-state plasma level depends only on the

   (A) dose of the drug
   (B) volume of distribution of the drug
   (C) half-life of the drug
   (D) dosing interval
   (E) fraction of dose absorbed (bioavailability)

30. A specific drug has a first-order biologic half-life of 4 hours. This half-life value will

   (A) be independent of the initial drug concentration
   (B) increase when the concentration of the drug increases
   (C) decrease when the concentration of the drug increases
   (D) decrease if the patient has renal impairment
   (E) be the same whether the drug level is determined in the blood or by observing the pharmacologic action

31. Assuming complete absorption and an elimination half-life of 4 hours, how much of a drug will remain in the body 12 hours after administering a 400-mg dose? Assume linear pharmacokinetics (ie, first order).

   4 8 16   8
   ½ ¼ ⅛ ⅙   5)40

   (A) 200 mg
   (B) 100 mg
   (C) 50 mg
   (D) 25 mg
   (E) Almost no drug will remain.

32. The biologic half-life of a drug

   (A) is a constant physical property of the drug
   (B) is a constant chemical property of the drug
   (C) is the time for one half of the therapeutic activity to be lost
   (D) may be decreased by giving the drug by rapid IV injection
   (E) depends entirely on the route of administration

33. The biologic half-life of a drug that is eliminated by first-order kinetics is mathematically represented by _____ where k is the first-order rate constant for elimination.

   (A) 1/k
   (B) log k
   (C) 0.693/k
   (D) 2.303/k
   (E) peak serum concentration/2k

34. The biologic half-life of many drugs is often prolonged in newborn infants because of

   (A) a higher degree of protein binding
   (B) microsomal enzyme induction

   (C) more complete absorption of drugs
   (D) incompletely developed enzyme systems
   (E) incompletely developed barriers to the distribution of drugs in the body

35. A certain drug appears to be eliminated from the body at a rate constant of 20% per hour. Estimate the drug's half-life assuming first-order kinetics.

   (A) 1 hour
   (B) 2.5 hours
   (C) 3.5 hours
   (D) 5 hours
   (E) 10 hours

   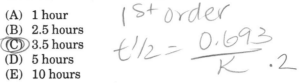
   1st order
   $t_{1/2} = \dfrac{0.693}{k} \quad \dfrac{}{.2}$

36. The volume of distribution of a drug is

   (A) a mathematical relationship between the total amount of drug in the body and the concentration of drug in the blood
   (B) a measure of an individual's blood volume
   (C) a measure of an individual's total fluid volume
   (D) an expression of total body volume
   (E) none of the above

37. The volume of distribution (V_d) of a particular drug will be

   greater in tissues b/c means less in plasma

   (A) greater for drugs that concentrate in tissues rather than in plasma
   (B) greater for drugs that concentrate in plasma rather than in tissues
   (C) independent of tissue concentration
   (D) independent of plasma concentration
   (E) approximately the same for all drugs in a given individual

38. Estimate the plasma concentration of a drug when 50 mg is given by IV bolus to a 140-lb patient if her volume of distribution is 1.6 L/kg.

   (A) 0.1 mg/L
   (B) 0.5 mg/L
   (C) 1 mg/L
   (D) 5 mg/L
   (E) 31 mg/L

39. A knowledge of volume of distribution (V_d) for a given drug is useful because it allows us to

   (A) estimate the elimination rate constant
   (B) determine the biologic half-life
   (C) calculate a reasonable loading dose
   (D) determine the best dosing interval
   (E) determine the peak plasma concentration

40. Which of the following is NOT a desirable characteristic of an effective urinary tract antimicrobial drug?

(A) high activity against gram-negative bacilli
(B) high volume of distribution in the body
(C) low level of protein binding
(D) short biologic half-life
(E) all of the above are desirable characteristics

Questions 41 through 45

The following graph represents drug blood level curves. Answer the next five questions based upon this graph.

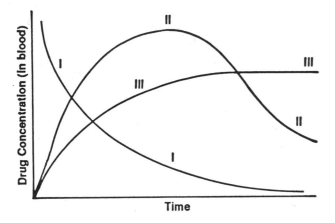

41. Curve I represents the blood level concentration of a drug administered by
  I. the oral route
  II. intramuscular injection
  III. intravenous injection

(A) I only
(B) III only
(C) I and II only
(D) II and III only
(E) I, II, and III

42. The upward slope of curve II could represent
  I. increased absorption of drug from a capsule dosage form
  II. absorption of drug from an intramuscular injection
  III. absorption of drug from a sustained-release tablet

(A) I only
(B) III only
(C) I and II only
(D) II and III only
(E) I, II, and III

43. Which one of the following statements concerning the graph is completely true?

(A) Once the peak in curve II has been reached, no further drug absorption is likely to occur.
(B) Doubling the administered dose will double the height of curve II. NO 1st order Independent

(C) The Y axis (concentration of drug in the blood) should be expressed as a log function.
(D) The X axis (time) should be expressed as a log function.
(E) None of the above are completely true.

44. Curve III would best illustrate a drug administered by

(A) intravenous push
(B) intravenous infusion
(C) intramuscular injection
(D) intrathecal injection
(E) either intravenous push or infusion

45. The time needed to reach maximum drug blood levels (the plateau portion of curve III) during constant-rate intravenous infusion is

(A) directly proportional to the rate of infusion
(B) inversely proportional to the rate of infusion
(C) independent of the rate of infusion
(D) independent of the biologic half-life
(E) not related to either the infusion rate or the biologic half-life

$4\ t_{1/2}$

46. Compartmental models are often used to illustrate the various principles of pharmacokinetics. A compartment is best defined as

(A) any anatomical entity that is capable of absorbing drug
(B) a kinetically distinguishable pool of drug
(C) specific body organs or tissues that can be assayed for drug
(D) any body fluid—such as blood or urine—that may contain drug
(E) any component of the blood, including blood proteins, that would have a tendency to absorb drug

47. At diffusion equilibrium, the concentrations of a drug in the various body compartments (body fluids, tissues, organs) are usually NOT equal because

(A) all body compartments are not equal in size and weight
(B) those compartments closest to the absorption site(s) will absorb most of the drug
(C) the CNS is a body compartment that usually does not accumulate drugs
(D) most drugs end up in the urine
(E) the various body compartments are not equally accessible to the drug, nor do they have equal affinities for it

48. The pharmacokinetic parameter known as clearance is essentially the

(A) rate at which the plasma is cleared of all waste materials and foreign substances (eg, drugs)
(B) volume of blood that passes through the kidneys per unit of time

(C) volume of blood that passes through the liver per unit of time

(D) rate at which a drug is removed (cleared) from its site of absorption

(E) volume of blood that is completely cleared of drug per unit of time

49. A knowledge of the clearance (Cl) of a given drug is useful because it allows us to

(A) calculate the maintenance dose required to sustain a desired average steady-state plasma concentration

(B) determine the volume of distribution

(C) determine the ideal dosing interval

(D) decide whether or not a loading dose is necessary

(E) determine whether the drug is metabolized or excreted unchanged

50. The difference between peak and trough concentrations is greatest when a drug is given at dosing intervals

(A) much longer than the half-life

(B) about equal to the half-life

(C) much shorter than the half-life

(D) equal to the half-life times serum creatinine

(E) equal to the time it takes to reach peak concentration following a single oral dose

51. A prolonged-release tablet delivers 20 mg of drug every hour. The percentage of drug remaining to be released in the 250-mg tablet after 3 hours is approximately

(A) 12

(B) 24

(C) 60

(D) 76

(E) 190

52. In dosing drugs that are primarily excreted by the kidneys, one must have some idea of the patient's renal function. A calculated pharmacokinetic parameter that gives us a reasonable estimate of renal function is the

(A) blood urea nitrogen (BUN)

(B) serum creatinine (Sr_{Cr})

(C) creatinine clearance (Cl_{Cr})

(D) urine creatinine (U_{Cr})

(E) free water clearance (Cl_{fw})

53. If the rate of elimination of a drug is reduced because of impaired renal function, the

(A) half-life and the time required to reach steady-state plasma levels will be increased

(B) half-life and the time required to reach steady-state plasma levels will be decreased

(C) half-life will be increased and the time required

to reach steady-state plasma levels will be decreased

(D) half-life will be decreased and the time required to reach steady-state plasma levels will be increased

(E) half-life and the time required to reach steady-state plasma levels will remain the same

54. When comparing a highly protein-bound drug to its less- or nonprotein-bound analog, the highly bound drug will probably have

(A) a longer biologic half-life

(B) delayed elimination from the body

(C) a more uniform distribution throughout body tissues

(D) all of the above characteristics

(E) none of the above characteristics

55. Which one of the following drugs does NOT bind to plasma protein to any significant extent?

(A) allopurinol (Zyloprim)

(B) amitriptyline (Elavil)

(C) lidocaine (Xylocaine)

(D) propranolol (Inderal)

(E) warfarin (Coumadin)

56. The metabolism of drugs generally results in

(A) less acidic compounds

(B) more acidic compounds

(C) compounds having a higher oil/water partition coefficient

(D) more polar compounds

(E) compounds with lower aqueous solubility

57. Most drugs are metabolized or eliminated from the body by first-order kinetics. This implies that the amount of drug metabolized or eliminated

(A) is constant

(B) changes with time but is NOT dependent on the concentration of drug in the blood

(C) changes with time and is dependent only on the concentration of drug in the blood

(D) is independent of drug concentration in the blood

(E) none of the above

58. The transfer of drugs from the blood to the urine and the biotransformation of drugs to inactive metabolites are usually both

(A) related to creatinine clearance

(B) irreversible processes

(C) competitive processes

(D) dependent on the rate constant for absorption

(E) functions performed primarily by the kidneys

59. The transfer of most drugs across biological membranes occurs by

(A) active transport from a region of high concentration to one of low concentration

(B) active transport from a region of low concentration to one of high concentration

(C) passive diffusion from a region of high concentration to one of low concentration

(D) passive diffusion from a region of low concentration to one of high concentration

(E) facilitated diffusion regardless of concentration gradient

60. When considering drug transport, a "passive transport process" implies that

(A) all of the drug will pass from one compartment to another

(B) the drug is highly lipid soluble

(C) the net transfer of drug is from an area of high concentration to an area of low concentration

(D) the net transfer of drug is from an area of low concentration to an area of high concentration

(E) the rate of drug transfer is constant

61. The rate of diffusion of drugs across biological membranes is most commonly

(A) independent of the concentration gradient

(B) directly proportional to the concentration gradient

(C) dependent on the availability of carrier substrate

(D) dependent on the route of administration

(E) directly proportional to membrane thickness

62. Which one of the following statements concerning carrier-mediated transport is NOT correct? Carrier-mediated transport systems

(A) consume energy *True*

(B) may be adversely affected by certain chemicals

(C) are structure specific *True*

(D) reach equilibrium faster than passive transport systems

(E) can become saturated *True*

63. When the active transport system described in the previous question becomes saturated, the rate process will be

(A) zero order

(B) pseudo-zero order

(C) first order

(D) pseudo-first order

(E) second order

64. The term prodrug refers to a

(A) chemical substance that is part of the synthesis procedure in preparing a drug

(B) compound that liberates an active drug in the body

(C) compound that may be therapeutically active but is still under clinical trials

(D) drug that has only prophylactic activity in the body

(E) drug that is classified as being "probably effective"

65. An example of a commercial product that is a prodrug is

(A) Dalmane

(B) Lasix

(C) Norpramin

(D) Chlorazepate

(E) Prostaphlin

66. The rectal route of administration may be preferred over the oral route for some drugs because

(A) the drug does not have to be absorbed

(B) absorption is predictable and complete

(C) a portion of the absorbed drug does not pass through the liver before entering the systemic circulation

(D) inert binders, diluents, and excipients cannot interfere with absorption

(E) the dissolution process is avoided

67. If a drug appears in the feces after oral administration,

(A) the drug cannot have been completely absorbed from the GI tract

(B) the drug must not have completely dissolved in the GI fluids

(C) the drug must have complexed with materials in the GI tract

(D) parenteral administration of the drug may determine the contribution of the biliary system to the amount of drug in the feces

(E) parenteral administration of the drug will be useful to determine the bioavailability of the oral formulation

68. Drugs that are poorly lipid soluble or extensively ionized at the pH of blood generally

(A) penetrate the CNS very slowly and may be eliminated from the body before a significant concentration in the CNS is reached

(B) penetrate the CNS very slowly but are centrally active in much lower concentration

(C) achieve adequate CNS concentrations only if given IV

(D) must be metabolized to a more polar form before they can gain access to the CNS

(E) can gain access to the CNS if other drugs are used to modify blood pH

69. Which of the following objectives is desirable when developing a new antibiotic drug?
    I. increasing the minimum inhibitory concentration
    II. increasing the minimum toxic concentration
    III. decreasing the tendency for protein binding

    (A) I only
    (B) III only
    (C) I and II only
    (D) II and III only
    (E) I, II, and III

70. The properties of a drug may preclude its formulation into a sustained-release dosage form. Drugs with which of the following characteristics probably should NOT be so formulated?
    I. poor water solubility
    II. very long half-life
    III. very short half-life

    (A) I only
    (B) III only
    (C) I and II only
    (D) II and III only
    (E) I, II, and III

Answers and Explanations

1. **(C)** For most drugs, a dose-response relationship can be correlated with the amount of drug that gains access to the general circulation. In many cases, the amount of drug that is present in the blood (blood level) is directly related to the intensity and duration of the pharmacologic effect. The relative amount of drug that is biologically available compared to the total amount of drug in the dosage form administered is a measure of bioavailability. *(30:3)*

2. **(C)** Although the blood levels of various drugs are often used to compare different formulations of the same drug, it must be remembered that to exert a pharmacologic effect, a drug must reach its site(s) of action in an adequate concentration. Some drugs (eg, urinary tract anti-infectives) do not necessarily have to achieve high blood concentration to reach their site(s) of action. *(1:697)*

3. **(E)** The surface area of a drug is so limited in the intact tablet that dissolution of drug from the intact tablet is negligible except for very water-soluble drugs. Therefore, although a drug must dissolve before it can be absorbed, a tablet must generally disintegrate before the drug can dissolve. *(27:65; 31:123)*

4. **(C)** While differences in bioavailability of various drug products might be anticipated with any route of administration that requires the drug to be absorbed into the blood compartment, the oral route is most often involved because it is the most common route of administration and it presents the most difficult conditions in terms of chemical and biologic obstacles. *(1:746; 30:145)*

5. **(C)** The availability of a drug from a specific formulation is compared to a reference standard that is administered at the same dose level. The standard for oral drugs is usually a solution of the pure drug. The relative bioavailability is then calculated by dividing either the AUC of the drug or the total amount of the drug excreted in the urine by respective values for the reference standard. The absolute bioavailability can be calculated by comparing similar data for the drug product to an IV bolus dose. *(31:43)*

6. **(D)** The area under the curve (AUC) can be calculated mathematically by the use of equations or evaluation of a graph when concentration (drug wt/volume) is plotted on the Y axis and time is plotted on the X axis. Usually the calculation involves the use of the trapezoidal rule. Units for AUC are weight and time/volume. *(31:459)*

7. **(A)** F values are calculated for drugs in their dosage forms by comparing AUCs, or total amount of drug excreted, to the control reference of an IV bolus dose as outlined in question 5. An ideal F value would be 1.0, which indicates complete absorption of the drug and no losses from other mechanisms such as hepatic first-pass effect. *(31:43)*

8. **(C)** As outlined in question 7, the F value can be estimated by using the equation:

$$F = \frac{AUC_{cap}}{AUC_{iv}} = \frac{20}{25} = 0.8$$

Since in this example the comparison of AUCs relates to the absolute standard of an IV bolus dose, the drug's absolute bioavailability was calculated. If the comparison had been to another standard, such as to an oral solution or another product of the same drug, the F value would be the relative bioavailability. *(31:43)*

9. **(A)** This problem is similar to question 8, except that a correction factor is necessary since different doses of the drug were administered. *(31:43)*

By proportion, $\dfrac{50 \text{ mg IV}}{40 \text{ (AUC)}} = \dfrac{100 \text{ mg IV}}{x \text{ AUC}}$

$x = $ AUC of 80 μg/mL/h

$$F = \frac{AUC_{tab}}{AUC_{iv}} = \frac{20}{80} = 0.25 \qquad (31:43)$$

10. **(C)** Peak concentrations and times of peak concentrations can be easily read from the graph. AUCs involve complex calculations. *(1:733; 30:183)*

11. **(B)** Prior to the peak time, the rate of absorption is greater than the rate of elimination, and the curve ascends. After the peak, the rate of elimination is

greater than the rate of absorption, and the curve descends. If these rates are equal for some time interval, the curve will show a plateau rather than a distinct peak.   *(27:9)*

12. **(A)** For a given drug product the time interval between oral administration (zero time) and the time of the peak in the serum concentration vs time curve represents the time required for most of the drug to be absorbed into the blood. The shorter this interval is for a particular drug product, the faster the rate of absorption for the drug. While the distribution, metabolism, and elimination processes all influence the shape of the curve, we cannot distinguish these processes directly from the curve because they are all postabsorptive phenomena.   *(27:151)*

13. **(D)** Since the serum concentration-time curve is a quantitative representation of the concentration of drug in the serum over a specific period of time, the area under the curve is a mathematical function of the amount of drug that has entered the blood. The total area under the curve, then, represents the amount of drug that has been absorbed. By comparing the areas under the curves of two formulations of the same drug, we can determine the relative amount of drug that is available from each formulation.   *(27:8)*

14. **(B)** Although equal areas indicate that the same total amount of drug was made available to the body, the areas alone give no information regarding the rate at which the drugs were made available. Two formulations of a drug can yield radically different serum concentrations vs time curves that have approximately equal areas. It should be emphasized that the concept of bioequivalence involves not only the amount of drug that is available but also the rate at which it becomes available.   *(1:1453)*

15. **(B)** If the areas under the respective curves are equal, it can be concluded that the total amount of drug delivered to the body by each dosage form was equal. Since the intravenous administration did not involve an absorption process, the fact that the same amount of drug administered in a capsule formulation delivered the same total amount of drug indicates that the absorption of the drug from the oral capsule was essentially complete.   *(1:711,747)*

16. **(C)** If the therapeutic performance and/or toxicity of a particular drug is related to rather specific blood levels of the drug (eg, digoxin), relatively minor differences in bioavailability may be extremely important. Under these circumstances, small differences observed in the area under the curves, the time of the peak concentration, and the height of the peak concentration may be significant enough to produce a therapeutic failure and/or toxic responses to the drug.   *(27:146)*

17. **(B)** While in vitro dissolution rate studies may be useful in quality control procedures to evaluate batch-to-batch variability, they are of little value in bioavailability evaluations unless they can be correlated with in vivo studies in humans. More commonly, when several formulations of a particular drug are found to be biologically inequivalent through studies in humans, in vitro dissolution studies are performed to establish the basis of their inequivalence.   *(27:159)*

18. **(A)** The ionic equilibrium that is established in the acid contents of the stomach will favor a relatively higher concentration of unionized drug in solution. The unionized molecule, because of the absence of a charge, is more lipid soluble than the ionic species and will be able to cross biological membranes more easily. If the drug reaches the more alkaline contents of the intestines before absorption is complete, the higher pH will then favor the ionic form of the drug, which has considerably less lipid solubility and is much less readily absorbed. It should be pointed out, however, that because of the extremely large surface area of the intestine, weakly acidic drugs can be absorbed from the intestine in spite of the unfavorable ion/molecule ratio.   *(27:40)*

19. **(B)** When a drug is administered by the intravenous route, an absorption step is bypassed because the drug is injected directly into the bloodstream. All other routes of administration present the drug with various biological barriers through which the drug must pass to reach the blood.   *(27:3)*

20. **(C)** It is generally true that a drug must be in solution before it becomes available for absorption. An aqueous solution presents the drug in the dissolved state to the absorption site(s). Even if the drug precipitates upon contact with fluid in the GI tract, it will do so in the form of very small particles that are eventually completely wetted and ready to be redissolved. Suspensions, while having larger particles of drug, are also wetted and ready for dissolution. A powder formulation must disperse in the GI fluids and become wetted prior to dissolution. The gelatin shell of a capsule formulation must dissolve before the powder can disperse. Tablets must not only disintegrate from the tablet form, but they must also disintegrate from the smaller granulation particles before the GI fluids have access to the drug. Coated tablets have the additional barrier of the coating material.   *(27:61)*

21. **(B)** Making a drug dissolve faster (eg, by particle size reduction) will not increase the rate of its absorption if the absorption process itself is the rate-limiting step in the overall transport of the drug from its intact dosage form to the blood. Furthermore, there are some circumstances in which particle size reduction may actually reduce the amount of drug absorbed. For example, for drugs such as penicillin G that are unstable in gastric fluids, more rapid dissolution would enhance degradation by in-

creasing residence time of dissolved drug in the stomach and thereby result in reduced availability.

(27:51)

22. **(D)** When a drug is administered orally in a solid dosage form such as a tablet or capsule, it is frequently observed that the rate of absorption is controlled by the rate at which the drug dissolves in the fluids at the absorption site(s). When absorption is controlled by dissolution in this manner, absorption is said to be dissolution rate limited. If the dissolution step is eliminated by administering the drug in the form of a solution, it is quite likely that absorption will proceed more rapidly and/or more completely.

(27:45)

23. **(A)** Drugs are generally absorbed from the GI tract through capillaries that empty into the portal vein. This vessel carries the absorbed drugs to the liver, where they are subjected to varying degrees of metabolism before they are carried into the general circulation. This initial passage through the liver is therapeutically significant primarily for drugs that are metabolized to a less active or inactive form by the liver.

(27:154)

24. **(A)** The term first pass refers to the first passage of drug molecules through a designated organ such as the lungs or the liver. Biotransformation will often occur at this site, thereby altering the absolute bioavailability of a drug. Commercial preparations of such drugs are formulated to contain sufficient quantities of drug to compensate for loss due to first-pass biotransformation. While acetylsalicylic acid does not appear to undergo a significant first-pass hepatic biotransformation, some drug loss does occur in the intestinal lumen or during absorption through the GI mucosa.

(1:747; 31:120)

25. **(D)** Gastric emptying appears to be an exponential process with a normal half-life of between 20 and 60 minutes. However, many factors can influence the rate of this process. It is slowed by the A, B, C, and E choices and is speeded by hunger, mild exercise, cold meals, dilute solutions, and lying on the right side. Since some drugs and some dosage forms (eg, enteric coated tablets) are absorbed at rather specific sites along the GI tract, alterations in the rate of gastric emptying may lead to erratic and unpredictable absorption. For example, if an acid-labile drug that is preferentially absorbed from a portion of the small intestine is consumed as an enteric coated tablet, a greatly reduced gastric emptying rate may permit the tablet to dissolve in the stomach and be degraded by the acid fluids of the stomach. Similarly, if the gastric emptying rate is greatly increased, the tablet may not dissolve before it reaches its primary site of absorption.

(1:714; 30:160)

26. **(C)** After a drug gains access to the systemic circulation, it may be metabolized to varying degrees and/or be excreted unchanged. For most drugs and their metabolites, the kidneys are the primary organ of excretion. The presence of a drug and/or its metabolites in the urine must be preceded by the presence of drug in the blood. When an appreciable amount of drug is excreted in the urine, it is often possible to use urinary excretion data—such as cumulative amount of drug in the urine and maximum urinary excretion rate—to evaluate the systemic availability of various drug formulations.

(27:146)

27. **(C)** Urinary excretion studies require complete urine collection so that the total quantity of drug that is excreted in the urine can be determined. Normal or near-normal renal function is also a prerequisite for accurate urinary excretion studies because sufficiently impaired renal function can alter the composition of various body fluids which, in turn, can alter the pharmacokinetic properties of many drugs. Although urinary excretion studies are usually conducted on drugs that are primarily excreted unchanged by the kidney, it is not necessary that a drug be completely excreted unchanged by the kidney.

(7:195,801; 31:44)

28. **(C)** Just as shifting the ionic equilibrium in favor of the ionic species reduces the probability that a weakly acidic drug will be absorbed from the alkaline fluids of the intestines, it also reduces the probability that the drug will be reabsorbed from the renal tubules into the blood. Consequently, a greater fraction of drug in the tubules cannot be reabsorbed and will be excreted in the urine.

(30:359)

29. **(C)** For any drug that is eliminated by first-order kinetics, the time required to achieve steady-state plasma levels is dependent only on the biologic half-life of that drug in a given individual. As a drug is repeatedly administered in constant dosage and at constant time intervals (that are short enough to preclude complete elimination of the drug), the elimination rate of the drug increases as the concentration of drug in plasma increases. The tendency of a drug to accumulate on repeated dosing is, therefore, balanced by increased amounts of drug being eliminated. Eventually, a steady state will be reached in which the amount of drug absorbed will equal the amount of drug being eliminated. The time to reach steady state corresponds to about four to five half-lives and is more completely described in the following table:

Time (half-lives)	Plasma Concentration (% of steady-state level)
1	50
2	75
3	88
4	94
5	97
6	98
7	99

(7:10)

30. (A) Most drugs have biologic half-lives that follow first-order kinetics. A basic characteristic of first-order kinetics is that the rate constants for metabolism or excretion are independent of the initial drug concentration. That is, a specific fraction of drug will be lost in a given time period. Doubling the drug concentration will not change the rate constant, even though the amount of drug lost in a given time period would increase.

(D–incorrect) Renal impairment may affect the biologic half-life of drugs eliminated by the kidneys. However, the half-life would be expected to increase (not decrease) since the drug remains in the circulation for longer periods of time.

(E–incorrect) Two methods for determining half-life are (1) to determine drug blood levels with respect to time and (2) to quantify with respect to time actual biologic responses to the drug. Ideally, the half-life values by each method should be identical. However, they will be identical only when there is a direct and measurable relationship between drug blood concentrations and the biologic response. *(30:57)*

31. (C) One half (200 mg) of the administered dose will be eliminated in 4 hours. Of the remaining 200 mg, one half (100 mg) will be eliminated in the second 4-hour period. In the next 4-hour span, an additional 50 mg of drug will be lost. Therefore, after 12 hours (or three half-lives), only 50 mg of drug remains. *(30:59)*

32. (C) Generally, when a particular drug has a half-life of 6 hours, there is reasonable certainty that in spite of as much as a one- to twofold intersubject variation, the mean biologic half-life in any group of subjects will approximate 6 hours. Alterations in biologic half-life can be expected when a particular drug is primarily excreted unchanged by the kidneys. The presence of renal impairment slows the process of excretion and thereby increases the biologic half-life of the drug in the blood. *(1:729; 29:230)*

33. (C) *(31:21)*

34. (D) The metabolic pathways of newborn infants are incompletely developed at birth; most notably, the oxidative and conjugative mechanisms that are known to metabolize many drugs. The reduced capacity to metabolize certain drugs will therefore result in prolonged biologic half-lives of these drugs in newborn infants. Because of inadequate metabolic inactivation, the plasma concentration of chloramphenicol is higher in infants under 2 weeks of age than in older infants. *(19:78–3)*

35. (C) A rate constant of 20% per hour refers to a fraction loss of 0.2 per hour. The equation for determining half-lives for first-order reactions is

$$t_{50} = 0.693/k$$
$$= 0.693/0.2$$
$$= 3.5 \text{ hours}$$

(31:173)

36. (A) Volume of distribution (V_d) is an "apparent volume" measured in terms of a reference compartment, usually the blood, because of the accessibility of this compartment to sampling. This relationship, which is calculated by the expression:

$V_d = A_b/C_b$ where A_b = total amount of unchanged drug in the body and C_b = concentration of drug in the blood

is the total volume necessary to account for all of the absorbed drug, if the concentration of drug in this volume were equal to C_b. Knowledge of the volume of distribution for a particular drug permits calculation of the total amount of drug in the body (A_b) at any time by measuring the drug concentration in the blood (since $A_b = V_d \times C_b$). *(1:727; 29:2; 31:20)*

37. (A) Following a given dose of a drug, the greater its concentration in various tissue compartments, the smaller its concentration in plasma. Therefore, according to the relationship $A_b = V_d \times C_b$ (see previous commentary), the volume of distribution of a particular drug will be greater for those drugs that tend to concentrate in tissues as opposed to plasma. *(1:727; 31:21)*

38. (B) The simple relationships is: LD = (C_o) × (V) [loading dose = C_o (plasma concentration) × (volume of distribution)]

step 1: convert the patient's pound weight to kg

$$140 \text{ lb} \times \frac{1 \text{ kg}}{2.2 \text{ lb}} = 64 \text{ kg}$$

step 2: 50 mg = × (1.6 L/kg) (64 kg)
step 3: 50 mg = (10 μg/L) (V)

39. (C) Since the volume of distribution is a parameter that allows accountability for all of the drug in the body, it can be used to calculate the loading dose that would rapidly result in a desired plasma concentration (C_p).

$$\text{Loading dose} = \frac{(V_d)\ (C_p)}{(S)\ (F)}$$

where S = portion of the salt form that is active drug (eg, aminophylline is 80% to 85% theophylline, S = 0.8 to 0.85); F = fraction of dose absorbed. *(1:765; 19:1–3)*

40. (B) A high volume of distribution implies that the antimicrobial drug is being distributed in a large portion of the body or concentrated in body tissue. Since better antimicrobial activity would be anticipated if the drug was concentrated primarily in the urinary tract, a low volume of distribution would be preferred.

(A–incorrect) High activity against common gram-negative microorganisms (*Escherichia coli, En-*

terobacter aerogenes, Pseudomonas aeruginosa, and Proteus mirabilis) is desirable

(C–incorrect) Drugs that are bound to plasma protein are usually not available for therapeutic activity. It is generally the free form of the drug that is active.

(D–incorrect) For systemic antibiotics, a long biologic half-life may be useful to maintain satisfactory blood or tissue levels. Urinary tract antibiotics, however, appear to be more effective if they reach the site of action (urinary tract) quickly and in a high concentration. A drug with a short half-life is more likely to have these properties.

(19:43–2; 27:194; 31:20)

41. **(B)** Curve I shows an initial high concentration of drug in the blood with a steadily decreasing concentration. This curve is characteristic of drugs administered by rapid intravenous injection.   *(27:14; 31:18)*

42. **(E)** Any of the listed dosage forms could exhibit blood level curves similar to curve II. The first portion of the curve shows an increasing concentration of drug in the blood. This pattern would be expected whenever there is steady drug absorption (ie, when absorption is greater than elimination), either from the GI tract or from a tissue injection site. Curve III is also a good representation for a sustained-release product as it illustrates a plateau effect.

(1:733; 27:3; 31:42)

43. **(E)**
(A–incorrect) Two critical factors that affect the height and shape of a blood level curve are the rates of absorption and rates of elimination. Blood levels increase until a peak occurs where the rate of absorption equals the rate of elimination. Drug absorption will usually continue to occur even after the peak blood level has been reached. However, the blood level curve then begins to descend since the rate of elimination is greater than the rate of absorption.

(B–incorrect) Since most of the factors affecting pharmacokinetics are first order, doubling a drug dose will seldom double the height of a blood level curve. However, the total area under the drug curve can be expected to double since the area under the curve is directly proportional to the dose.

(C–incorrect) The pharmacokinetics of most drugs follow a first-order pattern. Therefore, if the concentration of drug in the blood is plotted as a log function on the Y axis, a straight line will be obtained rather than a curve, as shown.

(D–incorrect) The time factor is a constant variable plotted at regular intervals (hours, days, etc). It is very seldom expressed as a log function.   *(27:3,10)*

44. **(B)** Administration of drugs by intravenous infusion, which implies slow administration into a vein, will result in a plateau effect in respect to drug blood levels. The resulting steady-state levels are directly proportional to the infusion rate.

(A–incorrect) An intravenous push (bolus dose) will give a curve similar to I.

(D–incorrect) The blood level curve for an intrathecal (spinal) injection will probably resemble curve II as the drug slowly diffuses into the blood.

(1:726; 27:10; 35:214)

45. **(C)** The time in which the maximum drug blood level is obtained is independent of the infusion rate. It is dependent only on the biologic half-life of the particular drug. The time required to reach the plateau (steady state) is approximately four to five half-lives.   *(31:65,81)*

46. **(B)** While various organs, tissues, and fluids in the body can be considered to be compartments for a specific drug, a compartment does not necessarily have to be an anatomical entity. Any body site or fluid that appears to contain drug may be described as a compartment or "pool" in the model.   *(27:14)*

47. **(E)** *(27:2)*

48. **(E)** This is the definition of total systemic (whole body) clearance, which is the sum of all the separate clearances (ie, renal, hepatic, etc).   *(19:1–4)*

49. **(A)** When the clearance (Cl) of a drug is known, the maintenance dose required to sustain a desired average steady-state plasma concentration can be calculated by:

$$\text{Maintenance dose} = \frac{(Cl)\,(C_p)\,(\tau)}{(S)\,(F)}$$

Where C_p = average steady-state plasma concentration
  τ = dosing interval
  S = portion of salt that is active drug
  F = fraction of dose absorbed   *(19:1–7)*

50. **(A)** Drugs (eg, aminoglycosides) given at intervals that are much longer than one half-life are almost completely eliminated from the body before the next dose is given. This results in large differences between peak and trough drug concentrations; timing of blood sample(s) becomes crucial to interpretation of results. At the other extreme, drugs given at intervals that are much shorter than one half-life (eg, phenobarbital) are slowly cleared from the body; consequently, their peak-to-trough concentration differences are relatively small.   *(1:755; 19:1–6)*

51. **(D)** A zero order rate constant refers to a system in which the same quantity of drug is being changed or lost per unit of time. In this problem 20 mg of drug is being released from the tablet every hour. In three hours, 20 mg × 3 = 60 mg has been released. Therefore, the amount of drug remaining in the tablet is 250 mg – 60 mg = 190 mg or 76%.

52. **(C)** Drug elimination by the kidney can often be correlated with blood urea nitrogen (BUN), serum creatinine (S_rC_r), and creatinine clearance (CL_{cr}).

The BUN and S_rC_r, however, are less useful indices of renal function than the CL_{cr} because they are influenced by other factors (eg, state of hydration, age, etc). For example, as patients age, both the production and clearance of creatinine decrease. Therefore, an elderly patient with a normal serum creatinine of 1 mg/dL may have a creatinine clearance of much less than 100 mL/min (normal CL_{cr} is 100 to 120 mL/min for a 70-kg adult). There are a number of methods used to calculate CL_{cr}. An example of a useful equation is:

$$\text{Male } CL_{cr} = \frac{(40 - \text{age}) \, (\text{weight})}{72 \, (S_rC_r)}$$

Age is in years, weight is in kilograms, and serum creatinine is in mg/dL. For females, multiply the CL_{cr} by 0.85. *(19:1–7)*

53. **(A)** If the biologic half-life of a drug is increased in patients with impaired renal function, the time required to reach steady-state plasma levels will also be increased. The time required to reach steady-state plasma levels is dependent only on the biologic half-life of a given drug in a given individual. *(7:11)*

54. **(D)** Binding of drugs to blood components leads to a more even distribution throughout body tissues, thereby decreasing selective accumulation in specific body areas. Also, since only the unbound fraction of drug is available for biotransformation and excretion, protein-bound drugs have a tendency to remain in the body longer (ie, delayed elimination and longer half-lives). *(4:15; 27:200)*

55. **(A)** When administered in therapeutic doses, allopurinol does not appear to bind to plasma proteins. The pharmacist should carefully monitor drug therapy when two or more drugs that exhibit significant protein-binding properties are prescribed. Relatively small changes in the degree of protein binding caused by competition for binding sites can result in significant changes in plasma concentration of free drug and in the intensity of the clinical response. *(1:750)*

56. **(D)** Drug metabolites are usually more polar and less lipid soluble than the parent compound. Because of these changes, metabolites are usually not as tightly nor as extensively protein bound. They are ionized to a greater degree and are less likely to cross biologic membranes than the parent compound. Drug metabolism, therefore, is generally a process that inactivates a drug and changes it to a form that can be excreted more easily and rapidly. For some drugs, however, metabolism may result in activation of an inactive substance, or an active substance may be transformed into (an) active metabolite(s). In these cases, either further biotransformation takes place to inactivate the metabolite(s) or it (they) is (are) excreted unchanged. *(1:718)*

57. **(C)** A first-order process is one in which the rate is determined by a single factor. In this case, the single factor is the concentration of a drug in the blood. The general differential formula for a first-order process is

$$- dc/dt = kc$$

$- dc/dt$ is the rate of change of concentration with respect to time, k is the rate constant for the process, and c is the concentration of drug in the plasma. The rate of this process changes as the concentration of drug changes. *(1:742)*

58. **(B)** While a number of drugs can be reabsorbed into the systemic circulation from the kidney tubule, the elimination and biotransformation processes are irreversible for most drugs. *(27:1; 31:149)*

59. **(C)** Although some drugs are absorbed from the gastrointestinal tract by active transport mechanisms against a concentration gradient or by facilitated diffusion with a concentration gradient, most drugs are passively absorbed from a region of high concentration to a region of low concentration (ie, with a concentration gradient). *(27:25)*

60. **(C)** Passive transport is the most common type of drug transport. It occurs when a drug is unevenly distributed between two compartments that are separated by a membrane or barrier that is permeable to the drug. Since the drug can pass freely through the membrane, it will do so until equilibrium is reached. *(34:33)*

61. **(B)** The greater the difference between the drug concentrations on each side of a biologic membrane, the greater the rate of transfer from the side having the higher concentration to the side having the lower concentration. *(29:25; 30:134)*

62. **(D)** As the name implies, carrier-mediated or active transport involves active participation of a membrane in transferring molecules from one side to the other. The "carrier," such as an enzyme in the membrane, aids in transporting the molecules of drug across the membrane. Since this transfer process is continuous, it can work against a concentration gradient and continue until all of the drug has been transported. Therefore, equilibrium does not occur. (B–incorrect) Certain chemicals, known as poisons, can reduce active transport, probably by destroying or inactivating the drug carriers. (C–incorrect) Carriers are often very specific in respect to the drug they will transport. Only a certain chemical structure or similar chemical structures may be actively transported by a given carrier. (E–incorrect) Because of the chemical specificity and limited capacity of carriers, active transport systems may become saturated. When this occurs, the active transport rate becomes a constant value until the drug concentration is reduced. *(1:709; 30:38)*

63. (A) A characteristic of a zero-order process or reaction is a constant rate of change. When the active transport system is saturated, there are not enough carriers to handle the large number of transferable molecules. Therefore, the carriers work at maximum capacity, transferring molecules at a constant rate until the drug concentration is reduced to less than the capacity of the carrier system. At this time, the number of molecules transferred will be a fraction of those present for transfer (ie, a first-order rate).

(30:39)

64. (B) In order to take advantage of certain desirable characteristics, some drugs are marketed as prodrugs. These are chemical modifications of biologically active drugs and may not be active themselves. However, the active form of the drug is liberated in the body by some biotransformation. Prodrugs may possess better water solubility, be more stable, have a less objectionable taste, or give higher blood levels than the parent compound. *(29:54; 30:316)*

65. (D) Chlorazepate (Tranxene) is rapidly decarboxylated in the acidic stomach to an active metabolite that possesses antiepileptic properties. *(10; 11:863)*

66. (C) Although it is desirable for certain drugs rapidly metabolized by the liver to bypass absorption into the portal circulation, the value of using the rectal route for this purpose is limited. This is due to the fact that while the blood supply to the rectum is drained by three principal veins, only the middle and inferior hemorrhoidal veins actually bypass the liver. The superior hemorrhoidal vein enters the portal circulation via the inferior mesenteric vein.

(1:1581)

67. (D) If an orally administered drug appears in the feces, it might be desirable to determine whether this is the result of incomplete absorption or secretion of the drug into the GI tract via biliary excretion. The clinical significance of biliary excretion or enterohepatic cycling of the drug depends on the fraction of the dose excreted in the bile. By administering the drug parenterally, this fraction can be determined. *(1:721; 29:209)*

68. (A) The "blood–brain barrier" appears to behave as a lipoid membrane toward foreign compounds. This barrier may be due to a sheath of glial cells surrounding the capillaries of the brain. The rate of entry of a drug can often be correlated with its oil/water partition coefficient and degree of ionization at plasma pH. *(27:188; 31:135)*

69. (D) The minimum inhibitory concentration is the concentration of antibiotic that prevents the growth of microorganisms. The lower the value, the more effective the antibiotic is in respect to the concentration needed. Increasing the minimum toxic concentration will increase the safety of the drug and decrease the incidence of side effects. Binding of drug to plasma protein is generally undesirable since the bound fraction of drug is unavailable for therapeutic activity. *(30:288)*

70. (E) All of these drug characteristics are probably undesirable for a sustained-release dosage form. For a successful sustained-release product, the rate-limiting step must be drug release from the dosage form. If the drug has poor solubility, the dissolution rate may become the rate-limiting step. In this case, the patient may not absorb the quantity of drug needed for desired blood levels and therapeutic activity. Drugs with very long half-lives do not need to be formulated for sustained-release since they will be biologically present for a long period of time. Intelligent dosing, such as every 12 or 24 hours (depending on the actual half-life), ensures sufficient blood levels. The release of drug from most sustained-release dosage forms is subject to individual biologic variations. This patient to patient variability may result in the release of two or three times the normal dose in a particular patient. Therefore, a dangerous situation may develop if very large amounts of very potent drugs are formulated as sustained-release products. Conversely, a drug with a very short half-life is also a poor candidate for sustained release. A very large amount of drug would have to be included in the dosage form, and rapid release of the drug would be necessary. *(30:194)*

CHAPTER 6

Clinical Pharmacy

Clinical pharmacy is a term many have found difficult to define. A US Supreme Court Justice, when challenged to define pornography, is said to have replied that although he could not define it, he sure could recognize it if he saw it. With this example in mind, we have assembled a series of questions for this chapter that we believe fall under the category of clinical pharmacy; ie, they relate to patients, diseases, drugs, information, and pharmacists.

Questions

DIRECTIONS (Questions 1 through 206): Each of the numbered items or incomplete statements in this section is followed by answers or by completions of the statement. Select the ONE lettered answer or completion that is BEST in each case.

1. Which of the following drugs is generally considered the drug of choice in treating status epilepticus?

   (A) glutethimide (Doriden)
   (B) ethosuximide (Zarontin)
   (C) phenytoin (Dilantin)
   (D) paraldehyde
   (E) diazepam (Valium)

2. A syndrome strongly resembling systemic lupus erythematosus (SLE) is an adverse reaction associated with the use of

   (A) hydralazine (Apresoline) *+ procainimide*
   (B) reserpine
   (C) diazoxide (Hyperstat IV)
   (D) methyldopa (Aldomet)
   (E) guanethidine (Ismelin)

3. The antihypertensive effect of guanethidine (Ismelin) is inhibited by
   MAO
   Tricyclic
   BC
   (A) diazepam (Valium)
   (B) amitriptyline (Elavil)
   (C) hydrochlorothiazide (HydroDIURIL)
   (D) probenecid (Benemid)
   (E) nitrofurantoin (Furandantin)

4. In terms of its major pharmacologic effect, metoprolol (Lopressor) is most similar to   *B₁*

   (A) isoproterenol (Isuprel) *B₂*
   (B) metaproterenol (Alupent) *B₂*
   (C) guanethidine (Ismelin) *direct vasocon*
   (D) hydrochlorothiazide (HydroDIURIL) *Diuretic*
   (E) propranolol (Inderal) *B₁ & B₂*

5. When dispensing a new prescription, for which of the following drugs should the pharmacist advise the patient that he may experience a large fall in blood pressure following the first dose?

   (A) methyldopa (Aldomet)
   (B) prazosin (Minipress)
   (C) clonidine (Catapres)
   (D) reserpine (Serpasil)
   (E) propranolol (Inderal)

6. The ganglionic blocking agents are NOT extensively used as antihypertensive agents because

   (A) they cannot be administered orally
   (B) of their long duration of action
   (C) they do not selectively block sympathetic ganglia
   (D) their hypotensive effect is unpredictable and slow in onset
   (E) they may cause congestive heart failure

7. In the treatment of acute hypertensive crisis, diazoxide (Hyperstat IV) is administered

   (A) orally
   (B) intramuscularly
   (C) by infusion over 15 to 30 minutes
   (D) by slow infusion over 1 to 4 hours
   (E) by slow infusion for 6 to 24 hours

8. A physician has decided upon a course of tetracycline therapy for a patient with renal impairment. Which of the following drugs is LEAST likely to accumulate in the patient's blood?

   (A) demeclocycline *10-17*
   (B) doxycycline *22*
   (C) minocycline *11-12*
   (D) oxytetracycline *6-10*
   (E) tetracycline *6-17*

   not elim by kidney

9. Which of the following antihypertensive agents would probably be the BEST choice to use in combination with hydrochlorothiazide in a hypertensive patient who is severely depressed?

(A) reserpine (Serpasil)
(B) hydralazine (Apresoline)
(C) guanethidine (Ismelin)
(D) methyldopa (Aldomet)
(E) clonidine (Catapres)

10. Benztropine (Cogentin) is often given to patients taking the antipsychotic phenothiazine because benztropine

(A) reduces the dose of phenothiazine required
(B) is an anticholinergic drug that reduces the extrapyramidal side effects of the phenothiazine
(C) eliminates the unpleasant GI irritation caused by the phenothiazine
(D) is an antidepressant
(E) reduces gut motility to ensure that the phenothiazine is completely absorbed

11. Cholestyramine (Questran) will probably interfere with the gastrointestinal absorption of
    I. chlorothiazide
    II. warfarin
    III. phenobarbital

(A) I only
(B) III only
(C) I and II only
(D) II and III only
(E) I, II, and III

12. A clinically noticeable drug interaction resulting from the displacement of drug A by drug B from common plasma protein-binding sites is most often seen when

(A) drug A has a high association constant (K) for binding the protein
(B) drug B has a high association constant (K) for binding the protein and is given in large doses
(C) drug B has a low association constant (K) for binding the protein and is given in large doses
(D) drug B is more toxic than drug A
(E) drug B is rapidly absorbed

13. The metabolism of which of the following compounds is altered in patients taking anticonvulsants?

(A) pyridoxine
(B) folic acid
(C) riboflavin
(D) renin
(E) tyrosine

14. When valproic acid (Depakene) is prescribed for petit mal epilepsy (absence seizures) in a patient who is already receiving phenobarbital,

(A) the phenobarbital should be discontinued because phenobarbital will inactivate valproic acid
(B) the dose of phenobarbital may have to be decreased because valproic acid will increase phenobarbital blood levels
(C) ethosuximide (Zarontin) should also be prescribed
(D) the valproic acid should be given in the morning and the phenobarbital should be given at bedtime
(E) the dose of both drugs may have to be higher than usual because each drug enhances the metabolism of the other

15. A microorganism that is particularly dangerous to the eye is

(A) *Aspergillus niger*
(B) *Bacillus subtilis*
(C) *Escherichia coli*
(D) *Pseudomonas aeruginosa*
(E) *Streptococcus thermophilus*

16. Purulent boils in the ear are usually caused by species of

(A) *Aspergillus*
(B) *Candida*
(C) *Pseudomonas*
(D) *Staphylococcus*
(E) *Streptococcus*

17. The treatment of choice for herpes simplex infection of the eyelids and conjunctiva is

(A) thiabendazole (Mintezol)
(B) idoxuridine (Stoxil)
(C) amphotericin B (Fungizone)
(D) bacitracin (Baciguent)
(E) mupirocin (Bactroban)

18. Which of the following antifungal agents is ineffective against *Candida* organisms?

(A) nystatin (Mycostatin)
(B) clotrimazole (Lotrimin)
(C) tolnaftate (Tinactin)
(D) haloprogin (Halotex)
(E) miconazole (Micatin)

19. Methotrexate has been shown to be of clinical use in the management of

(A) psoriasis
(B) seborrhea
(C) acne
(D) ringworm infections of the skin
(E) warts

20. An important potential complication of corticosteroid therapy is
  I. dissemination of local infection
  II. masking symptoms of an infection
  III. increased susceptibility to infection

(A) I only
(B) III only
(C) I and II only
(D) II and III only
(E) I, II, and III

21. The primary advantage of piroxicam (Feldene) over other nonsteroidal anti-inflammatory drugs (NSAIDs) is that it

(A) is relatively inexpensive
(B) acts by a different mechanism of action that may be additive to other NSAIDs
(C) may be given on a once-a-day schedule
(D) has a cytoprotective effect
(E) has essentially no gastrointestinal side effects

22. Which of the following arylalkanoic acid derivatives might be particularly useful in an arthritic patient who has difficulty remembering to take his or her medication during the day?

(A) tolmetin (Tolectin)
(B) fenoprofen (Nalfon)
(C) ibuprofen (Motrin)
(D) naproxen (Naprosyn)
(E) diclofenac sodium (Voltaren)

23. When dispensing the fluorouracil solutions Fluoroplex or Efudex, the pharmacist should give the patient all of the following advice and warnings EXCEPT

(A) apply with a nonmetallic applicator or fingertips
(B) avoid prolonged exposure to sunlight
(C) avoid exposure to ultraviolet light
(D) cover infected area with an occlusive dressing after application
(E) burning sensation and inflammation may occur

24. Which of the following best described the condition known as hypoprothrombinemia?

(A) a diminished blood supply to the brain
(B) blood clot formation in a peripheral blood vessel

(C) a reduced capability for blood to clot
(D) a low level of iron in the blood
(E) a decrease in the production of red blood cells by the bone marrow

25. The reversal of anticoagulant-induced hypoprothrombinemia is most rapidly accomplished by the administration of
  I. phytonadione (AquaMEPHYTON)
  II. menadiol sodium diphosphate (Synkayvite)
  III. fresh blood or plasma

(A) I only
(B) III only
(C) I and II only
(D) II and III only
(E) I, II, and III

26. A patient complains of a reddish discoloration of his urine. Which of the following drugs would most likely produce such an effect?

(A) Gelusil
(B) Pyridium
(C) Gantrisin
(D) Darvon
(E) Mandelamine

27. Clomiphene citrate (Clomid) is used clinically in the treatment of

(A) psoriasis
(B) infertility
(C) nausea
(D) depression
(E) dysmenorrhea

28. The e.p.t. Stick Test, the home pregnancy test marketed by Warner-Lambert, assays for the presence of

(A) estradiol
(B) human chorionic gonadotropin
(C) progesterone
(D) prolactin
(E) estrogen

29. The clinical investigation of a new drug consists of four phases. Phase I of the clinical testing involves administering the drug

(A) to animals to determine the effectiveness of the drug
(B) to animals for toxicity studies
(C) by select clinicians to healthy volunteers
(D) by select clinicians to patients suffering from the disease
(E) by general practitioners to patients suffering from the disease

30. Which of the following best describes the common clinical manifestations of hypoparathyroidism?

(A) hypocalcemia and hypophosphatemia
(B) hypocalcemia and hyperphosphatemia
(C) hypercalcemia and hypophosphatemia
(D) hypercalcemia and hyperphosphatemia
(E) hypercalcemia and hypochlorhydria

31. Tubocurarine should NOT be used in patients who are taking

(A) aspirin
(B) morphine
(C) indomethacin
(D) levodopa
(E) gentamicin

32. Myxedema is what kind of state?

(A) hypothyroid
(B) hypoparathyroid
(C) hyperthyroid
(D) hyperparathyroid
(E) hypopituitarism

33. A person with normal thyroid function is called

(A) myxedematous
(B) basal
(C) euthyroid
(D) hypothyroid
(E) equithyroid

34. Which of the following should NOT be used in patients who are allergic to aspirin?

(A) Fiorinal
(B) Darvocet-N
(C) Excedrin PM
(D) Motrin
(E) Wygesic

35. Which of the following phrases best defines the clinical disorder known as hemochromatosis?

(A) a lack of circulating antibodies
(B) excessive storage of iron by the body
(C) abnormally shaped red blood cells
(D) diminished circulating blood volume
(E) absence of pigmentation in circulating red blood cells

36. A reversible cholestatic hepatitis with fever and jaundice has been observed as an adverse drug reaction in patients taking erythromycin

(A) stearate (Erythrocin Filmtab)
(B) ethylsuccinate (EES Granules)
(C) base (E-Mycitablets)
(D) estolate (Ilosone)
(E) gluceptate (Ilotycin)

37. The most important indication for vancomycin (Vancocin) is in the treatment of serious infections that do NOT respond to other treatment and that are caused by which of the following organisms?

(A) pneumococcal
(B) staphylococcal
(C) streptococcal
(D) gonococcal
(E) pseudomonal

38. Nizatidine (Axid) inhibits gastric acid secretion as a result of what kind of activity?

(A) anticholinergic
(B) antiadrenergic
(C) antihistaminic
(D) antianxiety
(E) anorectic

39. Benzylpenicilloyl-polylysine is a substance used to

(A) stabilize crystalline penicillin G preparations
(B) counteract allergic reactions to penicillin
(C) reduce the renal secretion of penicillin
(D) skin test patients for penicillin allergy
(E) manufacture the semisynthetic penicillins

40. A tricyclic amine that is used as an antiviral agent is

(A) desipramine (Norpramin, Pertofrane)
(B) amantadine (Symmetrel)
(C) 5-fluorouracil
(D) cytosine arabinoside (Cytarabine, Cytosar)
(E) idoxuridine (Herplex)

41. Ticarcillin may be preferred to carbenicillin for patients with congestive heart failure (CHF), renal failure, and hypertension because it

(A) contains less sodium than carbenicillin
(B) is usually given in smaller doses than carbenicillin
(C) does not induce hypokalemia
(D) stimulates renal blood flow
(E) has a broader spectrum than carbenicillin

42. Isoniazid (isonicotinic acid hydrazide, INH, Nydrazid) is an antitubercular agent. Which of the following statements is correct for isoniazid?

(A) should not be used in combination with other drugs
(B) one of the most effective antitubercular drugs
(C) pyridoxine antagonizes the antitubercular action
(D) not metabolized in the liver
(E) must be used alone; other antitubercular drugs are inhibitory

43. The purpose of combined drug treatment in tuberculosis is to
    I. reduce the duration of active therapy
    II. delay the emergence of drug resistance
    III. increase the tuberculostatic effects of the drugs

    (A) I only
    (B) III only
    (C) I and II only
    (D) II and III only
    (E) I, II, and III

44. Patients taking the antitubercular drug rifampin (Rifadin) should be told that the drug

    (A) may impart an orange color to their urine and sweat
    (B) may cause them to sunburn more easily
    (C) may produce nausea and vomiting if alcoholic beverages are consumed
    (D) may cause diarrhea
    (E) should be swallowed whole (ie, not chewed) to prevent staining of the teeth

45. Chloramphenicol (Chloromycetin) is indicated primarily in
    (A) typhoid fever
    (B) rheumatic fever
    (C) tuberculosis
    (D) yellow fever
    (E) amebiasis

46. A penicillin derivative that is most closely related to ampicillin but has a much greater activity against *Pseudomonas* is

    (A) methicillin (Staphcillin)
    (B) ticarcillin (Ticar)   — pseud.
    (C) nafcillin (Unipen)
    (D) dicloxacillin (Dynapen)
    (E) oxacillin (Prostaphlin)

47. Antibiotic-induced pseudomembranous colitis is most commonly treated with

    (A) attapulgite (Kaopectate)
    (B) vancomycin (Vancocin)
    (C) loperamide (Imodium)
    (D) gentamicin (Garamycin)
    (E) sulfasalazine (Azulfidine)

48. A Fanconi-like syndrome has been associated with the use of outdated and degraded

    (A) ampicillin
    (B) doxycycline   → nephrotox
    (C) tetracycline
    (D) chloramphenicol
    (E) clindamycin

49. The aminoglycoside antibiotics are
    I. bactericidal for a wide range of gram-positive and gram-negative microorganisms
    II. suitable for long-term treatment of chronic urinary tract infections
    III. metabolized by the liver

    (A) I only   kidney
    (B) III only
    (C) I and II only
    (D) II and III only
    (E) I, II, and III

50. Which one of the following cephalosporins is available in both oral and parenteral dosage forms?

    (A) cefaclor (Ceclor) PO 2nd
    (B) cephradine (Velosef) PO IV 1st
    (C) moxalactam (Moxam)
    (D) cefazolin (Ancef, Kefzol) no IV only 1st
    (E) cefotaxime (Claforan) IV 3rd

51. A disadvantage of using cromolyn sodium powder for asthma is

    (A) its brief duration of action
    (B) the development of rebound bronchoconstriction
    (C) the rapid development of tachyphylaxis
    (D) that it is ineffective in treating acute attacks
    (E) its poor GI absorption after administration of the capsule dosage form

52. An asthmatic patient who is currently taking Tedral tablets (t.i.d.), prednisone 5 mg (q.i.d.), and Medihaler-Iso (p.r.n.) gives you a prescription for Vanceril Inhaler. The directions on the prescription are "one inhalation p.r.n. breathing difficulty." The most appropriate action for you to take is to

    (A) fill the prescription
    (B) consult with the physician, advising him that Vanceril (beclomethasone) is a prophylactic drug that should be taken regularly
    (C) consult with the physician, advising him that the prednisone should be discontinued before Vanceril therapy is initiated
    (D) consult with the patient, advising him to stop using the Medihaler-Iso
    (E) carefully observe the patient for obvious signs of corticosteroid toxicity and consult with the physician if necessary

53. A common name for the antidiuretic hormone elaborated by the posterior pituitary gland is

    (A) norepinephrine
    (B) renin
    (C) luteotropic hormone
    (D) vasopressin
    (E) secretin

54. Which of the following is true of lithium carbonate (Eskalith, Lithane)?

(A) indicated in the treatment of severe manic-depressive psychoses

(B) may only be administered by the intramuscular route

(C) onset of action occurs within 2 hours of the first administered dose

(D) should be administered with a diuretic to minimize edema formation

(E) usually given to adult patients in single daily doses

55. Patients on lithium carbonate therapy should be advised

(A) to limit water intake

(B) to stop taking the drug if they experience mild side effects

(C) not to restrict their normal dietary salt intake

(D) not to take the drug during the manic phase of their cycle

(E) not to take the drug with food

56. Hemolytic anemia due to erythrocyte deficiency of glucose-6-phosphate dehydrogenase (G 6 PD) would most likely be precipitated by

(A) primaquine

(B) ascorbic acid

(C) isoniazid (INH)

(D) phenytoin (Dilantin)

(E) gentamicin (Garamycin)

57. The anticoagulant action of heparin is monitored by the

(A) complete blood count

(B) activated partial thromboplastin time

(C) prothrombin time

(D) bleeding time

(E) antiplatelet clotting time

58. Two hours after receiving his last dose of heparin (9000 units IV), a patient begins bleeding from his gums after brushing his teeth. What is the most appropriate therapeutic action?

(A) inject 10 mg of phytonadione (AquaMEPHYTON) intravenously

(B) inject 60 mg of protamine sulfate intravenously

(C) inject 30 mg of protamine sulfate intravenously

(D) swab a small amount of epinephrine 1:100 onto the gum tissue to produce local vasoconstriction

(E) wait for the anticoagulant effect to subside

59. A 40-year-old woman with a history of deep vein thrombosis is stabilized on 5 mg of warfarin daily. She is again admitted to the hospital because of a suspected duodenal ulcer. In addition to the drug listed below, her warfarin is maintained at 5 mg daily. After several days her prothrombin time increases from 27 seconds to 80 seconds (control value is 11 seconds). Which of her medications may be responsible for this increase in PT time?

(A) acetaminophen (Tylenol) 650 mg q4h

(B) cimetidine (Tagamet) 300 mg q.i.d.

(C) milk of magnesia 30 mL hs

(D) diazepam (Valium) 5 mg q.i.d.

(E) ampicillin (Omnipen) 250 mg q.i.d.

60. Which of the following would be considered to be a blood sugar concentration within normal limits for a fasting adult?

(A) 100 mg/dL

(B) 200 mg/dL

(C) 300 mg/dL

(D) 400 mg/dL

(E) 500 mg/dL

61. Which of the following drugs can interfere with the diagnosis of pernicious anemia?

(A) pyridoxine

(B) menadione

(C) thiamine

(D) ascorbic acid

(E) folic acid

62. The direct van den Bergh test measures

(A) conjugated bilirubin in the blood

(B) unconjugated bilirubin in the blood

(C) total bilirubin in the blood

(D) unconjugated bilirubin in the urine

(E) total bilirubin in the urine

63. A white cell differential count is a laboratory procedure that

(A) determines the relative proportions of the various white blood cells

(B) determines the relative proportions of white cells to red cells

(C) differentiates between iron-deficient and folic acid-deficient anemia

(D) differentiates immature from mature white blood cells

(E) differentiates normal from abnormal white blood cells

64. A patient who has recently suffered a myocardial infarction will most likely have elevated serum levels of

(A) creatine kinase (CK)

(B) amylase

(C) acid phosphatase

(D) alkaline phosphatase

(E) cholinesterase

65. The hematocrit (HCT) measures the

    (A) total number of blood cells per volume of blood
    (B) number of red blood cells per volume of blood
    (C) percentage of red blood cells per volume of blood
    (D) weight of hemoglobin per volume of blood
    (E) weight of red blood cells per volume of blood

66. Which of the following is NOT a white blood cell (or leukocyte)?

    (A) basophil
    (B) eosinophil   *Immature erythrocyte*
    (C) monocyte
    (D) reticulocyte
    (E) lymphocyte

67. A unit-dose package is one that contains

    (A) one discrete pharmaceutical dosage form (eg, one tablet, one ampule, etc)
    (B) solid dosage forms only
    (C) the exact amount of medication necessary to fill a prescription (eg, 30 tablets in a sealed container)
    (D) the exact dose of a drug ordered for a given patient
    (E) a 24-hour supply of a specific drug that is sent to a nursing unit

68. Reagent strips impregnated with glucose oxidase, peroxidase, and orthotolidine are dipped into urine or blood as a test for the presence of glucose. The reaction(s) that occur are

    (A) glucose is oxidized to CO, which forms carbonic acid, which turns the orthotolidine a blue color
    (B) glucose oxidase is reduced to glucose reductase, which converts glucose to a blue color in the presence of orthotolidine and peroxidase
    (C) glucose is oxidized to gluconic acid and hydrogen peroxide, then hydrogen peroxide in the presence of peroxidase converts the orthotolidine to a blue substance
    (D) sucrose is oxidized by glucose oxidase to glucose, which is oxidized to glucuronic acid by peroxidase and orthotolidine to form a dye
    (E) glucose oxidase and atmospheric oxygen oxidize glucose to aldehyde, which undergoes a Schiff test reaction with orthotolidine and peroxidase to yield colored compounds

69. Which of the following is specific for the measurement of glucose?

    (A) Benedict's solution   *copper reduction*
    (B) Acetest tablets
    (C) Clinitest tablets
    (D) Tes-Tape
    (E) Ketostix   *Ketones*

70. The intentional administration of intravenous fluids into subcutaneous tissue is called

    (A) infiltration
    (B) venoclysis
    (C) hypodermoclysis
    (D) hemodialysis
    (E) hemolysis

71. Intermittent IV therapy is used to

    I. avoid anticipated or potential stability or compatibility problems
    II. reduce the potential of thrombophlebitis
    III. promote better diffusion of some drugs into tissues because of a greater concentration gradient

    (A) I only
    (B) III only
    (C) I and II only
    (D) II and III only
    (E) I, II, and III

72. Parenterally administered electrolytes are usually ordered in

    (A) equivalents
    (B) milliequivalents (mEq)   *Ionic*
    (C) milligrams percent (mg %, or mg/dL)
    (D) millimoles
    (E) micrograms (μg)

73. A drug information source that consists of microfiche copies of papers published in medical and pharmaceutical journals is

    (A) *Current Contents / Clinical Practice*
    (B) *de Haen Drug Information Systems*
    (C) *Index Medicus*
    (D) *International Pharmaceutical Abstracts*
    (E) *Iowa Drug Information Service*

74. Which of the following reference sources would be appropriate to use to find an American equivalent of a British drug?

    (A) *Facts and Comparisons*
    (B) *Martindale's Extra Pharmacopoeia*
    (C) *USPDI*
    (D) *AHFS Drug Information*
    (E) *United States Pharmacopoeia*

75. Generally, drug literature abstracts are most appropriately used to

    (A) provide the individual requesting the information with written documentation
    (B) provide detailed answers to specific questions
    (C) answer general questions
    (D) provide a rapid response to questions
    (E) identify those articles likely to contain the desired information

76. Kernicterus is a drug-induced disorder that may occur in the neonate following therapy with which of the following drugs?

  (A) isoniazid (INH)
  (B) sulfisoxazole (Gantrisin)
  (C) phenytoin (Dilantin)
  (D) gentamicin (Garamycin)
  (E) promethazine (Phenergan)

77. Generally, the presence of impaired renal function or overt renal failure in a patient reduces his requirements for
  I. all drugs
  II. drugs that are reabsorbed from the kidney tubules
  III. drugs that are directly excreted or whose active metabolites are excreted by the kidneys

  (A) I only
  (B) III only
  (C) I and II only
  (D) II and III only
  (E) I, II, and III

78. A common result of "slow metabolic acetylation" of isoniazid is

  (A) enhanced sensitivity to therapy and toxicity
  (B) peripheral neuropathy that is resistant to pyridoxine therapy
  (C) slow metabolism and reduced therapeutic response
  (D) slow metabolism and enhanced therapeutic response
  (E) slow acetylation but normal therapeutic response

79. Electrolytes should NOT be added to intravenous solutions of amphotericin B (Fungizone) because
  I. they will precipitate (salt out) the drug
  II. they will lower the pH and hasten the decomposition of the drug
  III. the solution is hypertonic by itself

  (A) I only
  (B) III only
  (C) I and II only
  (D) II and III only
  (E) I, II, and III

80. The level of which of the following enzymes would be elevated in acute pancreatitis?

  (A) alkaline phosphatase
  (B) acid phosphatase
  (C) lactic dehydrogenase
  (D) creatinine phosphokinase
  (E) amylase

81. The cation most prevalent in the extracellular fluid of the human body is

  (A) sodium
  (B) chloride
  (C) magnesium
  (D) phosphate
  (E) potassium

Extra Na
Intra K

82. The cation present in the highest concentration in intracellular water is

  (A) calcium
  (B) chloride
  (C) magnesium
  (D) potassium
  (E) sodium

83. The blood concentration of which of the following cations would normally rise if a patient became hypophosphatemic?

  (A) phosphorus
  (B) magnesium
  (C) potassium
  (D) iron
  (E) calcium

84. Pyrantel pamoate (Antiminth)
  I. may be used to treat trichinosis
  II. is available only as an oral suspension
  III. is taken for 7 days

  (A) I only
  (B) III only
  (C) I and II only
  (D) II and III only
  (E) I, II, and III

85. Large overdoses of acetaminophen are likely to cause

  (A) tinnitis
  (B) hepatic necrosis
  (C) agranulocytosis
  (D) renal tubular acidosis
  (E) seizures

86. An adult patient who ingested 30 acetaminophen tablets (325 mg/tablet) 6 hours ago should be treated with/by

  (A) careful observation for signs of central nervous system toxicity
  (B) ipecac syrup
  (C) activated charcoal
  (D) N-acetylcysteine
  (E) glutathione

87. Which of the following is(are) correct descriptions of sulfasalazine (Azulfidine)?
    I. available as oral tablets and injection
    II. poor absorption from GI tract
    III. used in treating ulcerative colitis and regional enteritis

    (A) I only
    (B) III only
    (C) I and II only
    (D) II and III only
    (E) I, II, and III

88. Asthmatic patients with a documented allergy to aspirin should NOT receive

    (A) propoxyphene (Darvon)
    (B) acetaminophen (Tylenol)
    (C) ibuprofen (Motrin)
    (D) pentazocine (Talwin)
    (E) nalbuphine (Nubain)

89. Patients who have a history of penicillin allergy should also be suspected of exhibiting a possible allergy to

    (A) sulfonamides
    (B) cephalosporins
    (C) tetracyclines
    (D) aminoglycosides
    (E) chloramphenicol

90. Which of the following agents would be most dangerous to use in a patient already receiving high doses of gentamicin?

    (A) ethacrynic acid (Edecrin)
    (B) tetracycline HCl
    (C) propantheline bromide (Pro-Banthine)
    (D) HydroDIURIL
    (E) pentobarbital sodium

91. A patient arriving in a hospital emergency room suffering from severe hypertensive crisis would most likely be treated initially with

    (A) guanethidine (Ismelin)
    (B) methyldopa (Aldomet)
    (C) reserpine (Serpasil)
    (D) hydrochlorothiazide (Esidrix)
    (E) diazoxide (Hyperstat IV)

92. Which of the following should be considered as part of the initial drug therapy of most hypertensive patients?

    (A) verapamil (Calan, Isoptin)
    (B) methyldopa (Aldomet)
    (C) a thiazide diuretic
    (D) hydralazine (Apresoline)
    (E) guanethidine (Ismelin)

93. Which of the following antihypertensive drugs should be administered by slow intravenous infusion?

    (A) minoxidil (Loniten)
    (B) clonidine (Catapres)
    (C) hydralazine (Apresoline)
    (D) prazosin (Minipress)
    (E) nitroprusside (Nipride)

94. Food containing tyramine should NOT be part of the diet of patients taking which of the following antihypertensive agents?

    (A) reserpine (Serpasil)
    (B) hydralazine (Apresoline)
    (C) isocarboxazid (Parnate)
    (D) methyldopa (Aldomet)
    (E) fosinopril (Monopril)

95. Which of the following symptoms would be LEAST likley to be exhibited by a patient suffering from diabetes mellitus?

    (A) urinary retention
    (B) excessive thirst
    (C) glycosuria
    (D) weight loss
    (E) weakness

96. Which of the following agents would most logically be given to a patient suffering from hypoparathyroidism?

    (A) alpha-tocopherol
    (B) pantothenic acid
    (C) ergocalciferol
    (D) nicotinamide
    (E) phytonadione

97. Which of the following therapeutic agents is specifically contraindicated for use in patients who have bronchial asthma?

    (A) propranolol (Inderal)
    (B) quinidine
    (C) procainamide (Pronestyl)
    (D) digoxin
    (E) chlorpromazine (Thorazine)

98. Which of the following phenothiazines is LEAST likely to produce extrapyramidal side effects?

    (A) chlorpromazine (Thorazine)
    (B) perphenazine (Trilafon)
    (C) prochlorperazine (Compazine)
    (D) thioridazine (Mellaril)
    (E) trifluoperazine (Stelazine)

99. Which of the following potential adverse effects of the phenothiazines is thought to be irreversible?

(A) akathisia
(B) muscular rigidity
(C) tremor
(D) orthostatic hypotension
(E) tardive dyskinesia

100. A middle-aged female patient is at the prescription counter to pick up her first refill on a chlorpromazine (Thorazine) prescription. She is also about to purchase a bottle of aspirin, which she says is for her fever. She asks you what you would recommend for a "sore throat" she has had for several days. Having this information you would

(A) tell the patient that she is allergic to chlorpromazine and contact the patient's physician
(B) recommend a cough-cold preparation that does not contain a sympathomimetic
(C) contact the patient's physician and discuss the possibility of chlorpromazine-induced agranulocytosis
(D) tell the patient to see her doctor if her fever and sore throat do not improve in a day or two
(E) inquire about these symptoms the next time the patient comes in to refill the prescription

101. The antiemetic effect of which of the following drugs is the result of increased gastric emptying?

(A) amitriptyline (Elavil)
(B) benztropine (Cogentin)
(C) codeine
(D) metoclopramide (Reglan)
(E) aluminum hydroxide gel (Amphojel)

102. A pharmacist should suggest that suppositories made with what substance as the base be moistened with water before insertion?
   I. Carbowax
   II. glycerinated gelatin
   III. theobroma oil

(A) I only
(B) III only
(C) I and II only
(D) II and III only
(E) I, II, and III

103. The expectorant dose of ipecac syrup for an adult would be approximately

(A) 1 mL
(B) 5 mL
(C) 10 mL
(D) 15 mL
(E) 30 mL

104. Which one of the following cough syrups should NOT be suggested to a diabetic patient?

(A) Cerose-DM
(B) Dimetane-DX
(C) Tussar SF
(D) Robitussin-PE
(E) Hycomine

105. A pharmacist tells a young mother about clinical (fever) thermometers. He advises her to report to the pediatrician both the degrees of temperature and whether the temperature was taken rectally or orally. This is good advice because

(A) oral temperature is about one degree Fahrenheit above rectal temperature
(B) oral thermometers have degree calibrations that differ from rectal thermometers
(C) rectal temperature is about one degree Fahrenheit above oral temperature
(D) the normal temperature (marked with an arrow) is 99.6° F on the rectal thermometer and 98.6° F on the oral one
(E) the bulb on the rectal thermometer is round and contains more mercury than in the thin cylindrical bulb of the oral thermometer

106. The best emergency advice that a pharmacist could give an individual who has just suffered a minor burn is to

(A) apply butter to the burn
(B) apply Vaseline to the burn
(C) contact a physician immediately
(D) immerse the burned area in warm water followed by cold water
(E) immerse the burned area in cold water

107. Angle-closure glaucoma is present in approximately what percentage of the total glaucoma population?

(A) 10
(B) 25
(C) 50
(D) 75
(E) 95

108. The miotic effect of pilocarpine after instillation into the eye is observed

(A) immediately
(B) within 1 minute
(C) in 2 to 4 hours
(D) in 15 to 30 minutes
(E) after 1 hour

109. The number 20 in Ocusert Pilo-20 refers to the

(A) duration of action of one Ocusert in days
(B) strength of the preparation as a percentage
(C) strength of the preparation in milligrams
(D) rate of release of drug from the Ocusert
(E) number of dosage units (Ocuserts) per original container

110. Which of the following should NOT be administered to a patient being treated for narrow-angle glaucoma?

(A) physostigmine
(B) pilocarpine
(C) phospholine iodide
(D) homatropine
(E) carbachol

111. Advantage(s) of timolol maleate (Timoptic) over pilocarpine for the reduction of elevated intraocular pressure include(s)

I. longer duration of activity
II. little or no effect on visual acuity or accommodation
III. little or no effect on pupil size

(A) I only
(B) III only
(C) I and II only
(D) II and III only
(E) I, II, and III

112. All of the following drugs are used to treat patients with open-angle glaucoma EXCEPT

(A) carbachol
(B) atropine
(C) demecarium
(D) physostigmine
(E) betaxolol

113. Epinephrine is a useful drug for lowering intraocular pressure in open-angle glaucoma because it

(A) increases outflow of aqueous humor and inhibits the formation of aqueous humor
(B) causes miosis
(C) causes mydriasis
(D) inhibits carbonic anhydrase
(E) dilates blood vessels in the eye

114. Scabies is a contagious skin disease caused by a

(A) flea
(B) fungus
(C) mite
(D) protozoa
(E) tick

115. Psoriasis is characterized by

(A) granulomatous lesions
(B) nodules

(C) silvery gray scales
(D) small red vesicles
(E) small water-filled blisters

116. A patient with a documented allergy to morphine should NOT receive which of the following analgesics?

(A) meperidine (Demerol)
(B) pentazocine (Talwin)
(C) codeine
(D) methadone (Dolophine)
(E) butorphanol (Stadol)

117. The number 5 in Transderm-Nitro 5 refers to the

(A) half-life of the preparation in hours
(B) surface area of the patch
(C) nitroglycerin content (mg) of the product
(D) amount of nitroglycerin released over a 24-hour period
(E) equivalent amount of nitroglycerin ointment in inches

118. The claimed purpose for including vitamin C in various hematinic preparations such as Fero-Grad-500, Fergon Plus, and Vitron C is to

(A) enhance iron absorption
(B) correct the vitamin C deficiency that accompanies iron deficiency
(C) prevent gastrointestinal side effects of iron
(D) prevent the unabsorbed iron from darkening the stool
(E) increase the rate of formation of hemoglobin

119. Which of the following antihypertensive agents is available in a transdermal patch dosage form?

(A) clonidine (Catapres)
(B) guanethidine (Ismelin)
(C) terazosin (Hytrin)
(D) lisinopril (Zestril)
(E) penbutolol (Levatol)

120. Ideally, an antacid should raise the pH of the stomach contents to a value of approximately

(A) 3.5
(B) 5.5
(C) 6.5
(D) 7.5
(E) 9.5

121. Which of the following drugs is used in conjunction with levodopa (Dopar, Larodopa), specifically to allow a reduction in the dose of levodopa?

(A) pyridoxine
(B) carbidopa
(C) tyrosine
(D) diphenhydramine (Benadryl)
(E) promethazine (Phenergan)

122. A patient with Parkinson's disease has been receiving levodopa (1 g four times daily) with fairly good response but excessive side effects. The patient's physician wishes to switch from levodopa to Sinemet. An approximate dose of Sinemet would be

(A) one 10/100 tablet daily
(B) one 10/100 tablet four times daily
(C) one 25/250 tablet daily
(D) one 25/250 tablet four times daily
(E) four 25/250 tablets four times daily

123. A patient is being effectively treated for Parkinson's disease with levodopa. Suddenly, all therapeutic benefits of the levodopa are lost and the adverse effects also disappear. Which of the following facts obtained from a medication history would most likely explain this phenomenon?

(A) the patient has forgotten to take two doses of the medication
(B) antacids were taken occasionally
(C) trihexyphenidyl was added to the drug regimen for 1 week
(D) over-the-counter multivitamins were taken toward off a cold that winter
(E) the patient occasionally drank some whiskey

124. If the patient in the preceding question was especially affected by early morning symptoms of stiffness and rigidity, which of the following anticholinergics might be of value?

(A) benztropine mesylate (Cogentin)
(B) trihexyphenidyl HCl (Artane)
(C) ethopropazine HCl (Parsidol)
(D) orphenadrine HCl (Norflex)
(E) procyclidine HCl (Kemadrin)

125. Which of the following drugs is associated with the "gray syndrome" in infants?

(A) phenytoin
(B) chloramphenicol
(C) demeclocycline
(D) amphotericin B
(E) kanamycin

126. Stomatitis refers to an inflammation of the

(A) eyelid
(B) nasal passages
(C) oral mucosa
(D) stomach wall
(E) tongue

127. An obese individual would most likely be suffering from

(A) alopecia
(B) hirsutism
(C) polyphagia

(D) urticaria
(E) nystagmus

128. Hypertrophy refers to

(A) an abnormal increase in the number of cells in a tissue
(B) an enlargement or overgrowth of an organ
(C) excessive perspiration
(D) increased motor activity
(E) excessive sensitivity of the skin

129. Dyspnea refers to

(A) difficult or labored breathing
(B) difficulty in swallowing
(C) impairment of digestive function
(D) painful or difficult urination
(E) restlessness

130. All of the following terms directly relate to body muscles EXCEPT

(A) myalgia
(B) myocardia
(C) myoclonus
(D) myopia
(E) myositis

131. Ischemia refers to

(A) a deficiency of blood in a part of the body
(B) excessive collection of blood in an area
(C) a jaundice condition
(D) nodules usually located on the back
(E) a red, inflamed patch of skin

132. Stenosis refers to

(A) hardening of tissues with a loss of elasticity
(B) inflammation of the sternum
(C) inflammation of the vertebrae
(D) narrowing or stricture of a duct or canal
(E) stoppage of blood flow in a part of the body

133. Phlebitis is most closely associated with which type of injections?

(A) intradermal
(B) intramuscular
(C) intravenous
(D) subcutaneous
(E) both intramuscular and intravenous

134. A 60-year-old patient with congestive heart failure who has been stabilized for 3 months on digoxin, hydrochlorothiazide, and potassium chloride is gradually placed on the following additional medicines. Which of these drugs may cause a problem?

    (A) quinidine
    (B) temazepam (Restoril)
    (C) captopril (Capoten)
    (D) aspirin
    (E) nitroglycerin

135. Which of the following diuretics would be LEAST likely to produce a hypokalemic effect in a patient?

    (A) hydrochlorothiazide (Esidrix)
    (B) amiloride (Midamor)
    (C) chlorthalidone (Hygroton)
    (D) furosemide (Lasix)
    (E) ethacrynic acid (Edecrin)

136. Mannitol is used therapeutically primarily as a(n)

    (A) cardiac stimulant
    (B) sucrose substitute
    (C) osmotic diuretic
    (D) antianginal agent
    (E) plasma expander

137. The tricyclic antidepressant imipramine (Tofranil) has been approved by the FDA for use in the treatment of

    (A) enuresis
    (B) Parkinson's disease
    (C) hypertension
    (D) peptic ulcer
    (E) mild anxiety states

138. Chenodiol (Chenix) has been approved for use in

    (A) reducing serum cholesterol levels
    (B) dissolving cholesterol gallstones
    (C) mobilizing heavy metal poisons
    (D) disintegrating kidney stones
    (E) quantifying urine cholesterol

139. Cyclosporin (Sandimmune) is a(n)

    (A) aminoglycoside antibiotic
    (B) third-generation cephalosporin
    (C) immunosuppressant
    (D) fungicide
    (E) prostaglandin analog

140. A potential problem of using nalbuphine (Nubain) in a patient who is dependent on codeine is

    (A) additive respiratory depression
    (B) precipitation of narcotic withdrawal symptoms
    (C) increased tolerance to codeine
    (D) impaired renal excretion of codeine
    (E) excessive central nervous system stimulation

141. The advantage naltrexone (Trexan) has over naloxone (Narcan) is

    (A) its more rapid onset of action
    (B) its longer duration of action
    (C) its availability as sublingual tablets
    (D) that it does not have to be reconstituted immediately before use
    (E) it is not addictive

142. Focal convulsions are usually associated with which of the following types of epilepsy?

    (A) grand mal
    (B) petit mal
    (C) Jacksonian
    (D) psychomotor
    (E) status epilepticus

143. Polycythemia refers to an elevated number of

    (A) leukocytes
    (B) erythrocytes
    (C) thrombocytes
    (D) reticulocytes
    (E) granulocytes

144. In treating excessive heparin therapy with protamine sulfate, caution must be exercised to avoid using more protamine than is necessary because

    (A) protamine sulfate is toxic in small amounts
    (B) protamine sulfate is also an anticoagulant
    (C) the production of endogenous heparin will be stimulated
    (D) the strongly basic protamine will produce alkalosis
    (E) protamine sulfate is a local anesthetic

145. If a patient on oral anticoagulant therapy experiences mild to moderate bleeding, the desirability of administering vitamin K should be carefully weighed against the underlying need for anticoagulant therapy because

    (A) the use of vitamin K will make it much more difficult to retitrate the patient on the oral anticoagulant
    (B) vitamin K will displace the oral anticoagulant from protein-binding sites and produce a transient increase in anticoagulant effect
    (C) it requires a minimum of 18 hours for vitamin K to become effective
    (D) rapid correction of vitamin K deficiency may precipitate thromboembolism
    (E) if anticoagulant therapy is to be resumed, an oral anticoagulant having a different mode of action will have to be used

146. Which of the following anticoagulants would be the best choice for use in a pregnant patient near the anticipated time of delivery?

    (A) bishydroxycoumarin (Dicumarol)
    (B) warfarin (Coumadin, Panwarfin)
    (C) heparin
    (D) aspirin
    (E) dipyridamole (Persantine)

147. Heparin Sodium USP should always be ordered by the physician in units rather than milligrams because

    (A) heparin syringes are calibrated in units only
    (B) it is difficult to measure milligrams accurately
    (C) a conversion table is difficult to use
    (D) many different strengths are available
    (E) the use of a standard units/mL of preparation gives a more reproducible dose

148. The prothrombin time of patients on anticoagulant therapy with coumarin derivatives will be decreased by

    (A) clofibrate (Atromid-S)
    (B) metronidazole (Flagyl)
    (C) heparin
    (D) phenylbutazone (Butazolidin)
    (E) vitamin K

149. The Schilling Test is useful for the detection of pernicious anemia. This test utilizes orally administered

    (A) vitamin B_{12} labeled with ^{59}Fe
    (B) intrinsic factor labeled with ^{59}Fe
    (C) vitamin B_{12} with ^{57}Co or ^{58}Co
    (D) red blood cells labeled with ^{59}Fe
    (E) intrinsic factor labeled with ^{57}Co

150. Which of the following drugs is a dopamine agonist used to treat hyperprolactinemia?

    (A) chlorpromazine (Thorazine)
    (B) bromocriptine (Parlodel)
    (C) benztropine (Cogentin)
    (D) diphenhydramine (Benadryl)
    (E) ascorbic acid

151. The only insulin preparation that can be given intravenously is

    (A) lente insulin
    (B) protamine zinc insulin
    (C) crystalline zinc (regular) insulin
    (D) isophane insulin
    (E) prompt insulin zinc

152. Which of the following insulins would be expected to exert the longest duration of action?

    (A) semilente
    (B) NPH
    (C) protamine zinc

    (D) lente
    (E) regular

153. The most common cause of diabetic ketoacidosis and coma in the diagnosed and treated diabetic is

    (A) insulin overdosage
    (B) failure of the patient to use insulin properly
    (C) electrolyte depletion
    (D) use of the wrong type of insulin
    (E) excessive physical activity

154. A diabetic patient has been taking cefaclor (Ceclor) 500 mg PO every 8 hours for a urinary tract infection. To determine whether this drug is interfering with the patient's urine glucose testing, a sample of urine is tested by both the Clinitest and the Tes-Tape methods. The results are 1% with Clinitest and 0.25% with Tes-Tape. The most appropriate conclusion from these data is that there is

    (A) no drug interference
    (B) a false-positive with Clintest
    (C) a false-positive with Tes-Tape
    (D) a false-negative with Clinitest
    (E) a false-negative with Tes-Tape

155. A mixture of regular insulin and PZI in a ratio of less than 1:1 would be expected to have about the same duration of action as

    (A) the individual components of the mixture because there is no interaction
    (B) NPH insulin because some free regular insulin will be present
    (C) PZI alone because the excess protamine in PZI will bind essentially all of the regular insulin, thereby converting it to PZI
    (D) lente insulin because lente insulin is made from these components in this specific ratio
    (E) PZI alone if neutral regular insulin is used

156. Which of the following benzodiazepines would be preferred as an anxiolytic drug for an elderly patient with a history of cirrhosis?

    (A) chlordiazepoxide (Librium)
    (B) diazepam (Valium)
    (C) clorazepate (Tranxene)
    (D) lorazepam (Ativan)
    (E) prazepam (Centrax)

157. Which of the following drugs is particularly useful for the treatment of acute hypoglycemic reactions when oral or intravenous administration of glucose is not possible?

    (A) adrenocorticotropic hormone
    (B) glucagon
    (C) protamine
    (D) pancreatin
    (E) norepinephrine

158. Doses of 6-mercaptopurine (Purinethol) should be reduced in patients taking allopurinol (Zyloprim) because allopurinol

(A) enhances the absorption of 6-mercaptopurine
(B) inhibits the renal excretion of 6-mercaptopurine
(C) releases 6-mercaptopurine from protein-binding sites
(D) inhibits the metabolism of 6-mercaptopurine
(E) inhibits tubular secretion of 6-mercaptopurine

159. A patient is admitted to the ER with marked hypotension and appears to be in shock. The drug of choice to treat the condition is probably

(A) dobutamine
(B) dopamine HCl
(C) epinephrine HCl
(D) nitroglycerine
(E) nitroprusside

160. When treating a patient with dopamine infusion, which of the following procedures should be followed if the patient's blood pressure increases to 165/100?

(A) Discontinue the infusion.
(B) Increase the infusion rate.
(C) Administer a hypotensive agent.
(D) Discontinue dopamine and start dobutamine.
(E) Continue the infusion while closely monitoring the patient.

161. The erythrocytes of an iron-deficient patient would be described as

(A) microcytic and hyperchromic
(B) macrocytic and hypochromic
(C) microcytic and hypochromic
(D) macrocytic and hyperchromic
(E) normocytic and hyperchromic

162. Which of the following is considered to be the drug of choice for treating trigeminal neuralgia (tic douloureux)?

(A) niacin (nicotinic acid)
(B) pentazocine (Talwin)
(C) isoniazid (INH)
(D) carbamazepine (Tegretol)
(E) hydroxyzine HCl (Atarax)

163. Parkinsonism is a disease characterized by four clinical features. Which one of the following is NOT typical of parkinsonism?

(A) tremor
(B) mental deterioration
(C) disturbances of posture
(D) bradykinesia
(E) rigidity

164. Lomotil should NOT be given to patients taking oral clindamycin because

(A) toxic effects of clindamycin may be enhanced
(B) adsorption of clindamycin will occur
(C) an insoluble complex will be formed
(D) the rate of hydrolytic destruction of clindamycin in the GI tract will increase
(E) none of the above

165. An advantage of loperamide (Imodium) over diphenoxylate (Lomotil) as an antidiarrheal is the fact that loperamide

(A) has a relatively short biologic half-life and is therefore not as likely to be abused
(B) has a direct effect on the central nervous system and therefore works more rapidly than diphenoxylate
(C) does not appear to have opiate-like effects
(D) is not a controlled substance
(E) can be given parenterally

166. Tricyclic antidepressants should NOT be used in patients also taking

(A) hydrochlorothiazide
(B) methyldopa (Aldomet)
(C) hydralazine (Apresoline)
(D) guanethidine (Ismelin)
(E) furosemide (Lasix)

167. Side effects of cyclobenzaprine (Flexeril) would be expected to be most similar to the side effects of

(A) amitriptyline (Elavil)
(B) dantrolene (Dantrium)
(C) diazepam (Valium)
(D) meprobamate (Equanil)
(E) methocarbamol (Robaxin)

168. Drug-induced neonatal jaundice can be treated with

(A) intravenous solutions to dilute the bilirubin
(B) calcium gluconate
(C) albumin
(D) dexamethasone (Decadron)
(E) phenobarbital

169. The initiation of therapy with which of the following agents would be LEAST likely to cause therapeutic problems in a patient already taking warfarin (Coumadin)?

(A) metronidazole
(B) chlorpheniramine maleate
(C) phenytoin
(D) aspirin
(E) cimetidine

170. A patient taking tranylcypromine (Parnate) wishes to have you recommend an over-the-counter cold remedy. Which of the following cold remedy ingredients should this patient avoid?

(A) chlorpheniramine maleate
(B) aspirin
(C) caffeine
(D) acetaminophen
(E) phenylephrine HCl

171. A nutritional product is said to contain 18 g of protein, 14 g of carbohydrate, and 10 g of fat in each 100-mL serving. The caloric content of a serving would be

(A) 218 kcal
(B) 198 kcal
(C) 238 kcal
(D) 168 kcal
(E) 378 kcal

172. Portagen is a dietary product used to treat patients with

(A) milk allergy
(B) diabetes mellitus
(C) steatorrhea
(D) calcium deficiencies
(E) kidney failure

173. An electrolyte supplement used to replenish electrolytes lost as a consequence of a diarrheal condition is

(A) Pedialyte
(B) K-Lyte
(C) Isomil
(D) Kaon
(E) Kayexalate

174. Parenteral administration of 1 L of 5% dextrose in water provides the patient with approximately how many kilocalories of energy?

(A) 100 to 125
(B) 170 to 200
(C) 400 to 450
(D) 800 to 850
(E) 1000

175. Lofenalac is a dietary product used in patients suffering from

(A) celiac disease
(B) pancreatic insufficiency
(C) steatorrhea
(D) phenylketonuria
(E) hyperlipidemia

176. Six weeks ago, a 32-year-old female patient with a history of recurrent urinary tract infections was treated with a 10-day course of ampicillin (250 mg q6h) for an *E. coli* urinary tract infection. She now presents with signs and symptoms of another UTI. Pending culture and sensitivity results, this patient should be started on

(A) gentamicin (Garamycin)
(B) trimethoprim-sulfamethoxazole (Bactrim)
(C) tetracycline (Achromycin)
(D) ampicillin (Omnipen)
(E) nitrofurantoin (Macrodantin)

177. Which of the following would be a good alternative to penicillin V in a pregnant patient allergic to penicillins?

I. demeclocycline (Declomycin)
II. trimethoprime (Trimpex)
III. erythromycin (Ilotycin)

(A) I only
(B) III only
(C) I and II only
(D) II and III only
(E) I, II, and III

178. Which of the following sulfonamides is best suited for the topical prophylactic treatment of burns?

(A) sulfacetamide (Sulamyd)
(B) sulfasalazine (Azulfidine)
(C) sulfisoxazole (Gantrisin)
(D) sulfamethoxazole (Gantanol)
(E) mafenide (Sulfamylon)

179. Which of the following drugs would be most appropriate to use for the treatment of gonorrhea in a poorly compliant patient with a documented penicillin allergy?

(A) amoxicillin (Polymox)
(B) spectinomycin (Spectrobid)
(C) tetracycline (Achromycin)
(D) clindamycin (Cleocin)
(E) piperacillin (Pipracil)

180. Which of the following drugs used in the treatment of gout does NOT affect urate metabolism or excretion?

I. allopurinol (Zyloprim)
II. probenecid (Benemid)
III. colchicine

(A) I only
(B) III only
(C) I and II only
(D) II and III only
(E) I, II, and III

181. A pharmacist wishes to dispense Opticrom 4% ophthalmic solution for use by a patient. Which of the following is true of this drug product?

    (A) It is used on a p.r.n. basis to control ophthalmic fungal infections.
    (B) It is administered at regular intervals to treat herpes simplex keratitis.
    (C) It is administered at regular intervals to treat cataracts.
    (D) It is administered on a p.r.n. basis to treat bacterial infections.
    (E) It is administered at regular intervals to treat allergic ocular disorders.

182. Thiazides may produce

    (A) reduced glucose tolerance
    (B) hyperkalemia
    (C) decreased blood levels of uric acid
    (D) hypernatremia
    (E) increased renal excretion of ammonia

183. An important advantage of using dopamine (Intropin) in cardiogenic shock is that dopamine

    (A) will not cross the blood–brain barrier and cause CNS effects
    (B) has no effects on alpha and beta receptors
    (C) produces dose-dependent increases in cardiac output and renal perfusion
    (D) will not increase blood pressure
    (E) can be given orally

184. A patient experiencing acute alcohol withdrawal is given 100 mg of chlordiazepoxide (Librium) intramuscularly. Because of an inadequate response, he is given another 100-mg IM dose in 30 minutes and a third 100-mg IM dose in another 30 minutes. Several hours later the patient becomes extremely ataxic and stuporous. These symptoms (ataxia and stupor) are most likely due to

    (A) the short duration of activity of the chlordiazepoxide
    (B) delayed absorption of relatively large amounts of drug
    (C) the combined effects of alcohol and chlordiazepoxide
    (D) the ineffectiveness of chlordiazepoxide in acute alcohol withdrawal
    (E) toxicity of the "special" diluent in which the drug is reconstituted

185. A patient who has been stabilized on 300 mg of Dilantin Kapseals once daily is having difficulty swallowing capsules. His physician writes a new prescription for Dilantin suspension 300 mg once daily. This change is likely to

    (A) reduce the phenytoin level because of decreased bioavailability from the suspension
    (B) increase the phenytoin level because of increased bioavailability from the suspension
    (C) have no impact on the phenytoin level
    (D) increase the phenytoin level because the 300-mg dose of suspension contains more of the active form of the drug
    (E) decrease the phenytoin level because the 300-mg dose of suspension contains less of the active form of the drug

186. Dobutamine (Dobutrex) is a(n)

    (A) general anesthetic drug
    (B) hypoglycemic drug
    (C) beta-adrenergic agonist
    (D) antihypertensive drug
    (E) antirheumatic drug

187. A patient for whom you dispensed a new prescription for amitriptyline (Elavil) (25 mg t.i.d.) 4 days ago returns to your pharmacy and complains that the drug makes him or her very sleepy, makes his or her mouth very dry, and has not helped his or her depression at all. These symptoms

    (A) indicate that amitriptyline is not effective for this patient and suggest you should inform the prescribing physician
    (B) strongly suggest that an anticholinergic drug is needed, which you should indicate to the prescribing physician
    (C) are expected effects of early treatment of the drug, which you should explain to the patient
    (D) indicate early signs of toxicity and suggest you should tell the patient to contact the prescribing physician
    (E) suggest that the patient is taking the entire daily dose at one time

188. A diabetic recovering from surgery receives insulin continuously by slow intravenous infusion in successive liter bottles of 5% dextrose in water. Urinary glucose tests indicate that blood glucose was markedly elevated after the first liter was administered. Similar testing after the second and third IVs were administered indicated noticeably improved control of blood glucose. Assuming that the insulin dose was initially adjusted for the stress of surgery, the hyperglycemia following the first IV was probably due to

(A) inadequate insulin dosing
(B) the initial loading of the circulatory system with glucose from the IV dextrose
(C) error in quantity of insulin added to the first IV
(D) adsorption of insulin on the bottle and tubing
(E) rapid diuresis in response to the initial fluid load followed by an apparent hyperglycemia

189. A diabetic patient tells you that he or she is planning a 4-week trip to Europe and will not have continued access to a refrigerator in which to store insulin. What information would you give him or her?

(A) store the insulin in a small styrofoam box that can be kept cold with several ice cubes
(B) be sure that insulin is available wherever you travel and purchase a fresh vial at least every third day
(C) the insulin will remain stable at room temperature during the time period in which a single vial will be used
(D) increase your insulin dose by 10% to account for any deterioration
(E) see your doctor to prescribe a mixture of insulins that will be more stable

190. The following "sliding scale" insulin coverage is ordered on a hospitalized diabetic:

4 +   10 units
3 +   8 units
2 +   6 units
1 +   4 units

Four additional units of insulin are added for large amounts of ketones, two units for moderate amounts of ketones, and no additional insulin for small amounts of ketones. The patient's urine testing results are as follows:

	7 AM	11 AM	4 PM	11 PM
Glucose	3+	2+	4+	1+
Ketones	Mod	Sm	Mod	0

The patient's 4 PM insulin dose would be

(A) 6 units of regular insulin
(B) 12 units of regular insulin
(C) 12 units of NPH insulin
(D) 42 units of regular insulin
(E) 42 units of NPH insulin

191. Peripheral veins are seldom used for the administration of total parenteral nutrition (TPN) fluids because

(A) TPN fluids tend to infiltrate surrounding tissue
(B) the blood flow in peripheral vessels is not great enough to protect the peripheral vessels from irritation
(C) large-bore needles must be used
(D) the hypotonic solution causes local hemolysis
(E) the vessels are easily occluded

192. An elderly insulin-dependent diabetic is about to be placed on a beta blocker for his hypertension. Which of the following beta blockers would be most appropriate for this type of patient?

(A) propranolol (Inderal)
(B) pindolol (Visken)
(C) timolol (Blocadren)
(D) nadolol (Corgard)
(E) atenolol (Tenormin)

193. When used to treat angina, nifedipine (Procardia) is much more likely than verapamil (Calan, Isoptin) and diltiazem (Cardizem) to cause

(A) hypokalemia
(B) tachycardia
(C) cardiac arrhythmias
(D) mental depression
(E) bronchospasm

194. Which of the following complications associated with the administration of total parenteral nutrition (TPN) solutions (composed of amino acids or protein hydrolysates, glucose, electrolytes, and vitamins) is most likely to occur after the infusions have been discontinued?

(A) alkalosis
(B) hyperchloremic metabolic acidosis
(C) hyperosmotic nonketotic hyperglycemia
(D) hypoglycemia
(E) pulmonary edema

195. Which one of the following provides the greatest number of calories per gram?

(A) ethanol
(B) fats
(C) anhydrous dextrose
(D) hydrous dextrose
(E) proteins

196. A patient requires high-dose cisplatin (Platinol) therapy for the treatment of advanced bladder cancer. During the cisplatin therapy, the patient develops severe nausea and vomiting. Which of the following drugs would be appropriate to administer to control these symptoms?

(A) neostigmine (Prostigmin)
(B) ganciclovir (Cytovene)
(C) danazol (Danocrine)
(D) asparaginase (Elspar)
(E) ondansetron (Zofran)

197. The mechanism of action of amiloride (Midamor) is most similar to that of

(A) spironolactone (Aldactone)
(B) hydrochlorothiazide (HydroDIURIL)
(C) metolazone (Zaroxolyn)
(D) triamterene (Dyrenium)
(E) chlorthalidone (Hygroton)

198. A 50-year-old hypertensive patient has been maintained on spironolactone with hydrochlorothiazide (Aldactazide), methyldopa (Aldomet), and potassium (K-Tabs). The patient is admitted to the hospital for elective surgery and is found to be hyperkalemic (serum K of 6.4; normal range is 3.5 to 5.5 mEq/L) with no symptoms and a normal electrocardiogram. This patient should be treated with

(A) IV calcium
(B) IV sodium bicarbonate
(C) IV glucose plus insulin
(D) rectal sodium polystyrene sulfonate (Kayexalate)
(E) hemodialysis

199. A 55-year-old patient with a 5-year history of angina and a recent myocardial infarction is admitted to the hospital because of malignant hypertension. Diazoxide should NOT be used in this patient because

(A) of its cardiostimulating effects
(B) of its slow onset of activity
(C) it tends to increase uric acid levels
(D) it is likely to cause orthostatic hypotension
(E) of its hepatotoxicity

200. Which of the following antihypertensives would be preferred in the patient described in question 199?

(A) propranolol (Inderal)
(B) nitroprusside (Nipride)
(C) trimethaphan (Arfonad)
(D) hydralazine (Apresoline)
(E) minoxidil (Loniten)

201. A 40-year-old male patient with a history of hypertension develops a moderately severe endogenous depression. His physician prescribes amitriptyline (Elavil) 25 mg t.i.d. The patient says that he cannot tolerate the drug because of dry mouth, constipation, and cardiac palpitations. The physician asks you whether there is another antidepressant that does not have the anticholinergic and cardiovascular side effects. Which of the following drugs would you suggest?

(A) imipramine (Tofranil)
(B) nortriptyline (Pamelor)
(C) trimipramine (Surmontil)
(D) maprotiline (Ludiomil)
(E) trazodone (Desyrel)

202. Considering the situation described in question 201 and assuming that the physician desires to use a drug that (like amitriptyline) primarily inhibits the reuptake of serotonin rather than of norepinephine, which of the following drugs would you now recommend?

(A) imipramine (Tofranil)
(B) nortriptyline (Pamelor)
(C) trimipramine (Surmontil)
(D) maprotiline (Ludiomil)
(E) trazodone (Desyrel)

203. A patient has been receiving 50 mg of hydrocortisone (Solu-Cortef) intravenously every 6 hours for an acute exacerbation of ulcerative colitis. After several days of IV therapy, the physician wishes to switch the patient to an equivalent dose of oral prednisone. The equivalent total daily dose of prednisone would be

(A) 10 mg
(B) 25 mg
(C) 50 mg
(D) 100 mg
(E) 200 mg

204. A 50-year-old patient with congestive heart failure is stabilized on digoxin 0.25 mg daily, hydrochlorothiazide 50 mg daily, and a low-sodium, high-potassium diet. The patient then develops polyarteritis, which requires corticosteroid therapy. Which of the following glucocorticoids would be more appropriate for this patient?

(A) hydrocortisone
(B) cortisone
(C) prednisolone
(D) prednisone
(E) dexamethasone

205. An asthmatic patient is stabilized to a therapeutic theophylline level on an IV aminophylline (dihydrate) infusion of 50 mg/h. The physician wishes to put the patient on an equivalent amount of sustained-release anhydrous theophylline (eg, Theo-Dur). An appropriate total daily dose of Theo-Dur would be

(A) 1500 mg
(B) 1200 mg
(C) 900 mg
(D) 600 mg
(E) 300 mg

206. A 20-year-old asthmatic patient has been treated with Theo-Dur 500 mg twice daily. Despite a good therapeutic steady-state serum concentration of 16 µg/mL, the patient has brief episodes of bronchospasm several times a week. The physician would like to give the patient additional bronchodilator therapy with an oral beta-adrenergic agonist. Which of the following drugs would be LEAST desirable?

(A) ephedrine
(B) metaproterenol (Alupent)
(C) terbutaline (Brethine)
(D) albuterol (Ventolin)
(E) isoetherine (Bronkosol)

DIRECTIONS (Questions 207 through 250): Each group of items in this section consists of lettered headings followed by a set of numbered words or phrases. For each numbered word or phrase, select the ONE lettered heading that is most closely associated with it. Each lettered heading may be selected once, more than once, or not at all.

Questions 207 through 211

MATCH the lettered meaning with the corresponding numbered prefix.

(A) apart
(B) below
(C) backward
(D) middle
(E) downward

207. cata
208. dis
209. infra
210. meso
211. retro

Questions 212 through 216

MATCH the lettered area or organ most closely associated with the numbered root.

(A) abdomen
(B) head
(C) heart
(D) large intestine
(E) rib

212. celi
213. cephal
214. col
215. cor
216. costa

Questions 217 through 219

MATCH the lettered body area or organ with the most closely related route of parenteral administration.

(A) artery
(B) heart
(C) joint
(D) joint fluid
(E) spinal fluid

217. intra-articular
218. intrasynovial
219. intrathecal

Questions 220 through 227

MATCH the lettered body part or organ with the most closely related numbered disease.

(A) adrenal cortex
(B) bones
(C) lymph nodes
(D) muscles
(E) thyroid

220. goiter
221. Cushing's syndrome
222. Hodgkin's disease
223. myasthenia gravis

(A) adrenal glands
(B) bones
(C) gastrointestinal tract
(D) heart
(E) kidneys

224. Addison's disease   A

225. Albright's syndrome   B

226. Bright's disease   E

227. Crohn's disease   C

Questions 228 through 231

MATCH each of the lettered diseases with the numbered description of symptoms.

(A) diabetes mellitus
(B) Graves' disease
(C) herpes simplex
(D) Ménière's disease
(E) Raynaud's disease

228. pallor or cyanosis of the fingers or toes   E

229. enlarged thyroid gland, exophthalmos   B

230. watery blisters on skin and mucous membranes, especially the lips   C

231. deafness, tinnitus, and dizziness   D

Questions 232 through 236

MATCH the lettered patient consultation most closely associated with the numbered drug brand name.

(A) take with a large volume of water
(B) take with milk, antacids, or meals
(C) take on an empty stomach
(D) do not take with mineral oil
(E) should be taken whole and not broken or chewed

232. Pentids   C

233. Indocin   B

234. Colace   D

235. Gantrisin   A

236. Dulcolax   E

Questions 237 through 245

A pharmacist must be fully acquainted with the contents of commonly used reference books so that drug information may be located quickly. Match the lettered reference book with the numbered piece of data that would most likely be found in that book.

(A) *Facts and Comparisons*
(B) *Handbook of Nonprescription Drugs*
(C) *Physicians' Desk Reference*
(D) *Drug Topics Red Book*
(E) *United States Pharmacopoeia*

237. comparison of sodium content of a group of antacid liquids   A

238. active drug in Sominex tablets   A

239. list of products manufactured by Elder Pharmaceuticals, Inc.   D

240. names of several vitamin tablets containing fluoride   A

241. NDC number for a commercial drug product   D

242. possible identification of a capsule having a distinctive color combination   C

243. qualitative identification of a drug powder suspected to be imipramine hydrochloride   E

244. relative costs of several commercial antacid liquids   B

245. table listing the solubility of drugs in several solvents   A

Questions 246 through 250

The following list of lettered organs is followed by numbered laboratory tests. Match the organ with the diagnostic test most closely associated with it.

(A) thyroid
(B) heart
(C) liver
(D) kidney
(E) pancreas

246. bilirubin   C

247. amylase   E

248. alkaline phosphatase   C

249. blood urea nitrogen (BUN)   D

250. lactate dehydrogenase (LDH)   B

Answers and Explanations

1. **(E)** When administered intravenously, diazepam (Valium) is a rapid-acting anticonvulsant with less tendency to produce respiratory depression than the barbiturates. Diazepam is effective in grand mal, focal motor, and petit mal seizures, and in status epilepticus. Because of its wide range of effectiveness, intravenous diazepam is probably the drug of choice for initial therapy of status epilepticus. Intravenous phenytoin is an important secondary drug but is likely to decrease heart rate and produce hypotension. Paraldehyde is also an effective drug but, like the barbiturates, is likely to cause respiratory depression. *(11:1104–5)*

2. **(A)** Chronic high-dose administration of hydralazine can produce an acute rheumatoid state in approximately 10% of patients taking the drug. A syndrome clinically indistinguishable from disseminated lupus erythematosis develops in a smaller percentage of users. This lupus-like syndrome (fever, arthralgia, splenomegaly, edema, and the presence of lupus erythematosus cells in the peripheral blood) has also been associated with procainamide use. *(11:525)*

3. **(B)** Following slow uptake by the adrenergic nerve, guanethidine replaces norepinephrine in storage granules and accumulates in the nerve in place of norepinephrine. After several days of guanethidine administration, the sympathetic nerves no longer contain sufficient amounts of norepinephrine to maintain normal venomotor tone. Tricyclic antidepressants inhibit the uptake of guanethidine into the adrenergic neuron, thereby inhibiting the antihypertensive effect of guanethidine. *(11:42)*

4. **(E)** Metoprolol (Lopressor) blocks beta-adrenergic receptors. It differs from propranolol (Inderal) primarily in that it has some preferential effect on beta-1 adrenoreceptors, which are chiefly located in cardiac muscle. This preferential effect is not absolute and, at higher doses, metoprolol also inhibits beta-2 adrenoreceptors, which are chiefly located in bronchial and vascular musculature. Although the mechanism of its antihypertensive effect is not known, the drug is indicated in the management of hypertension either alone or in combination with other antihypertensives. *(3:703)*

5. **(B)** Prazosin is believed to be a direct-acting vasodilator. Side effects of therapy may include a precipitous fall in blood pressure, possibly with tachycardia and loss of consciousness following the first dose. The drug is equivalent to and a possible alternative for hydralazine (Apresoline). The initial dose of prazosin is usually 1 mg two or three times a day and can be slowly increased to 10 mg twice daily. *(3:755–9)*

6. **(C)** The ganglionic blocking agents are very potent antihypertensive drugs. They block the transmission of impulses in the autonomic nervous system by interfering with the action of acetylcholine at both sympathetic and parasympathetic ganglia. They are not widely used because of the many unpleasant effects that result from their parasympatholytic action (eg, dryness of the mouth, constipation, impaired visual accommodation, urinary retention, etc). *(6:182)*

7. **(C)** Diazoxide has marked antihypertensive activity when given by rapid IV injection. It appears to lower blood pressure by a direct dilation of the arterioles, which minimizes the incidence of orthostatic hypotension. Both cardiac output and renal blood flow are increased. Initial doses of 1 to 3 mg/kg are used. Orally, the drug is used in the treatment of hypoglycemia. *(6:805)*

8. **(B)** Normal doses of doxycycline are not eliminated by the same pathways as the other listed tetracyclines. Since it does not appear to accumulate in the blood, it is one of the safest tetracyclines for treating extrarenal infections in patients with renal failure. *(6:1119)*

9. **(B)** Hydralazine (Apresoline) would be the best choice since depression is a major side effect of reserpine, guanethidine, methyldopa, and clonidine. The principal serious side effects of hydralazine are tachycardia and lupus erythematosus-like syndrome. *(11:599)*

10. **(B)** A significant and often dose-limiting side effect

of the phenothiazines is the development of extra-pyramidal symptoms that closely mimic Parkinson's disease (eg, akinesis, muscular rigidity, and tremor). These bothersome side effects can often be controlled by the anticholinergic drugs used to treat Parkinson's disease (eg, trihexyphenidyl, benztropine, etc).
(11:951–2)

11. **(E)** Cholestyramine is a basic anion exchange resin. This quaternary ammonium chloride compound exchanges the chloride ion for the cholate ion and, therefore, prevents the reabsorption of bile acids. Cholestyramine binds many organic acids, including all of the drugs listed in this question.
(11:615,723)

12. **(B)** If drug B has a greater affinity (ie, higher association constant) for specific protein-binding sites than drug A, it will have a tendency to displace drug A from these sites. Further, if drug B is given in large doses, the degree of this displacement will increase because there will be a greater amount of drug B competing with drug A for the binding sites.
(11:39)

13. **(B)** Each of the three major drugs used to treat convulsive disorders (phenobarbital, phenytoin, and primidone) can disturb folic acid metabolism. The hematologic problems associated with folic acid deficiency are relatively easy to detect. However, the abnormal mental states that may develop are considerably more difficult to diagnose. These symptoms may range from mild confusion to psychoses resembling schizophrenia.
(11:188,859)

14. **(B)** Valproic acid (Depakene) is an effective anticonvulsant for absence seizures and mixed types of epilepsy. This drug may be as effective as ethosuximide (Zarontin), which for many years had been considered to be the drug of choice for absence seizures. However, when valproic acid is added to a phenobarbital regimen, the serum levels of phenobarbital may increase by as much as 40%. Phenobarbital dosage may have to be reduced accordingly. It is not known whether this effect is due to modification of protein binding or diminished metabolism of phenobarbital.
(11:855–7)

15. **(D)** Penetration of the cornea by *Pseudomonas aeruginosa* will often lead to destruction of the cornea and interior portions of the eye. Blindness may result. This organism is a common contaminant in water. The need for sterility of ophthalmic products is well recognized.
(1:1588)

16. **(D)** Boils caused by *Staphylococcus* organisms form in the anterior portion of the external auditory meatus. They are usually self-limiting, and treatment with antibiotic ointments will prevent spreading.
(2:637)

17. **(B)** Idoxuridine is an antimetabolite that inhibits the replication of viral DNA with greater selectivity than that of the host cell. It is used primarily in the treatment of herpes simplex keratitis, a disease of viral origin that can cause blindness.
(6:1188)

18. **(C)** Although tolnaftate is effective against several types of fungi, it is ineffective against *Candida* organisms. Miconazole, clotrimazole, and haloprogin are relatively broad-spectrum antifungal agents with activity against some species of *Candida*.
(6:1176–8)

19. **(A)** Although methotrexate is not curative, it suppresses psoriatic lesions and induces prolonged remissions in up to 75% of psoriatic patients treated.
(6:1586)

20. **(E)** Complications of corticosteroid therapy are usually related to the length of time that they have been administered and the dosage used. Corticosteroids suppress normal tissue responses to infection (increasing susceptibility to infection) and allow further dissemination of existing infections. Since tissue responses to infection are suppressed, the subjective, objective, and laboratory manifestations of infection may be masked.
(6:1451–2)

21. **(C)** Although the NSAIDs are structurally different, they all possess similar pharmacologic properties and all inhibit prostaglandin synthesis. Furthermore, these drugs produce similar adverse effects, including gastrointestinal intolerance. Piroxicam has the longest half-life of the group (approximately 38 hours) and is recommended to be given on a once-a-day basis.
(6:668)

22. **(D)** Perhaps the most significant difference among these drugs is the prolonged biologic half-life of naproxen (13 hours). The other drugs have half-lives ranging from 1 to 3 hours. Because of this long biologic half-life, naproxen can be administered on a twice-a-day regimen. This may be of value to patients who have difficulty complying with dosing schedules that require more frequent dosing.
(11:489)

23. **(D)** Fluorouracil is used topically for the treatment of multiple premalignant actinic keratoses. It prevents further development of existing lesions and results in cosmetic improvement. If an occlusive dressing is applied, there may be an increased incidence of inflammatory reaction in the adjacent normal skin. However, even without an occlusive dressing, such responses occasionally occur in skin that appears clinically normal. This is due to the presence of subclinical actinic keratoses.
(E–incorrect) Normal progression of treatment includes erythema followed by scaling, tenderness, erosion, ulceration, necrosis, and re-epithelization. Treatment should be discontinued at the erosion stage.
(11:756)

24. **(C)** In the condition known as hypoprothrombinemia, there is a reduction in the levels of prothrom-

bin in the blood. This substance is essential in the blood clotting mechanism. *(6:1312)*

25. **(B)** Rapid reversal of drug-induced hypoprothrombinemia requires the use of a source of prothrombin such as fresh blood or plasma. The various vitamin K derivatives can be used if the situation is not urgent or as a supplement to one of the immediate sources of prothrombin (ie, blood or plasma). *(6:1565–6)*

26. **(B)** Pyridium is a red dye that commonly causes discoloration of the urine. It is used primarily as a urinary tract analgesic. *(6:1061)*

27. **(B)** Clomiphene citrate (Clomid) is an agent that has moderate antiestrogenic activity. It has been successfully used to induce ovulation in many patients with amenorrhea and other conditions that cause anovulatory cycles. *(6:1395–7)*

28. **(B)** Once conception has taken place, the body starts to produce chorionic gonadotropin. The e.p.t. Stick Test assays for the presence of this hormone in the urine. *(10)*

29. **(C)** Animal testing of a new drug is completed before the investigational new drug (IND) status is obtained for clinical testing. In Phase I of the study, healthy volunteers are tested to determine drug tolerance, dosing schedules, side effects, and pharmacokinetic data. This is followed by Phase II, in which actual patients suffering from the disease are tested with the drug. Drug efficacy is observed, and side effects not evident in healthy volunteers may occur. Phase III involves administration of the drug to large numbers of patients by private practitioners. Phase IV is the continuous investigation or monitoring of the drug after marketing. *(1:66)*

30. **(B)** Hypoparathyroidism usually presents itself as a disorder of calcium metabolism in which serum calcium levels of the patient decrease while levels of phosphate increase in an inversely proportional manner. Low serum calcium levels may precipitate a potentially serious condition known as tetany. To prevent the development of this disorder and to treat the hypoparathyroidism, calcium supplements such as calcium gluconate, calcium carbonate, calcium lactate, or calcium gluceptate are often prescribed. *(11:301–4)*

31. **(E)** Gentamicin and other aminoglycoside antibiotics (tobramycin, amikacin, etc) may produce neuromuscular blockade; this can enhance the blockade produced by skeletal muscle relaxants such as tubocurarine. *(6:1107)*

32. **(A)** The hypothyroid state is characterized by marked retardation of mental and physical activity, hoarseness, dry sparse hair, thickening of the skin and subcutaneous tissues, constipation, cold intolerance, anemia, and dry, pale, coarse skin. However, because of the nature of the general symptoms, hypothyroidism is usually recognized and treated before all the above symptoms develop. *(11:285–93)*

33. **(C)** *(19:71–5)*

34. **(A)** Fiorinal is the only agent listed that contains aspirin. *(3:1108)*

35. **(B)** Hemochromatosis is an iron storage disorder characterized by excessive amounts of iron in parenchymal tissues with resultant tissue damage. Such a condition may be caused by a number of factors, one of which is the prolonged use of excessive doses of iron preparations. *(11:177–8)*

36. **(D)** This syndrome generally occurs when erythromycin estolate is given to susceptible individuals for more than 10 to 14 days. It is more common after multiple exposures to the drug, the full recovery usually follows discontinuation of the medication. The reaction is unpredictable and is apparently due to individual hypersensitivity. It has not been observed with the use of erythromycin free base or with other derivaties of erythromycin. Since there is no established clinical superiority of the estolate salt, there is little justification for using it in light of the possibility of this potential toxicity. *(11:71)*

37. **(B)** Vancomycin is bactericidal for gram-positive bacteria. Most pathogenic staphylococci are killed by a plasma concentration of 10 µg/mL or less. However, since vancomycin is highly irritating to tissue, thrombophlebitis following IV injection is common. Also the drug is ototoxic and nephrotoxic. Consequently, it is used only for serious staphylococcal or enterococcal infections in patients who fail to respond to other drugs. *(6:1138–40)*

38. **(C)** Conventional antihistamines, or H_1-receptor antagonists, inhibit histamine-mediated contraction of the bronchi and gut. They do not, however, block the stimulatory effect of histamine on gastric acid secretion. Nizatidine (Axid), a selective H_2-receptor antagonist, blocks gastric acid and pepsin secretion in response to histamine, gastrin, food, distention, and caffeine. *(6:898–901)*

39. **(D)** In questionable cases of penicillin allergy, skin tests may be performed using benzylpenicilloyl-polylysine. Although a negative reaction to the test does not rule out the possibility of a hypersensitivity reaction, it does indicate that anaphylaxis is not likely to occur on administration of the drug. *(6:1084)*

40. **(B)** Amantadine (Symmetrel) inhibits the replication of certain myxoviruses (eg, influenza A, rubella, and some tumor viruses) in humans. A daily oral dose of 200 mg for 2 to 3 days before and 6 to 7 days after influenza A infection reduces the incidence and severity of symptoms and the magnitude of the serologic response to the infection. *(6:472–3)*

41. (B) Both carbenicillin and ticarcillin contain approximately 5 mEq/g of sodium and present a potential problem for patients with CHF, renal failure, and hypertension. Because of their high sodium content and the fact that they are nonabsorbable anions, carbenicillin and ticarcillin cause renal retention of sodium and excretion of potassium. Ticarcillin has an advantage over carbenicillin in that its usual dose is about one half that of carbenicillin. Thus, for equivalent therapeutic doses, ticarcillin will provide less sodium and a lower concentration of nonabsorbable ion than carbenicillin. *(6:1080–1)*

42. (B) Some authorities state that isoniazid is the best tolerated, most effective, and most economical drug used in the management of active TB. However, it is commonly used with a second or even a third drug to reduce the development of resistant strains. Combinations of INH with rifampin or ethambutol are very effective against pulmonary TB. Sodium PAS (given orally) and streptomycin (IM) are sometimes used with INH. *(6:1097–9)*
(A–incorrect) Isoniazid, without other drugs, is used prophylactically; it is given orally over a period of at least 1 year for this purpose.
(C–incorrect) Pyridoxine administered in doses of 50 mg daily will prevent development of peripheral neuritis, which is the most common adverse reaction caused by isoniazid. Pyridoxine does not interfere with the antitubercular action.
(D–incorrect) Isoniazid is converted to an acetylated form and to isonicotinic acid in the liver. These metabolic products and some unchanged drug are excreted by the kidneys. *(6:1147)*

43. (D) Combined drug treatment is usually required because of the rapid development of resistant organisms when a single agent is used. It has also been demonstrated that combined drug therapy enhances the tuberculostatic effects of the individual drugs. For example, a combination of streptomycin and isoniazid is significantly more tuberculostatic than either agent used alone. *(11:1096)*

44. (A) The color change imparted to urine and sweat is a predictable and harmless side effect. Patients should be told to expect this effect so that they are not alarmed by it. *(11:1099)*

45. (A) Because of adverse reactions associated with chloramphenicol (eg, bone marrow disturbances, aplastic anemia), it is currently indicated for only a few types of infections: (1) symptomatic salmonella infections (eg, typhoid fever); (2) *Hemophilus influenzae* that does not respond to ampicillin; (3) gram-negative bacteremias caused by organisms resistant to other drugs; (4) severe rickettsial infection; (5) bacteroides and other anaerobic infections; (6) meningococcal infections in patients hypersensitive to penicillin; and (7) certain ophthalmic infections (topically). *(11:70–6)*

46. (B) *(3:1606)*

47. (B) Pseudomembranous colitis is a severe and occasionally fatal complication of antibiotic therapy. One etiology appears to be the presence of an exotoxin produced by overgrowth of *Clostridium difficile* in the bowel. Clindamycin, lincomycin, and ampicillin have been the most commonly implicated antibiotics, although other antibiotics have also been implicated. Treatment is directed against the offending organism and its exotoxin. Oral vancomycin in doses of 125 to 500 mg three to four times daily for 7 to 14 days is most commonly used. Cholestyramine resin may also be used to bind the bacterial exotoxin. *(6:1139)*

48. (C) A clinical picture characterized by nausea, vomiting, polyuria, polydipsia, proteinuria, acidosis, glycosuria, and gross aminoaciduria (A Fanconi-like syndrome) can be produced by anhydro-4-epitetracycline, one of the degradation products of tetracycline. The syndrome is reversible with symptoms disappearing in about 1 month after termination of consumption of degraded drug. *(6:1122)*

49. (A) The aminoglycosides have activity against a wide range of microorganisms. After parenteral administration, they are excreted unchanged in the urine. Because of their well-established nephrotoxicity and ototoxicity, they are not suitable for long-term treatment of chronic tract infections. *(6:1102–4)*

50. (B) Moxalactam, cefazolin, and cefotaxime are not adequately absorbed from the gastrointestinal tract, and therefore must be administered parenterally for systemic therapy. Although both cefaclor and cephradine are adequately absorbed, only cephradine is commercially available in both oral and parenteral dosage forms. *(6:1088–90)*

51. (D) Cromolyn sodium is available as 20-mg capsules (Intal). The drug is administered by inhalation of the powder through a mechanical inhaler (Spinhaler). The particle size of the powder is small enough (2 to 6 μm in diameter) to reach the alveoli and may cause an initial bronchoconstriction severe enough to require that isoproterenol be administered concomitantly. It should be emphasized to the patient that the drug is not effective by the oral route and the capsules should not be swallowed. The more recently marketed solution (20 mg/2 mL ampule) is claimed to be as effective as the powder and to cause less bronchospasm. The solution is administered from a power-operated nebulizer equipped with a suitable face mask. Hand-operated nebulizers cannot be used. *(6:631)*

52. (B) A major advance in steroid therapy for asthma has been the development of corticosteroid aerosols such as beclomethasone (Vanceril). Like cromolyn (Intal), beclomethasone is a prophylactic agent that must be used regularly. It is not suitable for an acute asthmatic attack. The primary value of steroid therapy by inhalation is to avoid systemic side effects in patients who require steroids for the first time or to permit significant dosage reductions of oral steroids in patients on maintenance therapy. *(11:561)*

53. **(D)** Vasopressin, which is a purified preparation of antidiuretic hormone, is used therapeutically in the treatment of diabetes insipidus, a disease of pituitary origin. When administered in any one of a number of available dosage forms (IM, IV, SC, and nasal insufflation or spray), vasopressin will usually reverse the symptom of excessive urination (polyuria), which is the primary symptom of patients suffering from this disease. The initially observed action of the hormone was vasoconstriction, which led to the name vasopressin; this is still the official USP designation. *(11:106–7)*

54. **(A)** Lithium carbonate (Lithane, Eskalith) is primarily indicated for treating manic episodes in patients with manic-depressive illness. It is administered orally in daily divided doses of 600 mg to 1.8 g and generally should not be administered with diuretics, since retention of lithium may occur. *(6:936–40)*

55. **(C)** The rate of excretion of lithium carbonate is generally independent of urine flow and dietary sodium. However, in the presence of sodium deficiency, the excretion of lithium is markedly decreased and toxic levels can accumulate rapidly. Conversely, high sodium intake enhances lithium excretion. *(6:936–40)*

56. **(A)** Glucose-6-phosphate dehydrogenase controls the initial step in the pentose phosphate pathway, bringing about the oxidation of glucose-6-phosphate to 6-phosphogluconate, which reduces NADP to NADPH. Many oxidant drugs (eg, primaquine, sulfisoxazole, probenecid) increase the rate of oxidation of glutathione. This increases the intracellular demand for NADPH to maintain glutathione in the reduced form. In patients with a deficiency in erythrocyte G6PD, oxidized glutathione accumulates and, by some unknown mechanism, disrupts erythrocyte membrane integrity with subsequent hemolysis. *(11:205–7)*

57. **(B)** The anticoagulant effect of heparin is quantitated by the partial thromboplastin time (PTT). The usual therapeutic goal is to prolong the activated partial thromboplastin time to 2 to 2.5 times the laboratory control. *(6:313–17)*

58. **(E)** Because of heparin's brief duration of action, mild hemorrhaging is usually treated by simply withdrawing the drug. In the presence of severe hemorrhage, the use of a specific heparin antagonist (eg, protamine sulfate) is imperative. Usually 1 to 1.5 mg of protamine sulfate will neutralize 100 units of heparin. However, after the intravenous adminis-

tration of heparin, the quantity of protamine required decreases rapidly with time. Only 0.5 mg of protamine is required to neutralize 100 units of heparin 30 minutes after IV administration of heparin. *(6:313–17)*

59. **(B)** Cimetidine potentiates the effects of oral anticoagulants by decreasing the rate of hepatic metabolism of warfarin. Cimetidine causes a reversible but significant increase in plasma warfarin concentration and, consequently, in the prothrombin time. In this case, it is necessary to recognize this interaction and to decrease the dose of warfarin or use other ulcer therapy. It appears that ranitidine may be less likely to interact significantly with warfarin. *(11:41–4)*

60. **(A)** Normal fasting blood sugar values for adults range from 80 to 120 mg/dL (or 80 to 120 mg%). When the fasting blood sugar levels exceed 120 mg/dL, diabetes mellitus should be suspected. Levels below 60 mg/dL may suggest insulin overdosage, glucagon deficiencies, and/or hypoactivity of various endocrine glands. *(11:63–4)*

61. **(E)** The administration of pharmacologic doses (0.4 mg/day or more) of folic acid can stimulate reticulocytosis and improve the anemia associated with vitamin B$_{12}$ deficiency. However, folic acid administration does not prevent the development or progression of the neurologic manifestations of pernicious anemia. Consequently, the FDA has restricted the content of folic acid in over-the-counter products to a maximum of 0.1 mg. *(11:188–9)*

62. **(A)** The van den Bergh test is a serum test that can be used to differentiate between conjugated and unconjugated bilirubin. The direct test is performed in an aqueous medium and is a measure of the more soluble conjugated bilirubin. If alcohol is added, both the conjugated and the less soluble unconjugated bilirubin will react, giving a measure of total bilirubin. The total minus the direct reading will give the indirect level, a measure of unconjugated bilirubin. When the ability of the liver to excrete bilirubin is impaired by obstruction, it is believed that the excess bilirubin in the blood is relatively free of attached protein (ie, is unbound). When increased levels of bilirubin are due to increased red cell destruction (ie, hemolysis), it is believed that the bilirubin is attached to plasma protein (ie, bound). Since the direct van den Bergh test measures the amount of conjugated bilirubin (which is free of attached protein) and the indirect van den Bergh test measures the amount of unconjugated bilirubin (which is tightly bound to protein), a comparison of these values gives some indication as to whether a patient's illness is due to obstruction or hemolysis. *(11:69–70)*

63. **(A)** By revealing the relative proportions of the various white blood cells, the white cell differential

count may direct the physician's attention toward a particular disease or group of diseases. For example, eosinophils are increased in parasitic infections and allergic conditions; neutrophils are increased in most bacterial infections; basophils may be increased in certain blood dyscrasias; and monocytes are often greatly increased in chronic infections such as tuberculosis. *(19:3–15)*

64. **(A)** Creatine kinase (CK) is an enzyme that is found primarily in muscle tissue. It is released into the blood in response to muscle injury. Serum concentrations of CK are elevated in disorders involving muscle damage such as myocardial infarction, muscular dystrophy, muscle trauma, and muscular inflammation. However, no increase would be observed in CHF since CK is not present in the liver, which often undergoes damage in CHF. The normal values may vary with the assay method used. *(19:3–9)*

65. **(C)** Whole blood treated with anticoagulant is centrifuged in a calibrated hematocrit tube. The volume ratio of the packed red blood cells to total blood volume is determined. The hematocrit is normally 40 to 54 for men and 36 to 47 for women. It gives some indication of both the number and size of the red blood cells present in an individual. *(19:3–13)*

66. **(D)** A reticulocyte is an immature erythrocyte. *(19:3–14)*

67. **(D)** Choice A, known as a single-unit package, is also a unit-dose package if it contains the particular dose of drug that has been ordered for the patient. *(1:1753)*

68. **(C)** The glucose oxidase test is quite specific for glucose, in contrast to the Benedict's test, which relies on the reduction of cupric ions in alkaline solution to reddish-orange insoluble cuprous oxide. The latter reaction can be elicited by reducing substances such as ascorbic acid and by a number of drugs that may be eliminated in the urine. *(11:316)*

69. **(D)** Tes-Tape contains glucose oxidase and is therefore specific for glucose. Clinistix and Diastix also use the glucose oxidase method. Ascorbic acid, levodopa, salicylates, and phenazopyridine (Pyridium) may produce false-negative results with these atents. *(11:317)*
(A–incorrect; C–incorrect) Benedict's qualitative test and Clinitest tablets are based on the copper reduction method.
(B–incorrect; E–incorrect) Acetest tablets and Ketostix are used to detect the presence of ketones in the urine. Levodopa and phenazopyridine may interfere.

70. **(C)** Hypodermoclysis is used on rare occasions in infants or obese patients in whom veins are inaccessible. *(28:749)*

71. **(E)** The administration of a drug by intermittent (rather than continuous) intravenous injection is accomplished over a period of minutes (rather than hours). Stability and/or compatibility problems are less likely to occur because the drug does not remain in contact with a large-volume IV fluid for long periods of time. The potential for thrombophlebitis is reduced because the drug is not in constant contact with the blood vessel tissue at the site of the injection. Finally, the greater concentration gradient produced by a more rapid injection may promote better diffusion of some drugs into tissues. *(1:712)*

72. **(B)** The use of the milliequivalent unit takes into consideration the chemical-combining capacity of various ionic species. *(12:148)*

73. **(E)** Important papers from leading medical and pharmaceutical journals are microfilmed and sent to subscribers on a monthly basis. The microfiche cards are subdivided into drug and condition categories. Each paper is cross-indexed and descriptor terms are included to further define the paper's contents. *(1:1861)*
(A–incorrect) This weekly publication reproduces the tables of contents from journals devoted to clinical aspects of health care. By perusing this journal, the pharmacist will see the titles of all papers published in specific journals. Then, either the actual journal can be obtained for reading or a reprint request can be sent to the listed author. *(1:1861)*
(B–incorrect) The *de Haen Drug Information Systems* consist of several specialized services that present data from biomedical journals on microfiche. Microfiche are available on drugs in prospect, drugs in research, drugs in use, new drug releases, etc. *(1:1861)*

74. **(B)** *Martindale's Extra Pharmacopoeia* is probably one of the most comprehensive, international, single-volume references on drugs and drug products. *Martindale's* is divided into three parts. The first part consists of monographs on drugs and ancillary substances. Although drugs that are manufactured in the United Kingdom are stressed, generic and proprietary products from many other countries are included. The monographs includes physiochemical data, storage, incompatibilities, uses, doses, and toxic effects. The second part contains a supplementary discussion of new drugs, obsolete drugs, and miscellaneous substances. The third part lists formulas of OTC products sold in the United Kingdom. There is also a directory of worldwide pharmaceutical manufacturers. *(1:54)*

75. **(E)** Although literature abstracts often appear to provide sufficient detail to answer certain questions, it must be recognized that an abstract may contain statements taken out of context and that supporting detail and/or qualifications for such statements have been excluded. It is the obligation of the individual providing the information to retrieve the entire article to ascertain whether the information provided is accurate and complete. *(1:53)*

76. **(B)** Kernicterus is a neurologic syndrome in which damaging bile pigments are deposited in the basal ganglia in the central nervous system. It may develop in the neonate following therapy with the sulfonamides. Bilirubin is a normal breakdown product of hemoglobin; it is generally conjugated in the liver to a water-soluble glucuronide that is excreted in the bile. Because of a deficiency in the enzyme glucuronyl transferase, neonates have a limited capacity to metabolize bilirubin. Sulfonamides are implicated in this disorder because of their ability to displace unconjugated bilirubin from protein-binding sites. Sulfonamides should be avoided in pregnant women near term because these drugs cross the placenta, and by nursing mothers because they are excreted in breast milk. *(19:33–7)*

77. **(B)** Although the presence of impaired renal function or renal failure does not contraindicate the use of drugs that are directly excreted or whose active metabolites are excreted by the kidney, it does modify the dose required to produce a given therapeutic effect. Renal impairment or renal failure will allow these drugs or their metabolites to accumulate in the blood. Drug accumulation in these situations can be avoided by reducing the dose and/or the dosage schedule of the drug. Careful monitoring of drug concentrations in the blood and of remaining renal function should also be done. *(11:363–9)*

78. **(E)** No significant difference in clinical response can be identified between patients who acetylate isoniazid slowly and those who do so rapidly. *(6:1148)* (B–incorrect) Although slow acetylators of isoniazid are more likely to develop peripheral neuropathy from the drug, they respond equally well to pyridoxine therapy as rapid acetylators.

79. **(A)** For systemic use, amphotericin B is available as a colloidal dry powder combined with sodium deoxycholate. The colloidal solution is sensitive to heat, light, low pH, and substances (ie, additives) that will precipitate the drug. *(6:1167)*

80. **(E)** Amylase is an enzyme secreted by the pancreas that is involved in the breakdown of starches. In certain diseases of the pancreas such as acute pancreatitis, digestive enzymes of the pancreas escape into surrounding tissue, producing pain and inflammation, and into the blood, producing elevated serum levels. *(11:68–9)*

81. **(A)** The relative concentration of different anions and cations varies considerably between intracellular and extracellular fluids of the body. Intracellular body fluids contain high concentrations of potassium (a cation) and phosphate (an anion), whereas extracellular fluid contains high concentrations of sodium (a cation) and chloride (an anion). *(6:698)*

82. **(D)** The usual concentrations of cations in intracellular water are sodium 16, potassium 150, calcium 2, and magnesium 27. Anions include chloride 1, bicarbonate 10, phosphate 100, sulfate 20, and proteinate 63. *(19:28–2)*

83. **(E)** There is a reciprocal relationship between the concentration of calcium and phosphorus in the blood. For example, hypoparathyroidism is characterized by low serum calcium and high serum phosphorus, whereas hyperparathyroidism is characterized by low serum phosphorus and high serum calcium. *(11:301–4)*

84. **(C)** Pyrantel pamoate is used in the treatment of pinworms. It is available as an oral suspension. A single dose of 11 mg/kg is generally administered. The drug is well tolerated but may cause nausea, vomiting, diarrhea, or dizziness in some individuals. *(11:1224–6)*

85. **(B)** Acetaminophen is metabolized in the liver primarily by conjugation to glucuronide or sulfate metabolites. A small percentage is metabolized by the hepatic cytochrome P450 mixed-function oxidase system to a toxic intermediate metabolite. Normally, this metabolite is preferentially conjugated to glutathione and excreted in the urine. When large doses of acetaminophen are ingested, the glucuronide and sulfate pathways become saturated, and stores of glutathione become inadequate to conjugate the amount of toxic metabolite that is produced. The metabolite binds covalently to hepatocytes and produces hepatic necrosis. *(11:57–8)*

86. **(D)** Since the drug was ingested 6 hours ago, the likelihood of removing a large amount of drug from this patient's stomach with ipecac syrup is small. Activated charcoal effectively binds acetaminophen if given soon after ingestion, but its use here is also unlikely to be of value because of the elapsed time. Glutathione would seem a logical antidote (see commentary for question 85), but it does not enter cells readily and therefore will not prevent hepatic necrosis. N-acetylcysteine serves as a glutathione substitute that effectively binds the toxin and permits it to be excreted in the urine. N-acetylcysteine is given orally or by lavage tube. Cysteamine, a glutathione precursor, has also been used successfully. It is given intravenously. *(11:459)*

87. **(D)** Because of sulfasalazine's poor absorption from the GI tract, its localized activity is valuable as one of the first-line treatments for various forms of colitis and enteritis. The drug is available as oral tablets and as a suspension. *(6:650,1051)*

88. **(C)** Aspirin allergy in association with asthma is cause for serious concern. Asthma, rhinorrhea, and nasal polyps usually accompany this type of aspirin intolerance, which occurs in about 2% to 4% of asthmatic patients. These patients appear to exhibit a high degree of cross-reactivity to other nonsteroidal anti-inflammatory drugs such as ibuprofen. *(11:528)*

89. **(B)** Because of the structural similarity between the penicillins and the cephalosporins, cross-sensitivity may be a problem in these patients. Although the possibility exists, the incidence of cross-sensitivity is probably less than 5%. However, patients allergic to penicillin should be watched carefully when initiating cephalosporin therapy. *(11:1084)*

90. **(A)** Ethacrynic acid (Edecrin) is capable of producing ototoxicity, which would enhance the similar toxicity produced by gentamicin. *(19:17–9)*

91. **(E)** Diazoxide (Hyperstat IV) is a drug that is administered parenterally only in the emergency treatment of acute hypertensive crisis. It causes a rapid fall in blood pressure that may last from 3 hours to 7 or 8 days. *(6:804–5)*

92. **(C)** A thiazide diuretic should form the basis of antihypertensive therapy since it will potentiate the action of other antihypertensive agents and will often be sufficient to control many cases of mild to moderate hypertension. *(11:589)*

93. **(E)** Sodium nitroprusside is a powerful vasodilator that acts directly on the smooth muscle of blood vessels. Because of its rapid conversion to thiocyanate in the body, the effects of nitroprusside are quite transient. Following termination of the drug infusion, blood pressure begins to rise immediately and reaches the pretreatment level in 1 to 10 minutes. It is extremely important that the blood pressure and the flow rate of the solution be carefully monitored. Although the dose range is quite large, the average adult dose is 3 μg/kg/minute. Nitroprusside is used when short-term, rapid reduction in blood pressure is necessary *(6:803–4)*

94. **(C)** Isocarboxazid (Parnate), the only agent listed that is a monamine oxidase (MAO) inhibitor, may interact with pressor amines such as tyramine in some cheeses, wines, beers, etc, to produce a hypertensive crisis that may be life-threatening. *(6:415–7)*

95. **(A)** Frequent urination (polyuria) is a common symptom of diabetes mellitus. *(11:312–3)*

96. **(C)** Ergocalciferol or vitamin D is one of a number of active compounds collectively called vitamin D. Administration of vitamin D to a patient suffering from hypoparathyroidism is indicated since it will tend to elevate serum calcium levels and lower serum phosphate levels to acceptable ranges. *(6:1516)*

97. **(A)** Propranolol (Inderal) is used primarily for its ability to block beta-adrenergic activity, and is therefore useful in treating patients suffering from cardiac arrhythmias and angina pectoris. However, since beta-adrenergic blockage also tends to increase airway resistance, the drug is usually contraindicated for use in patients suffering from asthma or severe allergies. *(6:232–4)*

98. **(D)** The phenothiazine group of drugs can be subdivided into three groups according to chemical structure: dimethylaminopropyl derivatives (eg, chlorpromazine); piperazine derivatives (eg, perphenazine, prochlorperazine, and trifluoperazine); and the piperidyl derivatives (eg, thioridazine). Generally, the piperidyl group is the least likely to produce extrapyramidal symptoms and the piperazine group is the most likely to do so. *(6:387)*

99. **(E)** Tardive (late-occurring) dyskinesia (involuntary muscular movements) is a drug-induced neurologic disorder that appears to be irreversible and unresponsive to drug treatment. It is characterized by involuntary movement of the lips, tongue, or jaw and is commonly observed as a smacking of the lips, rhythmical movement of the tongue, or facial grimaces. This disorder may be due to hypersensitivity of dopaminergic receptors to endogenous dopamine after long-term blockade by antipsychotic drugs. (A–incorrect) Akathisia is a feeling of restlessness or a compelling need for movement. *(6:400)*

100. **(C)** Monitoring for phenothiazine side effects is best done by close observation rather than routine use of laboratory tests. Although it is a rare side effect, agranulocytosis characteristically occurs within the first 8 weeks of phenothiazine therapy. Sore throat with mucosal ulcerations, chills, and fever are among the early symptoms. Phenothiazine-induced agranulocytosis seems to be due to a direct toxic effect on bone marrow cells. It is particularly likely to occur in women over the age of 40. In the case outlined, the physician should be made aware of the patient's symptoms and the possible relationship to agranulocytosis. With early diagnosis and withdrawal of the drug, granulocyte recovery usually takes place in a week or more. *(6:400–1)*

101. **(D)** Metoclopramide exerts a potent antiemetic effect by inhibiting the chemoreceptor trigger zone (CTZ). It also stimulates gastrointestinal motility and increases the rate of gastric emptying. This enhances the antiemetic activity by eliminating stasis that precedes vomiting. All of the other drugs listed decrease the rate of gastric emptying. *(6:926–9)*

102. **(C)** Because of their hygroscopic nature, glycerinated gelatin and Carbowax suppositories may cause a stinging sensation when first inserted. This can be avoided by dipping the suppository into water just prior to insertion. *(1:1610–1)*

103. **(A)** The average adult expectorant dose is only 1 or 2 mL. The emetic dose of ipecac syrup is 10 to 30 mL. *(11:51–20)*

104. **(D)** All of the other listed syrups are sugar free. Robitussin-PE may contain sugar and does contain 1.4% alcohol, which would contribute calories. While a stablized diabetic could tolerate the additional calories, the brittle diabetic might not. *(3:993)*

105. (C) A satisfactory approximation of the temperature of the internal organs can be made by inserting a clinical thermometer into either the mouth or rectum. These are both closed cavities with good blood supply. The accepted average oral temperature is 98.6° F with recognition that both individual and diurnal variations regularly occur. The rectum is about 1° F warmer. Rectal and oral thermometers have the same temperature scales and markings, differing only in the shape of the bulb. To avoid the potential confusion and errors in subtracting or adding degrees from readings, physicians prefer that the actual temperature and the method be reported, ie, 102.5° F taken rectally. *(1:1882–3)*

106. (E) Immediate counteraction to the burn is recommended. Application of cold water will often reduce the severity of the burn. The burn area should be kept in cold water until no further pain is experienced whether in or out of the water. If necessary, a physician may then be contacted. *(11:776)*

107. (A) *(11:809)*

108. (D) Pilocarpine appears to be well absorbed through the cornea. Miosis occurs in 15 to 30 minutes with maximum reduction in ocular pressure in 2 to 4 hours. The duration of miotic action is usually 4 to 8 hours. *(6:127–30)*

109. (D) The Ocusert pilocarpine unit is a drug delivery system that has a centrally located reservoir of pilocarpine. The Ocusert is placed in the upper or lower cul-de-sac of the eye. Pilocarpine then diffuses across two outer polymeric layers that serve as rate-controlling membranes. The Ocusert is a clear oval device with a visible rigid white margin to aid in placement and removal. The unit is available in two strengths, Pilo-20 and Pilo-40, for use in chronic open-angle glaucoma. The numbers designate the rate of release of drug: 20 μg/h and 40 μg/h respectively. Each Ocusert unit contains sufficient drug for 1 week. *(6:129)*

110. (D) While each of the other choices will produce a constriction of the iris (miosis) and will most likely aid in reducing the patient's intraocular pressure, homatropine will produce mydriasis, which will further aggravate the patient's condition and possibly lead to blindness. *(6:812–3)*

111. (E) The usual categories of drugs used to treat glaucoma include cholinomimetics (eg, pilocarpine), sympathomimetics (eg, epinephrine), and carbonic anhydrase inhibitors (eg, acetazolamide). The most widely used cholinomimetic, pilocarpine, is relatively short-acting, causing accommodative spasm and miosis. Timolol maleate (Timoptic), a beta-receptor antagonist, represents a major advance in the treatment of chronic open-angle glaucoma. It is believed to reduce elevated intraocular pressure by decreasing the production of aqueous humor. Timolol exerts its maximal effect within 1 to 2 hours and maintains significant effects for as long as 24 hours following a single topical dose. There seems to be little or no effect on pupil size, visual acuity, or accommodation. *(11:816–21)*

112. (B) Atropine is a mydriatic used for retraction work and ophthalmoscopy. In a few instances, it has precipitated acute attacks of angle-closure glaucoma. *(11:813)*
(A–incorrect) Carbachol is used as a replacement when resistance or intolerance to pilocarpine occurs. *(11:817)*
(C–incorrect) Demecarium is a long-acting anticholinesterase used to treat primary open-angle glaucoma, glaucoma in aphakia, and accommodative esotropia. *(11:819)*
(D–incorrect) Physostigmine is a short-acting anticholinesterase used in the treatment of primary open-angle glaucoma and for emergency treatment of angle-closure glaucoma. *(11:819)*
(E–incorrect) Betaxolol (Alcon's Betoptic) is a beta-blocking drug similar to timolol. *(11:820)*

113. (A) Epinephrine effectively reduces intraocular pressure in open-angle (chronic) glaucoma by both increasing the outflow of aqueous humor from the anterior chamber of the eye and inhibiting the formation of aqueous humor. Because of its mydriatic action (pupillary dilation), epinephrine is contraindicated in narrow-angle glaucoma. Dilation of the pupils may precipitate acute-angle closure. *(11:821)*

114. (C) *(11:1227–8)*

115. (C) The distinctive lesion is a vivid red macule, papule, or plaque covered by silvery, lamellated scales. Usually the scalp, elbows, knees, and shins are affected first. *(11:764)*

116. (C) If morphine allergy is present, codeine should also be avoided because both codeine and morphine are structurally similar phenanthrene derivatives. Also, codeine is partially (10%) demethylated to morphine. *(6:489)*

117. (D) The labeling of the various transdermal nitroglycerin patches manufactured by Summit (Transderm Nitro), Key (Nitro-Dur), and Searle (Nitrodisc) was inconsistent and highly confusing when these products were first marketed. Ciba labeled its product in terms of the number of milligrams of nitroglycerin released over a 24-hour period. Key Pharmaceuticals labeled its product in terms of the surface area of the patch. Searle labeled its product in terms of the total amount of nitroglycerin contained in the patch. Now all companies identify their patches in terms of mg of nitroglycerin released in 24 hours. However, the physical and chemical properties of the delivery systems differ among the various products. Consequently, these products should not be considered interchangeable and dosing should be titrated for each patient. *(11:681)*

118. (A) Ascorbic acid is added to a number of iron preparations with the claim that it will enhance iron absorption. Ascorbic acid maintains iron in the ferrous state and forms a soluble and absorbable chelate with iron that is present in the ferric state. Doses of 500 of 1000 mg increase iron absorption by about 10%. Smaller doses present in the above preparations do not significantly increase the absorption of iron and are therefore not recommended. *(11:176)*

119. (A) Clonidine is a central alpha-adrenergic stimulant that reduces peripheral vascular resistance and heart rate. Patients who use oral clonidine are susceptible to rebound hypertension if they discontinue their use of the tablets. The transdermal dosage form (Catapres TTS) releases clonidine at a constant rate for about 7 days, thereby improving compliance and reducing the likelihood of rebound hypertension. *(11:598)*

120. (A) Raising the intragastric pH from 1.0 to 3.5 neutralizes 99% of the acid and greatly reduces the proteolytic activity of pepsin, thus attenuating the two primary factors known to overwhelm gastric mucosal resistance. Buffering to higher pHs serves no useful puprose. *(6:904)*

121. (B) Carbidopa inhibits dopa decarboxylase peripherally but does not cross the blood–brain barrier. Inhibiting the peripheral metabolism of levodopa leaves a greater fraction of intact levodopa available to cross the blood–brain barrier where metabolism to dopamine is desired. If a larger fraction of a given dose of levodopa reaches the brain, then a smaller original dose can be used with a reduction in side effects of therapy. This combination of carbidopa and levodopa is commercially available as Sinemet tablets. *(6:471)*

122. (D) Sinemet is a combination product containing carbidopa and levodopa in a ratio of 1:10. Because carbidopa inhibits the peripheral decarboxylation of levodopa, much smaller doses of levodopa can be used. This, in turn, generally reduces the peripheral side effects associated with high doses of levodopa. Dosage levels of levodopa can be decreased by approximately 75%. *(6:472)*

123. (D) The administraton of pyridoxine even in the small doses (5 mg or more) contained in ordinary vitamin preparations is equivalent to a reduction in dosage of levodopa. Pyridoxine is believed to be a cofactor for the enzyme dopa decarboxylase, which is responsible for the peripheral metabolism of levodopa. The decarboxylated metabolic product cannot enter the brain, which is the desired site of action. *(6:471)*

124. (A) While the anticholinergic agents are qualitatively similar in their actions and side effects, a desirable feature of benztropine mesylate is its long duration of action. This property makes the drug very useful as bedtime medication to reduce the early morning symptoms. *(6:160)*

125. (B) The gray syndrome occurs in premature and term newborn infants when chloramphenicol is administered during the first few days of life. The syndrome results from the inability of the infant to metabolize the drug because of a deficient enzyme, glucuronyl transferase, which is required to detoxify the drug by changing it to the glucuronide. Symptoms consist of cyanosis, vascular collapse, and elevated chloramphenicol levels in the blood. *(6:1128–9)*

126. (C) *(28:1481)*

(A–incorrect) Inflammation of the eyelid is blepharitis. *(28:193)*
(D–incorrect) Gastritis is an inflammation of the stomach wall. *(28:635)*
(E–incorrect) Inflammation of the tongue would be known as glossitis. *(28:655)*

127. (C) Polyphagia is defined as an excessive craving for food. *(28:1237)*
(A–incorrect) Alopecia is baldness. *(28:49)*
(B–incorrect) Hirsutism is abnormal hairiness. *(28:717)*
(D–incorrect) Urticaria is commonly called hives. *(28:1676)*
(E–incorrect) Nystagmus is an involuntary rapid movement of the eyeball that may be horizontal, vertical, rotatory, or mixed. *(28:1074)*

128. (B) *(28:746)*

(A–incorrect) An abnormal increase in cell number in a tissue is hyperplasia. *(28:744)*
(C–incorrect) Excessive sweating is hyperhidrosis. *(28:740)*
(D–incorrect) Increased motor activity (excessive movement) is called hyperkinesia. *(28:741)*
(E–incorrect) Excessive sensitivity to stimulation is hyperesthesia. *(28:739)*

129. (A) *(28:480)*

(B–incorrect) Difficulty in swallowing is dysphagia. *(28:478)*
(C–incorrect) Impairment of digestive functioning is dyspepsia. *(28:478)*
(D–incorrect) Painful or difficult urination is dysuria. *(28:482)*
(E–incorrect) Restlessness is dysphoria. *(28:479)*

130. (D) Myopia is the condition of nearsightedness. *(28:1017–8)*

(A–incorrect) Myalgia is pain in a muscle. *(28:1009)*
(B–incorrect) Myocardia pertains to the heart muscle. *(28:1015)*
(C–incorrect) Myoclonus is muscular twitching or contraction. *(28:1015)*
(E–incorrect) Myositis is inflammation of a voluntary muscle. *(28:1018)*

131. (A) The deficiency is usually due to a constriction or actual obstruction of a blood vessel. For example,

myocardial ischemia is a deficiency of the blood supply to the heart muscle. *(28:803)*
(C–incorrect) Icterus is a synonym for jaundice. *(30:814)*

132. (D) For example, aortic stenosis is the narrowing of the aortic orifice of the heart. Pyloric stenosis is obstruction of the pyloric orifice of the stomach, caused by hypertrophy of the pyloric muscle. *(28:1473)*
(A–incorrect) Sclerosis is generally caused by overgrowth of fibrous tissue. *(28:1393)*
(C–incorrect) Refers to spondylitis. *(28:1456)*
(E–incorrect) Refers to stasis. *(28:1470)*

133. (C) Phlebitis indicates vein inflammation. It results from injury to the endothelial cells of a blood vessel, usually the vein at an intravenous injection site. The earliest sign is tenderness at the site. The area around the vein then becomes red, warm, and painful, often with edema and stiffness. In some instances thrombophlebitis occurs. This term implies that a clot (thrombus) has formed in the blood vessel at the site of the inflammation. Breakage of the thrombus from the site of formation may lead to an embolism (ie, obstruction or occlusion of a blood vessel at some site removed from the site of clot formation). *(28:1186)*

134. (A) Although digoxin and quinidine are frequently used together, it is well documented that administering quinidine to a patient previously stabilized on digoxin will cause serum digoxin levels to rise an average 2- to 2.5-fold. The mechanism of this interaction may involve both a displacement of digoxin from tissue-binding sites and a reduction in renal clearance of digoxin. Even though the significance of this interaction remains controversial, many clinicians suggest reducing the dose of digoxin by 50% when adding quinidine. In any case, the patient should be carefully monitored for signs of digoxin toxicity. *(6:857)*

135. (B) Under normal circumstances, diuresis induced by amiloride is accompanied by either no appreciable difference or only a slight increase in potassium excretion. However, a sharp reduction in potassium output is observed when either amiloride (Midamor) or triamterene (Dyrenium) is given with other natriuretic drugs. This potassium-sparing action is the rationale for concomitant drug therapy with amiloride. Because of the possibility of inducing serious hyperkalemia, potassium supplements should not be given to patients being treated with amiloride or triamterene. Spironolactone (Aldactone) is an aldosterone antagonist also used to decrease the potassium loss that occurs secondary to the use of other diuretics. *(6:727–8)*

136. (C) Mannitol is usually administered intravenously as a hypertonic 10% to 25% solution (an isotonic solution is about 5.5%). The introduction of a hypertonic solution provokes urine flow. Mannitol solutions are used in prophylaxis of acute renal failure,

in the evaluation of acute oliguria, and for the reduction of the pressure and volume of the intraocular and cerebrospinal fluids. *(6:714–6)*

137. (A) Since many patients who took imipramine for depression reported difficulty in urination, it was reasoned that the drug might be of value in treating enuresis. Now the drug is used routinely to treat nocturnal enuresis, especially in children. It is not recommended for children younger than 6 years of age. Doses of imipramine range from 25 to 75 mg, lower than those used for treatment of depression. Other brands besides Tofranil are Janimine and SK-Pramine. *(3:1228)*

138. (B) Chenodiol (Chenix) is the bile acid chenodeoxycholic acid, a naturally occurring normal hepatic metabolite of cholesterol. It is taken orally to dissolve gallstones. It should be used only in patients with radiolucent (cholesterol) stones in well-functioning gallbladders who refuse elective surgery or are poor surgical risks because of systemic disease or age. Therapy may be continued for as long as 24 months. Patients must comply with the dosage regimen and with the schedule of periodic liver function tests and oral cholescystograms or ultrasonograms for monitoring stone dissolution. Hepatotoxicity is the most serious toxic effect, and diarrhea is the most common side effect.
(A–incorrect) Serum levels of total cholesterol and low-density lipoprotein (LDL) cholesterol may increase by 10% or more during chenodiol therapy. Cholesterol levels should be monitored at 6-month intervals. *(3:1553)*

139. (C) Cyclosporine (Sandimmune) is a cyclic polypeptide immunosuppressive agent that prolongs survival of allogenic transplants (heart, kidney, liver, and other organs) in humans and other animals. Nephrotoxicity has been noted in 25% to 38% of organ transplant recipients using cyclosporine. Synergism with nephrotoxic drugs may occur. Hypertension, hirsutism, and gum hyperplasia are other adverse reactions. The oral solution (100 mg/mL) is taken immediately after mixing with milk, chocolate milk, or orange juice. Soft gelatin capsules and an intravenous dosage form are also marketed. Cyclosporine may be administered concurrently with adrenal corticosteroids but not with other immunosuppressants. *(3:2592–6)*

140. (B) Nalbuphine (Nubain) is a mixed narcotic agonist-antagonist capable of relieving moderate to severe pain. In subjects dependent on narcotics such as morphine and codeine, nalbuphine precipitates a withdrawal syndrome. Although it is capable of producing euphoriant effects similar to morphine, its effect on respiration seems to exhibit a ceiling effect, such that doses above 30 mg produce no further respiratory depression. *(6:512–3)*

141. (B) *(3:2508–10)*

142. (C) Jacksonian epilepsy consists of a focal convulsion during which consciousness is often maintained. The seizure itself may be motor, sensory, or autonomic in nature. It usually begins in part of a limb or the face as a localized clonic spasm, then spreads in a somewhat orderly fashion. *(11:847)*

143. (B) Mild polycythemia is normal in persons who exercise excessively and in persons who live at high altitudes. Polycythemia vera is a state in which the rate of red cell production is far greater than normal, even though there is no apparent physiologic need for the increased production. It is believed that this disease may result from some sort of tumor of the bone marrow. Phlebotomy whenever the hematocrit rises above 55% may suffice as the only treatment for patients who do not have severe thrombocytosis. Drugs used to treat polycythemia include busulfan (Myleran) and radioactive phosphorus ($_{32}$P). *(11:73)*

144. (B) Protamine is a strongly basic substance that combines with the strongly acidic heparin to produce a stable salt and a loss of anticoagulant activity. Because protamine itself possesses anticoagulant properties, it is unwise to administer more than 100 mg of protamine over a short period of time unless it is known that there is a definite need for a larger amount. *(6:1317)*

145. (A) Administration of vitamin K_1 (phytonadione) will correct oral anticoagulant-induced bleeding within a few hours. This form of treatment, however, should only be used in severe cases of hemorrhage since the patient may beocme temporarily refractory to renewed oral anticoagulant therapy. *(6:1563)*

146. (C) Althogh the risk of hemorrhage in the fetus can be minimized by closely monitoring the prothrombin time of the mother, it is probably best to use heparin if anticoagulant therapy is necessary under these circumstances. Since heparin is a high-molecular-weight mucopolysaccharide, it does not cross the placenta. *(6:1313–7)*

147. (E) Heparin is not a uniform molecular species, and therefore should be prescribed in units rather than milligrams. The old equivalent of 100 mg = 10,000 units is a poor approximation because the USP specifies that the potency must be not less than 120 U/mg when derived from lung tissues and not less than 140 U/mg when derived from other tissues. Potency must be within 90% to 110% of what is stated on the label. If a physician orders 100 mg of heparin, it is not clear whether he means 10,000 units, 12,000 units, or some other quantity. Other nations use an international unit that is not identical to the USP heparin unit. *(6:1313–7)*

148. (E) Prothrombin time (PT) is a measure of the time it takes for fibrin to gel in plasma after addition of calcium and thromboplastin. The PT of patients on coumarin drugs is prolonged because of the reduced activity of several blood factors. Vitamin K antagonizes the action of these anticoagulants and therefore shortens PT. The other drugs will increase PT. *(11:80)*

149. (C) In normal individuals, over 50% of an oral dose of vitamin B_{12} is absorbed from the gastrointestinal tract. This absorption only occurs in the presence of the intrinsic factor of Castle, with which the vitamin must presumably combine in order to pass through the intestinal walls. By means of radioactive cobalt-labeled cyanocobalamin, it has been shown that over half of an oral dose soon appears in the blood. Normally, only a small amount of radioactivity appears in the urine. However, if a large "flushing" dose (1000 µg) of vitamin B_{12} is given parenterally within an hour of the tagged oral dose, the renal threshold for B_{12} is exceeded and radioactivity is observed in the urine. In patients with pernicious anemia, there is a deficiency in intrinsic factor that results in poor absorption of the radioactive B_{12}. Most of the radioactivity in these patients will be detected in the feces. *(11:181–7)*

150. (B) Bromocriptine is an ergot alkaloid derivative that acts on the anterior pituitary gland to suppress prolactin secretion. The drug may be indicated in the treatment of amenorrhea and galactorrhea associated with hyperprolactinemia. It is available as 2.5-mg tablets, and the usual therapeutic dose is one tablet two or three times daily. *(11:876)*
(A–incorrect) Chlorpromazine is a dopamine antagonist.
(C–incorrect) Benztropine is an anticholinergic drug.
(D–incorrect) Diphenhydramine is an antihistaminic drug.

151. (C) Insulin injection (regular or crystalline zinc) is used in situations where rapid onset and brief duration of action are desired. It is the only preparation that can be given intravenously; it is so used in the treatment of diabetic ketoacidosis. In this emergency situation, the drug is often used in conjunction with subcutaneously administered, longer-acting insulin preparations. *(11:324)*

152. (C) Protamine zinc insulin exerts an action for as long as 24 to 36 hours. The shortest duration is exhibited by regular insulin, which may act only for 6 to 8 hours. *(11:324–5)*

153. (B) Diabetic ketoacidosis is a direct result of the lack of insulin. The omission of insulin doses or errors in adjusting the insulin dosage in response to changes in food intake or physical activity is probably the most common cause of diabetic ketoacidosis. Other common causes include infections and myocardial infarctions. *(11:330–1)*

154. (B) Although copper reduction tests (eg, Clinitest) are more quantitative measures of glucosuria than the glucose oxidase tests (eg, Tes-Tape), they are less specific for glucose. It is well documented that the cephalosporin antibiotics may cause false-positive readings with copper reduction tests. To enable a patient to use the copper reduction method of urine testing while taking cefaclor, it is desirable to determine whether or not the drug is interfering with the test. In this example, the fact that the tests yielded different results indicates that there is an interference. The fact that cephalosporins do not interfere with Tes-Tape indicates that the interference is a false-positive with Clinitest. *(11:316–7)*

155. (C) *(11:329)*

156. (D) Chlordiazepoxide, diazepam, clorazepate, and prazepam are all metabolized by oxidation in the liver to desmethyldiazepam, an active metabolite with a very long half-life. This process is impaired in the elderly and in the presence of liver disease (eg, cirrhosis) resulting in drug accumulation and the risk of oversedation. Lorazepam and oxazepam (Serax) are metabolized by glucuronidation, a process that is much less dependent on liver function than oxidation. Furthermore, the metabolites of lorazepam and oxazepam are inactive. *(11:911–2)*

157. (B) The usual method of treating an acute hypoglycemic reaction is to give glucose orally or, in unconscious patients, intravenously in concentrated solutions. If, however, these routes cannot be used, 0.5 to 1 mg of glucagon may be given subcutaneously or intramuscularly as well as intravenously. Glucagon is an endogenous hormone produced by the alpha cells of the pancreatic islets of Langerhans. Glucagon increases blood glucose by stimulating hepatic gluconeogenesis and glycogenolysis. *(6:1488–9)*

158. (D) Since 6-mercaptopurine is metabolized by the enzyme xanthine oxidase, concomitant administration of allopurinol, which is a xanthine oxidase inhibitor, will decrease the rate of metabolism of 6-mercaptopurine. This will potentiate the effects and toxicity of 6-MP unless the dose of 6-MP is reduced to 25% to 30% of its usual therapeutic level. *(11:518)*

159. (B) Dopamine exerts a positive inotropic effect by direct action on beta-adrenergic receptors and causes a release of norepinephrine from storage sites. A major advantage of the drug is that its hemodynamic effects can be varied by controlling the infusion rate. *(6:200–1)*

160. (E) Significant increases in blood pressure can be controlled by either reducing the infusion rate or discontinuing the infusion until the blood pressure has been stabilized. Among the major drug interactions of dopamine is concurrent use of the monoamine oxidase inhibitors. Since dopamine is metabolized by monamine oxidase enzymes, doses of dopamine may have to be reduced to 10% of normal when the patient has been medicated with a monoamine oxidase inhibitor drug. *(6:200–1)*

161. (C) In the iron-deficient state, the iron storage compartment becomes depleted. This is followed by a reduction in plasma transferrin saturation. Subsequently, the number and size of the erythrocytes as well as their hemoglobin content will be decreased. *(11:171–2)*

162. (D) Trigeminal neuralgia is a disorder characterized by sudden attacks of severe pain along the distribution of the fifth cranial nerve. Attacks are often precipitated by stimulation of a "trigger zone" in the area of the pain. Carbamazepine (Tegretol) is remarkably effective in both relieving and preventing the pain of trigeminal neuralgia. Anticonvulsants such as phenytoin (Dilantin) may also be beneficial in some cases. Other drugs that have been effective are vitamin B_{12} in massive doses (1 mg) and injection of alcohol into the ganglion or the branches of the trigeminal nerve. *(6:443,449)*

163. (B) Although aged people with parkinsonism may have impairment of memory and judgment or mental disturbances due to other disease states or social isolation, these effects are not caused by the disease per se.
(A–incorrect) Tremor is a rhythmical alternating contraction of a given muscle group and its antagonist.
(C–incorrect) Posture disturbances include difficulty in maintaining an upright position of the trunk while standing or walking. Also, retropulsion (tendency to walk backward) or festination (an involuntary increase or hastening in gait, generally in a stooped position) may be present.
(D–incorrect) Bradykinesia is slow or retarded movement. In parkinsonism, there is diminished spontaneous movement, loss of normal associative movement, and slowness in initiation of all voluntary movements.
(E–incorrect) Rigidity is an increased muscle tone that is resistant to passive movement of an extremity. *(11:868–78)*

164. (A) The development of inflammatory conditions of the colon (eg, nonspecific colitis or a more severe pseudomembranous colitis) has been associated with antibiotic therapy. Although many antibiotics have been implicated, there have been a disproportionate number of reports specifically involving clindamycin and lincomycin. Colitis has been associated with both oral and parenteral administration of these drugs, and no clear predisposing conditions have been identified. Since antimotility drugs (eg, diphenoxalate) used to treat the resulting diarrhea seem to prolong the disease, they should not be used. *(19:40–7)*

165. (C) Loperamide (Imodium) inhibits peristaltic activity by a direct effect on the musculature of the intestinal wall. Loperamide appears to be devoid of opium-like effects. Even after chronic administration of loperamide, the injection of the narcotic antagonist naloxone does not produce pupillary dilation.   *(3:1589)*

166. **(D)** Tricyclic antidepressants such as imipramine (Tofranil) and amitriptyline (Elavil) may block the uptake of guanethidine by adrenergic nerves, thereby inhibiting its antihypertensive action.

    (3:1223)

167. **(A)** Cyclobenzaprine (Flexeril), an analogue of amitriptyline, is available for the treatment of acute voluntary muscle spasm. Because they are so alike in chemical structure, cyclobenzaprine and amitriptyline have essentially the same side effects and toxicity.   *(3:1439–41)*

168. **(E)** Although exchange transfusions have traditionally been used to manage hyperbilirubinemia, this treatment rarely decreases the bilirubin level to even half its pretransfusion level and exposes the neonate to the hazards of blood transfusion. More recently, phenobarbital has been found to be effective in lowering serum bilirubin levels. Apparently, phenobarbital enhances glucuronidation by stimulating synthesis of hepatic microsomal enzymes and by inducing production of bilirubin-binding Y protein. The dosage of phenobarbital is 5 mg every 8 hours (beginning 6 to 8 hours after delivery) for 3 to 5 days until serum bilirubin levels fall to below 10 mg/dL. Complete failure of this treatment can probably be attributed to discontinuing the drug prematurely.

    (6:364)

169. **(B)** Chlorpheniramine maleate will not displace warfarin from its protein-binding sites, and therefore has less of a tendency to cause a therapeutic problem in this patient. All of the other choices have a high affinity for plasma proteins.   *(6:1320)*

170. **(E)** Phenylephrine is an adrenergic stimulant normally metabolized in the liver by the enzyme monoamine oxidase (MAO). In the presence of an MAO inhibitor such as pargyline, much higher and more toxic blood levels of phenylephrine will result, thereby causing an elevation in the patient's blood pressure.   *(3:1251–2)*

171. **(A)** Each gram of protein supplies about 4 kcal, each gram of carbohydrate supplies about 4 kcal, and each gram of fat supplies about 9 kcal. It is obvious, therefore, that strictly on a weight basis, fats are better caloric sources than other nutrients.   *(11:122–3)*

172. **(C)** Portagen is a product used when conventional dietary fats may not be well absorbed, digested, or used. Its fat content consists of more than 95% medium-chain triglycerides, which are more rapidly absorbed than the triglycerides of long-chain fatty acids present in conventional food fats. Patients suffering from steatorrhea (excessive loss of fats in the feces) are ideal candidates for dietary supplementation with Portagen.   *(11:1419,3:183)*

173. **(A)** Pedialyte is an orally administered electrolyte solution containing dextrose, potassium chloride, and sodium, calcium, and magnesium salts. It is used to supply water and electrolytes in a balanced proportion in order to prevent serious deficits from occurring in patients suffering from mild to moderate fluid loss. The product does not contain protein or fats.   *(3:50)*

174. **(B)** Each gram of carbohydrate supplies 4 kcal of energy to a patient. Since a liter of dextrose 5% solution contains 50 g of dextrose, the administration of the liter will supply the patient with approximately 200 kcal.   *(11:122)*

175. **(D)** Phenylketonuria (PKU) is an inherited metabolic disorder characterized by high plasma phenylalanine hydroxylase, which converts phenylalanine to tyrosine. Routine testing of newborns for PKU is common in the US. Treatment consists of following a low-phenylalanine diet that is started early in life and continued perhaps indefinitely. Lofenalac, a complete nutritional product except for its low phenylalanine content, is used in place of the usual milk in the diet of children with PKU. Untreated PKU results in mental retardation. Foods and beverages containing aspartame (NutraSweet) must bear label warnings for people with PKU, since aspartame is metabolized to phenylalanine (and aspartic acid and methanol).   *(19:32–5,32–6)*

176. **(D)** Because this patient has a history of recurrent infections, the present symptoms probably indicate a reinfection. Therefore, ampicillin would be the most reasonable choice pending culture and sensitivity results. If this patient had been initially treated with a sulfonamide or a tetracycline, it would be desirable to switch to a different drug because bacteria frequently develop resistance to these drugs.

    (11:1109–22)

177. **(B)** Of the drugs listed, erythromycin has the lowest degree of toxicity and the spectrum of action most similar to penicillin. Demeclocycline may inhibit skeletal growth in the fetus. Deposition of tetracyclines in the teeth of the fetus has been associated with enamel defects and staining of the teeth. Trimethoprim is a teratogenic drug.   *(6:1131)*

178. **(E)** Sulfamylon cream applied topically to burns has been found to be quite effective in inhibiting the invasion of the affected site by both gram-positive and gram-negative bacteria. The cream is usually applied to a thickness of about 1/16 inch twice daily over the entire burned surface. Silver sulfadiazine is also used topically for the same purpose.   *(6:1051)*

179. **(B)** Spectinomycin is an aminocyclitol antibiotic related to the aminoglycosides. While active against many gram-positive and gram-negative organisms, it is generally reserved for the treatment of gonorrhea in patients who fail treatment with penicillin,

ampicillin, amoxacillin, or tetracycline; it may also be given to patients who are allergic to penicillin and are unable to tolerate, or are unlikely to comply with, a 5-day regimen of tetracycline. It is given as a single 2-g IM injection and produces a cure in 90% of cases. *(6:1137)*

180. (B) Colchicine is one of the most valuable drugs available for the treatment of an acute attack of gout. The mechanism of action is not known but is believed to be interference with the inflammatory response of gout. Colchicine may alter other inflammatory states, but the effects are less dramatic. The uricosuric drugs used for gout act by either increasing the rate of uric acid excretion by the kidney (ie, probenecid and sulfinpyrazone) or by decreasing the rate of synthesis of uric acid (ie, allopurinol).

(6:674–6)

181. (E) Opticrom ophthalmic solution contains cromolyn sodium 4%. It is used to treat ocular allergic disorders such as vernal conjunctivitis. It is only effective if it is used at regular intervals. *(3:2081)*

182. (A) Glucose tolerance is impaired by the thiazides, even though certain other sulfonamide derivatives are hypoglycemic agents. The degree of hyperglycemia induced by the thiazides is unimportant in patients with normal carbohydrate tolerance but may intensify the hyperglycemia of diabetes or precipitate glycosuria in persons predisposed to diabetes.

(6:721)

183. (C) Dopamine (Intropin) is a sympathomimetic drug that acts directly on alpha and beta receptors and produces indirect effects due to release of norepinephrine. Dopamine also dilates renal and mesenteric vessels through a dopamine receptor effect. The hemodynamic effects of dopamine are dose related. At low infusion rates (1 to 5 μg/kg/min) dopamine increases renal blood flow without much change in cardiac output or total peripheral resistance. In higher doses (5 to 20 μg/kg/min), cardiac output and heart rate increase, the increase in renal perfusion persists, and total peripheral resistance is variable. At higher infusion rates, renal vasoconstriction occurs, total peripheral resistance rises, and blood pressure increases. Consequently, the infusion rate must be adjusted and carefully monitored to achieve the desired response. *(6:200–1)*

184. (B) Because of the relatively poor aqueous solubility of chlordiazepoxide, the drug is reconstituted in a "special" diluent that consists primarily of propylene glycol. When injected intramuscularly, the drug is believed to precipitate at the injection site, forming a depot from which it slowly redissolves and becomes available for absorption. Compared to equal oral doses, intramuscular chlordiazepoxide is absorbed more slowly and produces lower blood levels. If large intramuscular doses of the drug are given repeatedly over a short period of time, it is quite likely that the patient will demonstrate symptoms of overdose several hours later when large amounts of the drug are absorbed from the multiple injections. Also, the drug and its metabolites have long half-lives. *(3:1202)*

185. (D) Although there are no reported differences in bioavailability between phenytoin capsules and suspension, this patient's phenytoin level is most likely going to increase because the milligram-for-milligram conversion is equivalent to an increase in dose. The capsule form of Dilantin is the sodium salt and as such contains only 92% phenytoin. The suspension is the free acid and contains 100% phenytoin. In this situation, the patient would be going from a daily dose of 276 mg phenytoin (as 300-mg phenytoin sodium) to 300 mg phenytoin. *(3:1376–7)*

186. (C) Dobutamine (Dobutrex) is a beta-adrenergic agonist that is available for intravenous use as an inotropic drug. Although dobutamine is similar to isoproterenol (Isuprel) in terms of its inotropic effect, dobutamine is relatively less potent than isoproterenol as a stimulator of peripheral beta receptors that mediate vasodilation. Consequently, dobutamine produces an inotropic effect with comparatively little effect on preload, afterload, or heart rate.

(6:202–3)

187. (C) The full therapeutic effect of the tricyclic antidepressants often takes several weeks to develop. During this period, many patients subjectively feel that their depression has worsened. On the other hand, the side effects of these drugs, sedation and anticholinergic effects, usually begin shortly after therapy is initiated. The pharmacist should discuss these anticipated effects with the patient. The pharmacist should also consult with the prescribing physician if it is apparent that an intensified depression may be serious enough to lead to suicide. *(6:404–14)*

188. (D) The theoretical advantage of administering insulin in IV glucose is that both insulin and glucose are delivered in constant proportions. Administration of insulin in this manner, however, can result in undesirable fluctuations in blood glucose levels. As much as 20% of the insulin added to an IV is bound to the container and tubing. Proportionally greater binding occurs with lower doses of insulin. If the same administration set is used for subsequent infusions, the binding sites on the set may be saturated with insulin. This would be observed clinically as some improvement in control of blood glucose, since subsequent binding would be to the IV container alone. Furthermore, even if the insulin dose is adjusted for binding by the container, hyperglycemia may still occur after the administration set is changed. This, of course, does not mean that insulin should not be administered by IV infusion, but that the adsorption of insulin by IV bottles and tubing should be considered in accounting for unusual changes in blood glucose levels and in determining insulin doses, especially when low doses are contemplated.   *(19:72–30)*

189. **(C)** In general, all insulins are reasonably stable at room temperature (75° F). Regular insulin may lose 10% of its activity at room temperature after 18 months. Modified insulins will coagulate within a few days if they are stored at temperatures above 75° F. Although this does not result in a total loss in potency, it is markedly more difficult to withdraw a uniform dose and to predict the onset of action and duration of response. Traveling diabetics should be advised to avoid prolonged exposure of their insulin to very high temperatures, and told that it is not necessary to refrigerate the vial in use. Insulin vials stored in pharmacies are required to be refrigerated since they may be kept in stock for a long time.
                                                              (19:72–25)

190. **(B)** The sliding scale (or rainbow scale) is a method of determining insulin dosing based on periodic determinations of glucose and ketones in the urine. The physician prescribes the regular insulin dosage as a function of the number of pluses determined by the copper reduction (Clinitest) glucose determination and the presence of urinary ketones. The physician may prescribe a fixed number of units for each plus (eg, 4 units for each plus) or a more variable schedule (as in the problem). At 4 PM the patient had a 4+ for glucose, for which 10 units of regular insulin are ordered. The patient also had moderate (Mod) amounts of ketones present, for which 2 units of regular insulin are ordered.

> Total 4 PM dose: 10 units
>   2 units
>   ─────────
>   12 units of regular insulin

(C–incorrect; E–incorrect) Since the "sliding scale" is generally used to determine the 24-hour insulin requirements of a ketotic diabetic, the modified insulins (eg, NPH) are not used.   *(19:72–20)*

191. **(B)** Fluids employed in total parenteral nutrition are generally very hypertonic and hyperosmotic. Until the technique of subclavian vein catheterization was perfected, it was too irritating and inflammatory to use the usual sites of intravenous administration. Peripheral veins are seldom used in the administration of hypertonic nutrient solutions; this is because blood flow is insufficient to provide the necessary dilution of the fluid to protect the intima of the vessel. The exception occurs when the slightly hypertonic amino acid solutions containing limited amounts of dextrose are administered.   *(11:155–6)*

192. **(E)** Although all beta blockers are likely to mask the symptoms of acute hypoglycemia (eg, rapid pulse, tachycardia, tremor) the cardioselective beta blockers atenolol (Tenormin) and metoprolol (Lopressor) are more appropriate in diabetics; these drugs have much less of an effect on the metabolic and cardiovascular responses to hypoglycemia than the nonselective beta blockers. They are therefore less likely to intensify hypoglycemia, precipitate hypertensive crises during hypoglycemia, and compromise peripheral circulation. Atenolol does not potentiate insulin-induced hypoglycemia and, unlike the nonselective beta blockers, does not delay recovery of glucose to normal levels.   *(3:710)*

193. **(B)** Inhibition of calcium entry into arterial smooth muscle is associated with decreased arteriolar tone and systemic vascular resistance, resulting in decreased arterial pressure. This reduction in arterial pressure, in turn, causes a significant reflex tachycardia. Because other calcium channel blockers such as verapamil (Calan, Isoptin) and diltiazem (Cardizem) also significantly decrease intracardiac conduction, they are much less likely to cause tachycardia.   *(3:645)*

194. **(D)** Suddenly discontinuing dextrose solution may cause a rebound hypoglycemia in response to the sudden elimination of the sustained glucose load of the TPN solution. It is best to maintain the patient on a nominal amount of dextrose such as D5W or to slowly wean the patient from the TPN solution.
(B–incorrect) Hyperchloremic metabolic acidosis may occur during TPN therapy when the total chloride ion content is high. The amino acids in the protein salts are usually chloride or hydrochloride salts. Additional amounts of chloride are obtained when sodium or potassium chlorides are added to the TPN solutions. It may be useful to supply either sodium or potassium as acetate salts.
(C–incorrect) Hyperosmotic nonketotic hyperglycemia is a result of infusing an overload of glucose. Causes include an overly rapid infusion rate, dextrose solutions that are too concentrated, and malfunction of pancreatic secretion of insulin.   *(11:155–61)*

195. **(B)** Fats provide approximately 9 kcal/g. Because of their isotonicity, fat emulsions can be safely administered through peripheral veins. A commercial example of a fat emulsion is Intralipid, a 10% soybean emulsion.
(A–incorrect) Ethanol provides 7 kcal/g. Disadvantages associated with ethanol are the fact that excessively rapid infusion can cause heartburn and/or intoxication, and the fact that it cannot be used in patients with GI disease such as pancreatitis.
(D–incorrect) Hydrous dextrose provides 3.4 kcal/g. It is the usual source of calories in TPN formulations because of its safety, economy, and availability to the body.
(E–incorrect) Proteins provide 3 to 4 kcal/g.
                                                              (11:156–8)

196. **(E)** Ondansetron (Zofran) is a selective 5-HT$_3$ receptor antagonist used to prevent nausea and vomiting associated with cancer chemotherapy. It is particu-

larly useful in treating nausea and vomiting accompanying cisplatin therapy. Ondansetron is administered by IV infusion beginning 15 to 30 minutes prior to initiating emetogenic chemotherapy. Additional doses are administered 4 and 8 hours after the initial dose. *(10)*

197. (D) Amiloride is a potassium-sparing diuretic with a mechanism of action similar to that of triamterene. Both drugs exert a diuretic effect by promoting the exchange of sodium for potassium in the distal portion of the renal tubule. In contrast to spironolactone, neither of these drugs inhibits aldosterone. Metolazone and chlorthalidone are thiazide-like diuretics. *(6:727–8)*

198. (D) Treatment of hyperkalemia can be approached by three methods. First, in the presence of ECG changes, calcium should be given to counteract the effects of excess potassium on the heart. Secondly, bicarbonate or glucose plus insulin can be used to rapidly shift potassium from extracellular to intracellular fluid compartments. Thirdly, exchange resins (eg, Kayexalate) or dialysis can be used to remove potassium from the body. In this case, since there are no symptoms of ECG changes, the rectal administration of Kayexalate (enemas containing 50 g in 70% sorbitol solution) is the most appropriate option. *(6:703–4)*

199. (A) The hypotensive activity of diazoxide is caused by a reduction in peripheral vascular resistance via direct arteriolar relaxation. As arterial pressure is lowered, baroreceptor reflexes are activated; this leads to cardiac stimulation with increased heart rate, stroke volume, and cardiac output. This, in turn, will increase myocardial oxygen demand, a potentially dangerous situation in a patient with ischemic heart disease. *(6:804–5)*

200. (B) Nitroprusside and trimethaphan both decrease total peripheral resistance rapidly, with minimal effects on myocardial oxygen consumption. Nitroprusside dilates both venous (capacitance) and arterial (resistance) vessels, therefore reducing preload and afterload on the heart. Nitroprusside is preferred over trimethaphan because tolerance develops rapidly to trimethaphan's hypotensive activity. Propranolol is not effective in hypertensive emergencies. Hydralazine and minoxidil are both likely to cause cardiac stimulation. *(6:181–4,803–4)*

201. (E) Although none of the cyclic antidepressants are totally without anticholinergic and cardiovascular side effects, trazodone (Desyrel) has much less of this activity and would be more appropriate for this patient. *(6:406)*

202. (E) Trazodone (Desyrel) is the only drug listed that acts primarily on the reuptake of serotonin. Imipramine, nortriptyline, and trimipramine affect reuptake of both serotonin and norepinephrine. Maprotil-

ine selectively inhibits the reuptake of norepinephrine with no effect on serotonin. *(11:931–2)*

203. (C) Prednisone is approximately four times more potent than hydrocortisone. Since this patient was receiving a total daily dose of 200 mg of hydrocorticone, an equivalent anti-inflammatory dose of prednisone would be 50 mg/day. *(11:258)*

204. (E) Glucocorticoids associated with a lesser degree of mineralocorticoid activity should be used in patients with conditions such as congestive heart failure in which sodium retention can be an aggravating factor. Because all glucocorticoids induce potassium loss regardless of their mineralocorticoid activity, even dexamethasone should be used with caution in this patient. *(6:1439–40)*

205. (C) At the infusion rate of 50 mg/hr the patient is receiving a total daily dose of 1200 mg (50 mg/hr × 24 hr) of aminophylline dihydrate. Since aminophylline dihydrate contains the equivalent of 79% anhydrous theophylline, this patient is receiving a total daily dose of 948 mg anhydrous theophylline (0.79 × 1200 mg/day). The most practical dose of TheoDur would be 900 mg/day given in doses of 300 mg every 8 hours. *(6:626)*

206. (A) Although a number of beta-adrenergic agonists are available for clinical use, only ephedrine, metaproterenol, terbutaline, and albuterol are available in oral dosage forms. Metaproterenol, terbutaline, and albuterol selectively stimulate beta$_2$-adrenergic receptors to a greater degree than beta$_1$- adrenergic receptors. They therefore are somewhat less likely to cause cardiac stimulation. Ephedrine has both weak alpha as well as beta$_1$- and beta$_2$-activity. When compared to these other agents, ephedrine has a shorter duration of action, a lower peak effect, and more adverse effects. Ephedrine also adds little to the bronchodilation produced by therapeutic doses of theophylline; such a combination is likely to produce synergistic toxicity. *(6:201–5)*

207. (E) Downward–*cata*bolism indicates any destructive process by which complex substances are converted by living cells into more simple compounds. *(28:256)*

208. (A) Apart–*dis*articulation is amputation or separation at a joint. *(28:442)*

209. (B) Below–*infra*orbital refers to lying under or on the floor of the orbit. *(28:782)*

210. (D) Middle–*meso*bronchitis indicates inflammation of the middle coat of the bronchi. *(28:949)*

211. (C) Backward–*retro*grade means to retrace a former course. *(28:1354)*

212. (A) *Celi*ac refers to the abdomen. For example, *celi*otomy is an incision into the abdominal cavity. *(28:264)*

213. (B) *Cephal*gia is a headache. *(28:277)*

214. (D) A *colo*proctitis is an inflammation of the colon and rectum. *(28:328)*

215. (C) *Cor* refers to the muscular organ that maintains blood circulation. The pre*cor*dium is the region over the heart. *(28:351)*

216. (E) The term inter*costal* means located between two ribs. *(28:362)*

217. (C) *(28:795)*

218. (D) *(28:796)*

219. (E) *(28:796)*

220. (E) Goiter is a condition characterized by the enlargement of the thyroid. *(28:662)*

221. (A) Cushing's syndrome is a series of clinical symptoms related to the excessive secretion of cortisol by the adrenal cortex. *(11:245)*

222. (C) Hodgkin's disease affects lymphoidal tissue. There is progressive enlargement of lymph nodes, spleen, and other lymphoid tissue. *(11:1291)*

223. (D) Myasthenia gravis is characterized by fatigue and exhaustion of muscles. Although progressive paralysis of muscles occurs, there are no sensory changes or atrophy. *(6:145–6)*

224. (A) Addison's disease is due to hypofunction of the adrenal glands. It is characterized by a bronze pigmentation of the skin, progressive anemia, low blood pressure, diarrhea, and severe prostration. *(11:255–9)*

225. (B) Albright's syndrome is a disorder of bone and cartilage characterized by fibrous dysplasia. *(28:1532)*

226. (E) Bright's disease is a term used to describe kidney disease charcterized by proteinuria and glomerulonephritis. *(28:445)*

227. (C) Crohn's disease is characterized by inflammation of layers of the intestinal tract. *(11:406–12)*

228. (E) *(11:454)*

229. (B) Graves' disease is a thyroid disorder of unknown etiology. Other symptoms include acceleration of pulse rate, sweating, nervousness, psychic disturbances, emaciation, and increased metabolic rate. *(11:273–5)*

230. (C) *(11:1196)*

231. (D) This is a nonsuppurative disease of the labyrinth. *(28:450)*

232. (C) In order to limit destruction by acid hydrolysis, penicillin G tablets should be taken on an empty stomach when gastric acid is at its lowest level. Pentids should be taken 1 hour before or 2 hours after meals. *(3:1612)*

233. (B) Indocin should be taken with food, immediately after meals, or with antacids to reduce gastric irritation. *(3:1117)*

234. (D) Colace is a surfactant and may increase the absorption of mineral oil if given concurrently. *(3:1564)*

235. (A) Sulfonamides are taken with a large volume of water to ensure a volume of urine adequate to keep the excretory products in solution. Crystalluria has occurred with some sulfonamides. *(3:1807)*

236. (E) Dulcolax tablets are enteric coated to prevent gastric irritation. *(3:1564)*

237. (B) The chapter that discusses antacids lists commercial products, with the sodium content of each where the data were available. *(2:282–92)*

238. (B) Each of the chapters in the Handbook covers a specific group of OTC products. Usually, the anatomy and physiology of the body area affected are discussed. Also, the pharmacologic action of ingredients commonly included in the OTC products is considered. Tables are present that list commercial products, manufacturers, ingredients, and levels of ingredients when known. For example, the active drug in Sominex is listed in the section discussing sleep aids. *(2)*

239. (C) The *Physicians' Desk Reference* is divided into several sections, one of which lists pharmaceutical companies with the products manufactured by each. *(25)*

240. (A) *Facts and Comparisons* lists prescription and some nonprescription drug products by pharmacologic classifications. Those prescription-only vitamins that contain fluoride are listed together so that the pharmacist can compare formulas and levels of ingredients. *(3)*

241. (D) The National Drug Code is a number which is often used for computer identification of drug products. The *Red Book* lists commercially available products alphabetically with wholesale prices, AWPs, and NDCs. *(1:54)*

242. (C) The *Physicians' Desk Reference (PDR)* has a color-plate reference section with photographs of products for easy identification. The section is subdivided by individual manufacturers. *(25)*

243. (E) Most drug monographs list identification tests that will aid in the qualitative identification of a drug. For example, the USP monograph for imipramine HCl describes three identification tests. *(1:55)*

244. (A) *Facts and Comparisons* features a cost index, which indicates the relative cost of similar products based upon cost per mL, per tablet, or other common dosage base. *(3)*

245. (E) The approximate solubilities of USP/NF articles are listed in table form. Among the solvents listed are water, boiling water, alcohol, chloroform, and ether. *(18c)*

246. (C) *(11:69–70)*

247. (E) *(11:68)*

248. (C) *(11:68)*

249. (D) *(11:63)*

250. (B) *(11:66–7)*

CHAPTER 7

Patient Profiles

The pharmacist, whether practicing in a community or institutional setting, must constantly refer to patient profiles for information regarding the medical history of a specific patient. Analysis of profile data requires a strong knowledge base in the pharmacy disciplines already reviewed in this book.

In this section, there are thirty patient medication profiles. Some are related to community pharmacy practice and some to institutional practice. Two facing pages have been used for each profile and questions that often relate to the information provided on the profile.

Questions

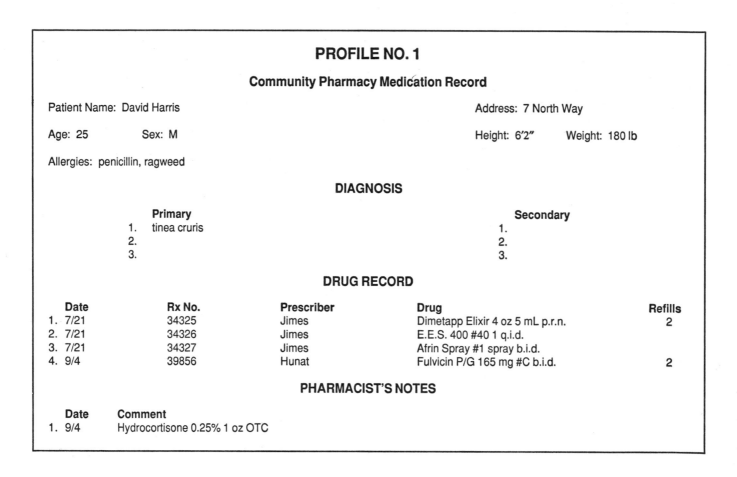

PROFILE NO. 1

Community Pharmacy Medication Record

Patient Name: David Harris

Address: 7 North Way

Age: 25   Sex: M

Height: 6'2"   Weight: 180 lb

Allergies: penicillin, ragweed

DIAGNOSIS

	Primary		Secondary
1.	tinea cruris	1.	
2.		2.	
3.		3.	

DRUG RECORD

	Date	Rx No.	Prescriber	Drug	Refills
1.	7/21	34325	Jimes	Dimetapp Elixir 4 oz 5 mL p.r.n.	2
2.	7/21	34326	Jimes	E.E.S. 400 #40 1 q.i.d.	
3.	7/21	34327	Jimes	Afrin Spray #1 spray b.i.d.	
4.	9/4	39856	Hunat	Fulvicin P/G 165 mg #C b.i.d.	2

PHARMACIST'S NOTES

	Date	Comment
1.	9/4	Hydrocortisone 0.25% 1 oz OTC

DIRECTIONS (Questions 1a through 1i): Each of the numbered items or incomplete statements in this section is followed by answers or by completions of the statement. Select the ONE lettered answer or completion that is BEST in each case.

1a. Tinea cruris is also known as

(A) thrush
(B) athlete's foot
(C) candidiasis
(D) jock itch
(E) coccidioidomycosis

1b. Tinea cruris is caused by a

(A) virus
(B) fungus
(C) gram-negative bacterium
(D) protozoan
(E) gram-positive bacterium

1c. The active ingredient in Fulvicin P/G is

(A) desiccated
(B) macrocrystalline
(C) ultramicrosized

(D) efflorescent

(E) deliquescent

1d. Fulvicin P/G contains

(A) polyethylene glycol

(B) propylene glycol

(C) polyoxyethylene guaiacolate

(D) phenolated glycerin

(E) glycolated protein

1e. Patients receiving Fulvicin P/G should be advised to

I. prevent excessive exposure to ultraviolet light

II. continue medication for entire course of therapy

III. avoid dairy products when using the medication

(A) I only

(B) III only

(C) I and II only

(D) II and III only

(E) I, II, and III

1f. The pharmacist should advise Dr Hunat of

(A) Mr Harris' age

(B) Mr Harris' penicillin allergy

(C) Mr Harris' ragweed allergy

(D) the dosage error made in prescribing Fulvicin P/G

(E) all of the above

1g. Which of the following products is most similar to Fulvicin P/G?

(A) Grifulvin V

(B) Ancobon

(C) Mycostatin

(D) Grisactin Ultra

(E) Nizoral

1h. A topical product that would be appropriate for this patient to use is

(A) bacitracin ointment

(B) metronidazole

(C) nystatin cream

(D) gentian violet

(E) tolnaftate cream

1i. The use of fluorinated steroids on areas affected by tinea is likely to result in

(A) local ulceration

(B) spread of the organism

(C) loss of hair in the area to which the steroid is applied

(D) increased blood glucose levels

(E) yellowish skin discoloration

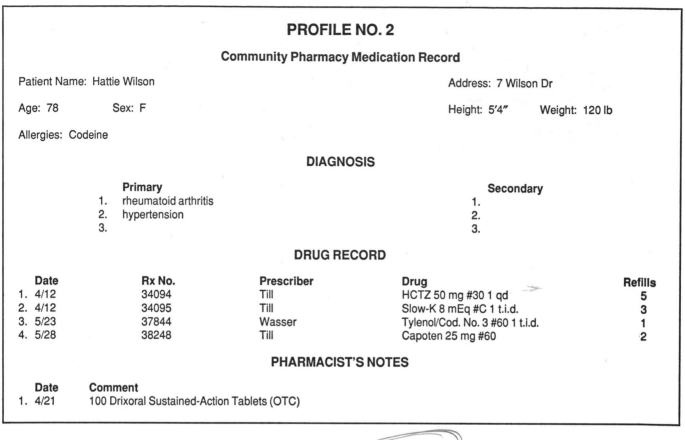

PROFILE NO. 2

Community Pharmacy Medication Record

Patient Name: Hattie Wilson

Address: 7 Wilson Dr

Age: 78   Sex: F

Height: 5'4"   Weight: 120 lb

Allergies: Codeine

DIAGNOSIS

	Primary		Secondary
1.	rheumatoid arthritis	1.	
2.	hypertension	2.	
3.		3.	

DRUG RECORD

	Date	Rx No.	Prescriber	Drug	Refills
1.	4/12	34094	Till	HCTZ 50 mg #30 1 qd	5
2.	4/12	34095	Till	Slow-K 8 mEq #C 1 t.i.d.	3
3.	5/23	37844	Wasser	Tylenol/Cod. No. 3 #60 1 t.i.d.	1
4.	5/28	38248	Till	Capoten 25 mg #60	2

PHARMACIST'S NOTES

	Date	Comment
1.	4/21	100 Drixoral Sustained-Action Tablets (OTC)

DIRECTIONS (Questions 2a through 2k): Each of the numbered items or incomplete statements in this section is followed by answers or by completions of the statement. Select the ONE lettered answer or completion that is BEST in each case.

(A) 592
(B) 296
(C) 312
(D) 872
(E) 740

2a. Which of the following products would be equivalent to the HCTZ prescribed?

I. Diuril
II. Esidrix
III. Oretic

(A) I only
(B) III only
(C) I and II only
(D) II and III only
(E) I, II and III only

2b. Which of the following best describes Slow-K?

(A) microencapsulation
(B) wax matrix
(C) enteric coating
(D) spansule
(E) chewable tablet

2c. Each Slow-K dosage unit contains 8 mEq of potassium as potassium chloride. How many mg of potassium chloride are in each Slow-K tablet? (atom. wt. K = 39; Cl = 35)

2d. Capoten can best be described as a(n)

(A) non-narcotic analgesic
(B) alpha$_1$-adrenergic blocker
(C) nonspecific beta-adrenergic blocker
(D) angiotensin-converting enzyme inhibitor
(E) direct-acting vasodilator

2e. Which of the following agents is most similar to HCTZ?

(A) bumetanide
(B) furosemide
(C) chlorthalidone
(D) acetazolamide
(E) ethacrynic acid

2f. When requesting Drixoral from the pharmacist the patient should be informed that Drixoral

(A) may interact with the Slow-K
(B) is contraindicated in hypertensive patients
(C) is contraindicated in patients allergic to codeine
(D) may not be sold without a prescription
(E) is contraindicated in patients with rheumatoid arthritis

2g. When Capoten is added to this patient's regimen, there is an increased likelihood of

(A) hypokalemia
(B) hypoglycemia
(C) hyperkalemia
(D) xanthine oxidase inhibition
(E) hypocalcemia

2h. Capoten is most similar in action to

(A) Monopril
(B) Lanoxin
(C) Ismelin
(D) Lopressor
(E) Capitrol

2i. Dysgeusia is a reported adverse effect related to the use of Capoten. Dysgeusia can best be defined as

(A) involuntary muscle movement
(B) hearing difficulty
(C) visual impairment
(D) taste impairment
(E) drooling

2j. The dose of codeine found in each dose of Tylenol/Codeine No. 3 is

(A) 3 mg
(B) 3 grains
(C) 30 mg
(D) 30 grains
(E) 0.3 mg

2k. The therapeutic category of brompheniramine maleate in the Drixoral product is

(A) H_1-receptor agonist
(B) H_2-receptor agonist
(C) H_1-receptor antagonist
(D) H_2-receptor antagonist
(E) alpha$_1$-adrenergic agonist

ACE ↑ K levels
+ K supplement
↓↓
hyperkalemia

PROFILE NO. 3

Community Pharmacy Medication Record

Patient Name: Carolyn Mann

Address: 45 No. High St

Age: 27   Sex: F

Height: 5'3"   Weight: 120 lb

Allergies: aspirin

DIAGNOSIS

Primary
1. grand mal seizures since age 8
2.
3.

Secondary
1. constipation
2.
3.

DRUG RECORD

	Date	Rx No.	Prescriber	Drug	Refills
1.	2/2	34568	Mazur	Micronor	5
2.	3/1	34568	Mazur	Refill	
3.	3/21	35908	Wilson	Dilantin Kap. 0.1#C 3 daily	2
4.	4/2	38998	Mazur	Theragran-M #C 1 daily	2

PHARMACIST'S NOTES

	Date	Comment
1.	4/2	Semicid 1 pk (OTC)
2.	4/9	Colace 100 mg #100 (OTC)

DIRECTIONS (Questions 3a through 3m): Each of the numbered items or incomplete statements in this section is followed by answers or by completions of the statement. Select the ONE lettered answer or completion that is BEST in each case.

3a. Micronor can best be described as a(n)

(A) triphasic oral contraceptive
(B) "minipill" oral contraceptive
(C) biphasic oral contraceptive
(D) ovulation inducer
(E) vaginal deodorant product

3b. Semicid is employed as a vaginal

(A) douche solution
(B) suppository
(C) cream
(D) silicone implant
(E) lubricant

3c. A synonym for grand mal seizures is

(A) Jacksonian seizures
(B) absence seizures
(C) focal seizures
(D) status epilepticus
(E) tonic-clonic seizures

3d. The Dilantin product prescribed may be administered

I. on a p.r.n. basis
II. as a single daily dose
III. in three divided daily doses

(A) I only
(B) III only
(C) I and II only
(D) II and III only
(E) I, II and III

3e. In the course of receiving Dilantin the patient develops gingival hyperplasia. This is a disorder of the

(A) nasal mucosa
(B) lymph nodes
(C) gums
(D) liver
(E) vaginal lining

3f. The generic name of the Dilantin product prescribed is

(A) phenytoin sodium
(B) ethotoin
(C) phensuximide
(D) phenytoin
(E) mephenytoin

3g. A plasma phenytoin determination reveals a plasma concentration of 5 µg/mL. This indicates that

(A) the patient may not be taking all prescribed doses
(B) the patient may be taking more doses than prescribed
(C) the concentration is within the therapeutic range
(D) there is a drug interaction with the Micronor
(E) hepatic impairment may exist

3h. The prescriber should be called because of

(A) cross-sensitivity between aspirin and Dilantin
(B) reduction in Micronor effectiveness
(C) reduction in Dilantin effectiveness
(D) carcinogenicity with Dilantin
(E) improper Dilantin dose prescribed

3i. Which of the following is true of parenterally administered Dilantin?

I. IM administration should generally be avoided.
II. Precipitation is likely to occur when Dilantin is combined with promethazine HCl in an IV admixture.
III. Dilantin parenteral solutions must be kept refrigerated until just prior to administration.

(A) I only
(B) III only
(C) I and II only
(D) II and III only
(E) I, II, and III

3j. Patients receiving Dilantin may develop a morbilliform rash. Morbilliform refers to

(A) multicolored
(B) measles-like
(C) acne-like
(D) symmetrical
(E) pus-containing

3k. The active ingredient of Semicid is

(A) ethinyl estradiol
(B) oxyquinoline sulfate
(C) boric acid
(D) sodium lauryl sulfate
(E) nonoxynol 9

3l. The active ingredient in Colace is a(n)

(A) stimulant
(B) anionic surfactant
(C) cationic surfactant
(D) osmotic laxative
(E) bulk former

3m. Which of the following is true of Theragran-M?

(A) It is available without a prescription.
(B) It is a sustained-release capsule product.
(C) Its use should be avoided in patients on Dilantin.
(D) Its use should be avoided in patients on Micronor.
(E) It is only available as a liquid.

Do not refrig
Do not mix w/other drugs
IM painful & irratic

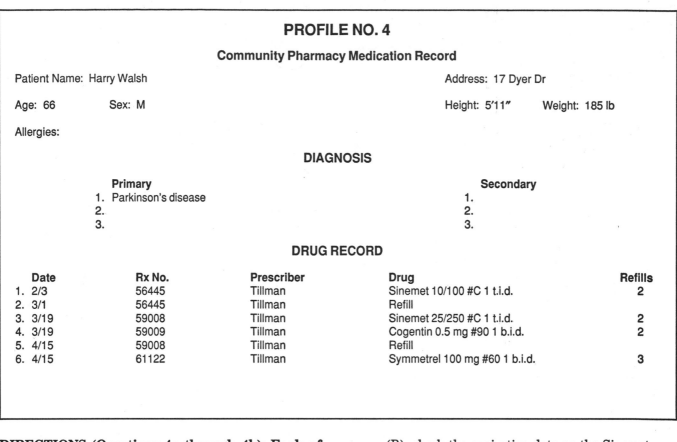

PROFILE NO. 4

Community Pharmacy Medication Record

Patient Name: Harry Walsh

Address: 17 Dyer Dr

Age: 66   Sex: M

Height: 5'11"   Weight: 185 lb

Allergies:

DIAGNOSIS

Primary	Secondary
1. Parkinson's disease	1.
2.	2.
3.	3.

DRUG RECORD

	Date	Rx No.	Prescriber	Drug	Refills
1.	2/3	56445	Tillman	Sinemet 10/100 #C 1 t.i.d.	2
2.	3/1	56445	Tillman	Refill	
3.	3/19	59008	Tillman	Sinemet 25/250 #C 1 t.i.d.	2
4.	3/19	59009	Tillman	Cogentin 0.5 mg #90 1 b.i.d.	2
5.	4/15	59008	Tillman	Refill	
6.	4/15	61122	Tillman	Symmetrel 100 mg #60 1 b.i.d.	3

DIRECTIONS (Questions 4a through 4k): Each of the numbered items or incomplete statements in this section is followed by answers or by completions of the statement. Select the ONE lettered answer or completion that is BEST in each case.

4a. The function of carbidopa in the Sinemet formulation is to

(A) act as a precursor for levodopa
(B) inhibit decarboxylation of peripheral levodopa
(C) act as a microsomal enzyme inhibitor
(D) act as a xanthine oxidase inhibitor
(E) increase the absorption of levodopa from the GI tract

4b. Patients receiving levodopa should avoid using vitamin supplements that contain

(A) folic acid
(B) thiamine
(C) ascorbic acid
(D) riboflavin
(E) pyridoxine

4c. A patient using Sinemet complains of an appreciable darkening of the urine beginning about 3 days after starting Sinemet therapy. The pharmacist should tell the patient to

(A) immediately stop taking the Sinemet and call the prescriber

(B) check the expiration date on the Sinemet container to make sure it has not expired
(C) disregard the discoloration since it is not harmful
(D) avoid the use of acidic foods while on Sinemet
(E) avoid the use of alkaline foods while on Sinemet

4d. Congentin has been prescribed because of its action as a(n)

(A) centrally acting skeletal muscle relaxant
(B) sedative
(C) anticholinergic
(D) memory enhancer
(E) peripheral vasodilator

4e. Which of the following is NOT employed in the treatment of Parkinson's disease?

(A) biperiden (Akineton)
(B) ethopropazine (Parisdol)
(C) trihexyphenidyl (Artane)
(D) bromocriptine (Parlodel)
(E) tranylcypromine (Parnate)

4f. Symmetrel is also employed in the treatment of

(A) hypertension
(B) psychoses
(C) gout
(D) viral infections
(E) bronchial asthma

4g. Diplopia is an adverse effect related to the use of levodopa. This can best be described as

(A) double vision
(B) impaired muscular coordination
(C) hearing loss
(D) focal seizures
(E) blood dyscrasias

4h. When a patient on levodopa is to be switched to Sinemet, which of the following is (are) true?

I. Reduce the dose of levodopa by 75% to 80%.
II. Permit at least 8 hours to elapse between the last dose of levodopa and the first dose of Sinemet.
III. Plasma levodopa levels must be measured each day for the first 5 days of Sinemet therapy.

(A) I only
(B) III only
(C) I and II only
(D) II and III only
(E) I, II and III only

4i. Levodopa can best be described as a(n)

(A) levulinic acid derivative
(B) dopamine antagonist
(C) dopamine precursor
(D) neurotransmitter
(E) anticonvulsant

4j. Which of the following products may be used in providing individually titrated doses of carbidopa?

(A) Tremin
(B) Lodosyn
(C) Larobec
(D) Dopar
(E) Disipal

4k. The prolonged use of which of the following drugs is associated with the development of Parkinson-like symptoms?

(A) tetracycline
(B) pentobarbital
(C) flecainide acetate
(D) enalapril maleate
(E) chlorpromazine

PROFILE NO. 5

Community Pharmacy Medication Record

Patient Name: Mildred North

Address: 721 Yager St

Age: 64   Sex: F

Height: 5'5"   Weight: 155 lb

Allergies: pollen, penicillin

DIAGNOSIS

Primary
1. open-angle glaucoma, primary
2. emphysema
3.

Secondary
1. wheezing
2.
3.

DRUG RECORD

	Date	Rx No.	Prescriber	Drug	Refills
1.	7/29	59083	Weber	Pilocarpine 1% 15 mL gtt 1 os t.i.d.	2
2.	8/20	59083	Weber	Refill	
3.	9/11	65002	Weber	Betoptic 0.5% 10 mL gtt 1 os b.i.d.	2
4.	10/21	65002	Weber	Refill	

PHARMACIST'S NOTES

	Date	Comment
1.	9/14	Ecotrin Maximum Strength (OTC)
2.	10/7	Visine (OTC)

DIRECTIONS (Questions 5a through 5k): Each of the numbered items or incomplete statements in this section is followed by answers or by completions of the statement. Select the ONE lettered answer or completion that is BEST in each case.

5a. The primary action of pilocarpine in the treatment of glaucoma is as a(n)

(A) mydriatic
(B) cycloplegic
(C) anesthetic
(D) vasoconstrictor
(E) miotic

5b. Pilocarpine is most similar in pharmacologic action to

(A) timolol
(B) isoflurophate
(C) physostigmine
(D) oxymetazoline
(E) carbachol

5c. Several weeks after using pilocarpine, the patient's intraocular pressure is measured as 14 mm Hg. This indicates that

(A) the dose of pilocarpine should be increased
(B) the intraocular pressure is under control
(C) an error in measurement must have occurred

(D) immediate surgery must be performed to relieve excessive intraocular pressure
(E) the dose of pilocarpine should be decreased

5d. Ocusert Pilo-20 is a system designed to release pilocarpine into the eye at a rate of

(A) 20 µg/hr
(B) 20 µg/day
(C) 20 mg/hr
(D) 20 mg/day
(E) 20 mg/week

5e. An Ocusert Pilo-20 system must be replaced

(A) every 7 days
(B) every 20 days
(C) every month
(D) when burning of the eye is experienced
(E) every day

5f. Betoptic is employed for the same purpose as
  I. Betagan
  II. Timoptic
  III. Miochol

(A) I only
(B) III only
(C) I and II only
(D) II and III only
(E) I, II, and III

5g. Betoptic is believed to act in reducing intraocular pressure by

(A) increasing the outflow of aqueous humor
(B) decreasing aqueous humor production
(C) causing miosis
(D) causing mydriasis
(E) causing cycloplegia

5h. Betoptic labeling indicates that the solution contains EDTA. This is used in this formulation as a(n)

(A) viscosity builder
(B) surfactant
(C) chelating agent
(D) antiseptic
(E) buffer

5i. The Visine purchased OTC by this patient contains

(A) phenylephrine
(B) tetrahydrozoline

(C) xylometazoline
(D) tropicamide
(E) pseudoephedrine

5j. The prescriber should be contacted by the pharmacist to discuss the possibility of

(A) respiratory distress
(B) interaction between pilocarpine and Betoptic
(C) increasing the Betoptic dose
(D) increasing the pilocarpine dose
(E) interaction between pilocarpine and Ecotrin

5k. The Ecotrin Maximum Strength formulation is most similar to which of the following?

(A) Bufferin
(B) Easprin
(C) Disalcid
(D) Dolobid
(E) Aspergum

PROFILE NO. 6

Community Pharmacy Medication Record

Patient Name: Lori Masters

Address: 34 Orchard St

Age: 21   Sex: F

Height: 5'2"   Weight: 119 lb

Allergies: penicillin

DIAGNOSIS

Primary	Secondary
1. acne vulgaris-severe	1.
2.	2.
3.	3.

DRUG RECORD

	Date	Rx No.	Prescriber	Drug	Refills
1.	6/7	45023	Thomas	Benzac 5 Gel 45 g ut dict	3
2.	6/22	48399	Wilson	Retin-A liquid 28 mL Apply p.r.n.	2
3.	7/13	45023	Thomas	Refill	
4.	8/24	45023	Thomas	Refill	
5.	9/17	57888	Wilson	Cleocin T Gel 30 g Apply topically	3
6.	10/5	59778	Thomas	Accutane 20 mg #60 1 b.i.d.	5

PHARMACIST'S NOTES

	Date	Comment
1.	7/1	Brasivol Medium
2.	7/30	Pernox Scrub 60 mL

DIRECTIONS (Questions 6a through 6l): Each of the numbered items or incomplete statements in this section is followed by answers or by completions of the statement. Select the ONE lettered answer or completion that is BEST in each case.

6a. The active ingredient in Benzac is

(A) benzopyrone
(B) benzyl alcohol
(C) benzyl penicillin
(D) benzoyl peroxide
(E) benzalkonium chloride

6b. Patients using Retin-A should avoid
  I. having product come in contact with the eyes
  II. excessive sunlight
  III. foods high in vitamin A

(A) I only
(B) III only
(C) I and II only
(D) II and III only
(E) I, II, and III

6c. Retin-A liquid contains butylated hydroxytoluene. The function of this ingredient is as a(n)

(A) viscosity builder

(B) antioxidant
(C) coloring agent
(D) chelating agent
(E) vehicle

6d. Which of the following adverse effects is associated with the use of Cleocin-T?

(A) hepatic impairment
(B) renal impairment
(C) diarrhea
(D) ataxia
(E) aplastic anemia

6e. The Cleocin-T product contains 10 mg of clindamycin per mL and is available in a 30-mL package size. This means that the solution has a strength of clindamycin of

(A) 10%
(B) 1%
(C) 0.1%
(D) 3%
(E) 0.3%

6f. Accutane is most closely related to

(A) vitamin B_{12}
(B) ascorbic acid

(C) vitamin D
(D) vitamin E
(E) vitamin A

6g. Which of the following are common adverse effects associated with the use of Accutane?

   I. cheilitis
  II. xerostomia
 III. conjunctivitis

(A) I only
(B) III only
(C) I and II only
(D) II and III only
(E) I, II, and III

6h. Upon dispensing Accutane, the pharmacist must provide the patient with a

(A) urine testing kit
(B) patient package insert
(C) "REFRIGERATE" auxiliary label
(D) UV lamp
(E) medicine dropper

6i. Prior to dispensing Accutane, the pharmacist should contact the prescriber to ascertain whether or not the patient is

(A) allergic to tetracycline
(B) pregnant

(C) a diabetic
(D) taking diuretics
(E) allergic to Novocaine

6j. Brasivol contains aluminum oxide. This ingredient is employed in this product as a(n)

(A) abrasive
(B) antimicrobial agent
(C) vehicle
(D) filler
(E) desiccating agent

6k. Pernox scrub contains salicylic acid. This ingredient is employed in this product as a(n)

(A) antiseptic
(B) buffer
(C) drying agent
(D) astringent
(E) keratolytic

6l. Patients with acne often secrete large amounts of

(A) cholesterol
(B) phosphodiesterase
(C) albumin
(D) bilirubin
(E) sebum

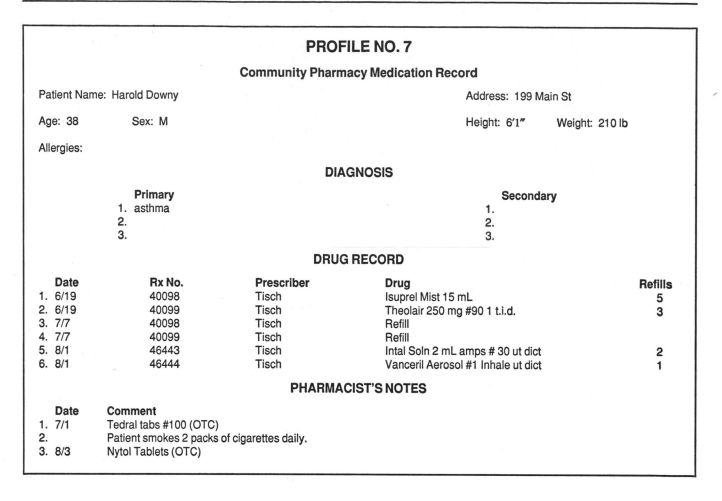

PROFILE NO. 7

Community Pharmacy Medication Record

Patient Name: Harold Downy   Address: 199 Main St

Age: 38   Sex: M   Height: 6'1"   Weight: 210 lb

Allergies:

DIAGNOSIS

Primary	Secondary
1. asthma	1.
2.	2.
3.	3.

DRUG RECORD

	Date	Rx No.	Prescriber	Drug	Refills
1.	6/19	40098	Tisch	Isuprel Mist 15 mL	5
2.	6/19	40099	Tisch	Theolair 250 mg #90 1 t.i.d.	3
3.	7/7	40098	Tisch	Refill	
4.	7/7	40099	Tisch	Refill	
5.	8/1	46443	Tisch	Intal Soln 2 mL amps # 30 ut dict	2
6.	8/1	46444	Tisch	Vanceril Aerosol #1 Inhale ut dict	1

PHARMACIST'S NOTES

	Date	Comment
1.	7/1	Tedral tabs #100 (OTC)
2.		Patient smokes 2 packs of cigarettes daily.
3.	8/3	Nytol Tablets (OTC)

DIRECTIONS (Questions 7a through 7m): Each of the numbered items or incomplete statements in this section is followed by answers or by completions of the statement. Select the ONE lettered answer or completion that is BEST in each case.

7a. The active ingredient in Isuprel Mistometer is isoproterenol. This agent can best be described as a(n)

(A) nonspecific alpha-adrenergic agonist
(B) selective beta receptor agonist
(C) nonspecific beta-adrenergic agonist
(D) alpha-adrenergic antagonist
(E) beta-adrenergic antagonist

7b. In an acute asthmatic attack, the patient uses one inhalation of Isuprel and, after 5 minutes, still has not been relieved. The patient should be advised to

(A) go to the local emergency room immediately
(B) administer a second inhalation about 2 to 5 minutes after the first if relief is not evident
(C) administer a double dose (2 inhalations) within 30 minutes after the first if relief is not evident
(D) breathe into a paper bag for 6 minutes to increase the respiratory concentration of carbon dioxide

(E) inhale steam in order to increase the penetration of the isoproterenol into the respiratory tract

7c. The active ingredient in Theolair is theophylline. This agent may be described as a

(A) phenothiazine
(B) prodrug
(C) xanthine oxidase inhibitor
(D) methylxanthine
(E) carbonic anhydrase inhibitor

7d. Which of the following is NOT a pharmacologic action of theophylline?

(A) increased diuresis
(B) central nervous system depression
(C) increased gastric acid secretion
(D) increased heart rate
(E) bronchodilation

7e. Which of the following theophylline derivatives is most appropriate to use in a rectal dosage form?

(A) aminophylline
(B) dyphylline
(C) oxtriphylline

(D) theophylline sodium glycinate
(E) theophylline anhydrous

7f. The Intal solution prescribed for this patient is administered

(A) intravenously
(B) intramuscularly
(C) subcutaneously
(D) by inhalation
(E) rectally

7g. The active ingredient found in Intal is

(A) ethylnorepinephrine
(B) oxtriphylline
(C) flunisolide
(D) dexamethasone sodium phosphate
(E) cromolyn

7h. The active ingredient in Vanceril can best be described as a(n)

(A) bronchodilator
(B) mucolytic
(C) respiratory surfactant
(D) corticosteroid
(E) anticholinergic

7i. Vanceril should be administered
   I. right after a bronchodilator has been inhaled
   II. as needed to control acute asthmatic attacks
   III. by IV infusion

(A) I only
(B) III only
(C) I and II only
(D) II and III only
(E) I, II and III

7j. The patient's heavy use of cigarettes may

(A) decrease the metabolism of theophylline
(B) increase the metabolism of isoproterenol
(C) increase the metabolism of theophylline
(D) decrease the metabolism of isoproterenol
(E) increase the metabolism of the Intal

7k. Which of the following is an ingredient of Tedral tablets?
   I. theophylline
   II. ephedrine HCl
   III. phenobarbital

(A) I only
(B) III only
(C) I and II only
(D) II and III only
(E) I, II, and III

7l. An advantage of terbutaline over isoproterenol is

(A) availability in a parenteral as well as inhalation dosage form
(B) more rapid onset of action when inhaled
(C) fewer cardiac effects
(D) no need for refrigeration prior to use
(E) asthmatic control with single daily dosing

7m. Vanceril is most similar to

(A) Atrovent
(B) Tornalate
(C) Sustaire
(D) Quibron
(E) Beclovent

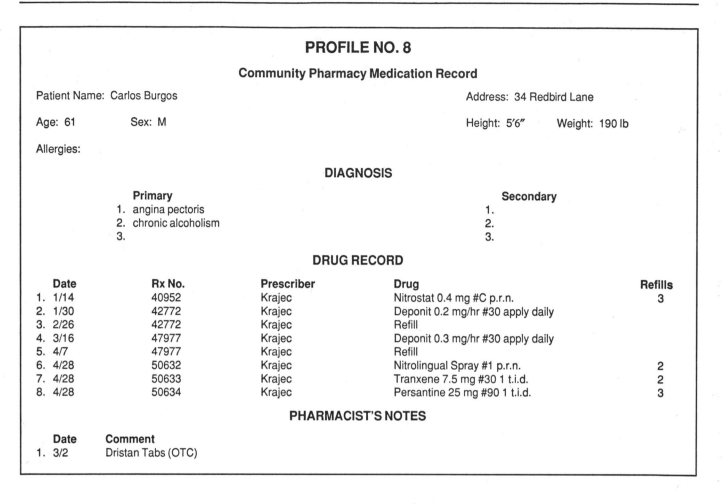

PROFILE NO. 8

Community Pharmacy Medication Record

Patient Name: Carlos Burgos

Address: 34 Redbird Lane

Age: 61   Sex: M

Height: 5'6"   Weight: 190 lb

Allergies:

DIAGNOSIS

Primary	Secondary
1. angina pectoris	1.
2. chronic alcoholism	2.
3.	3.

DRUG RECORD

	Date	Rx No.	Prescriber	Drug	Refills
1.	1/14	40952	Krajec	Nitrostat 0.4 mg #C p.r.n.	3
2.	1/30	42772	Krajec	Deponit 0.2 mg/hr #30 apply daily	
3.	2/26	42772	Krajec	Refill	
4.	3/16	47977	Krajec	Deponit 0.3 mg/hr #30 apply daily	
5.	4/7	47977	Krajec	Refill	
6.	4/28	50632	Krajec	Nitrolingual Spray #1 p.r.n.	2
7.	4/28	50633	Krajec	Tranxene 7.5 mg #30 1 t.i.d.	2
8.	4/28	50634	Krajec	Persantine 25 mg #90 1 t.i.d.	3

PHARMACIST'S NOTES

	Date	Comment
1.	3/2	Dristan Tabs (OTC)

DIRECTIONS (Questions 8a through 8k): Each of the numbered items or incomplete statements in this section is followed by answers or by completions of the statement. Select the ONE lettered answer or completion that is BEST in each case.

(A) I only
(B) III only
(C) I and II only
(D) II and III only
(E) I, II, and III

8a. An advantage of Nitrostat over other sublingual nitroglycerin products is that it is

(A) less subject to potency loss
(B) longer acting
(C) more rapidly absorbed
(D) effective when used orally as well as sublingually
(E) available in color-coded tablets

8b. Nitrostat should be dispensed

(A) in a tight, light-resistant plastic vial
(B) in quantities not greater than 25 tablets
(C) in its original container
(D) with a 6-month expiration date
(E) with a "REFRIGERATE" auxiliary label

8c. The patient should be advised to apply the Deponit to
  I. a hairless site
  II. the same application site each time it is applied
  III. the distal parts of the extremities

8d. When discontinuing therapy with Deponit

(A) headaches frequently occur
(B) the dosage should be gradually reduced over a 3-day period
(C) the number of hours/day that it is applied should be gradually reduced over 7 days
(D) the dosage and frequency of application should be gradually reduced over a 4- to 6-week period
(E) severe nausea and vomiting may occur

8e. An antianginal product administered by inhalation is

(A) pentaerythritol tetranitrate
(B) Nitrolingual Spray
(C) amyl nitrite
(D) isosorbide dinitrate
(E) erythritol tetranitrate

8f. In addition to being employed in the treatment of angina, dipyridamole (Persantine) is also used as a(n)

(A) antihypertensive agent
(B) antiarrhythmic agent
(C) analgesic
(D) antiplatelet agent
(E) nonsteroidal anti-inflammatory agent

8g. The reason why nitroglycerin products are generally NOT administered orally is because nitroglycerin

(A) will rapidly decompose in stomach acid
(B) is very irritating to GI membranes
(C) is rapidly decomposed by pepsin
(D) undergoes rapid first-pass deactivation
(E) is poorly absorbed from the GI tract

8h. Patients using nitroglycerin should be advised to AVOID the use of

(A) alcohol
(B) aspirin
(C) tyramine-containing foods
(D) foods with a high oxalate content
(E) dairy products

8i. Solutions of nitroglycerin intended for IV administration should be

(A) refrigerated until 30 minutes prior to administration
(B) given using the administration set provided by the manufacturer

(C) warmed for 15 minutes prior to infusion to dissolve crystalline material
(D) given only by direct IV injection
(E) kept covered with an opaque shield to protect it from decomposition

8j. When nitroglycerin topical ointment is administered
  I. the dose is measured in inches
  II. the area to which it is applied is covered with plastic wrap
  III. it should be rubbed into the skin until no further ointment is evident on the skin surface

(A) I only
(B) III only
(C) I and II only
(D) II and III only
(E) I, II, and III

8k. The most rapid onset of action is likely to occur with the use of

(A) Nitro-Dur
(B) Nitrolingual Spray
(C) Minitran
(D) Nitrogard
(E) Nitrodisc

PROFILE NO. 9

Community Pharmacy Medication Record

Patient Name: Maria Balou

Address: 845 Walton Ave

Age: 32   Sex: F

Height: 5'4"   Weight: 145 lb

Allergies: tetracyclines

DIAGNOSIS

Primary
1. Type I diabetes mellitus
2.
3.

Secondary
1.
2.
3.

DRUG RECORD

	Date	Rx No.	Prescriber	Drug	Refills
1.	9/11	29087	Madison	Humulin R 100 U 10 mL 24U qAM	5
2.	9/11	29088	Madison	Humulin N 100 U 10 mL 30 U mixed with Humulin R q AM	5
3.	9/11	29089	Madison	B-D Lo-Dose Syringes #100	5
4.	9/11	29090	Madison	AccuChek bG #1 as directed	

PHARMACIST'S NOTES

	Date	Comment
1.	9/1	Optilets-M-500 Filmtabs #100
2.	9/11	Clinitest Tabs #100
3.	9/20	Contac 12-Hour Caplets

DIRECTIONS (Questions 9a through 9l): Each of the numbered items or incomplete statements in this section is followed by answers or by completions of the statement. Select the ONE lettered answer or completion that is BEST in each case.

9a. The term "type I diabetes mellitus" is also referred to as

(A) diabetes insipidus
(B) brittle diabetes
(C) adult-onset diabetes
(D) insulin-dependent diabetes
(E) insulin-resistant diabetes

9b. Which of the following is (are) true of Humulin R?
   I. long-acting
   II. clear solution
   III. prepared by recombinant DNA technology

(A) I only
(B) III only
(C) I and II only
(D) II and III only
(E) I, II, and III

100u /mL

9c. In order to measure 24 U of Humulin R, the patient must withdraw what quantity of insulin from the vial?

(A) 0.24 mL
(B) 2.4mL

(C) It depends on the volume of the syringe.
(D) 0.024 mL

9d. In examining the patient, the physician notes that the patient complains of polydipsia. This refers to

(A) excessive urination
(B) excessive appetite
(C) excessive weight gain
(D) blurred vision
(E) excessive thirst

9e. Which of the following would be considered a normal fasting blood glucose level for this patient?

(A) 100 mg/L
(B) 100 µg/L
(C) 100 µg/dL
(D) 1 µg/mL
(E) 100 mg/dL

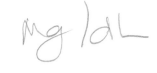

mg/dL

9f. The only insulin that is suitable for administration by IV infusion is

(A) lente
(B) regular
(C) PZI
(D) globin
(E) NPH

9g. In mixing the insulins prescribed, the patient should be advised

(A) to draw up the Humulin R first
(B) to draw up the Humulin N first
(C) that the mixture may be stored in the syringe for up to 1 month if kept refrigerated
(D) that the mixture may be stored in the syringe for up to 1 month if kept frozen
(E) that mixing these insulins is not advisable and the prescriber should be notified

9h. The patient's use of Optilets-M-500 Filmtabs may

(A) interfere with Clinitest testing
(B) cause a hyperglycemic episode
(C) cause a hypoglycemic episode
(D) increase the patient's insulin requirement
(E) decrease the patient's insulin requirement

9i. The Clinitest test operates by the same mechanism as

(A) Diastix
(B) Clinistix
(C) Benedict's test
(D) Chemstrip bG
(E) Chemstrip K

9j. The patient's use of Contac 12-hour Caplets may

(A) increase the patient's insulin requirement
(B) decrease the patient's insulin requirement
(C) increase the chance of lipodystrophy
(D) increase the chance of lipoatrophy
(E) precipitate ketoacidosis

9k. B-D Lo-Dose syringes have a capacity of

(A) 2 mL
(B) 0.5 mL
(C) 1.0 mL
(D) 0.25 mL
(E) 5 mL

9l. Which of the following antidiabetic agents is a second-generation sulfonylurea?

(A) glipizide
(B) chlorpropamide
(C) acetohexamide
(D) tolazamide
(E) tolbutamide

PROFILE NO. 10

Community Pharmacy Medication Record

Patient Name: Rowena Adams   Address: 99 East Ave

Age: 51   Sex: F   Height: 5'7"   Weight: 155 lb

Allergies:

DIAGNOSIS

Primary	Secondary
1. venous thrombosis	1.
2. hypothyroidism	2.
3.	3.

DRUG RECORD

	Date	Rx No.	Prescriber	Drug	Refills
1.	5/3	89322	Graves	Warfarin 5 mg #10 1 daily	
2.	5/12	90109	Graves	Warfarin 7.5 mg # 30 1 daily	
3.	5/21	91202	Graves	Warfarin 7.5 mg # 30 1 daily	5
4.	6/18	91202	Graves	Refill	
5.	7/15	91202	Graves	Refill	
6.	8/1	94388	Wilson	Synthroid 100 µg # 60 1 daily	5
7.	8/29	99733	Waxman	Empirin/Cod. No. 3 # 30 1 b.i.d.	

DIRECTIONS (Questions 10a through 10l): Each of the numbered items or incomplete statements in this section is followed by answers or by completions of the statement. Select the ONE lettered answer or completion that is BEST in each case.

10a. Warfarin is most closely related chemically to

(A) heparin
(B) alteplase
(C) streptokinase
(D) aminocaproic acid
(E) dicumarol

10b. Administration of which of the following drugs is likely to increase warfarin activity in this patient?

(A) phenobarbital *Inducer*
(B) chloral hydrate
(C) rifampin *inducer*
(D) phenytoin *— Inducer*
(E) glutethimide

10c. An appropriate antidote for the treatment of warfarin overdose is

(A) vitamin K
(B) EDTA
(C) protamine
(D) potassium permanganate
(E) zinc sulfate

10d. This patient asks the pharmacist for a recommendation for an OTC analgesic for her tennis elbow. Which of the following agents would be appropriate to recommend?

I. Ecotrin
II. Advil
III. Datril *—Tylenol*

(A) I only
(B) III only
(C) I and II only
(D) II or III only
(E) I, II, and III

10e. If the pharmacist wished to dispense a generic form of Synthroid, which of the following would be used?

(A) liotrix *T3 & T4*
(B) liothyronine *— T3*
(C) thyroglobulin
(D) levothyroxine
(E) propylthiouracil *hyper*

10f. A dose of 100 µg of Synthroid is approximately equivalent to

(A) 65 mg of Thyroid USP
(B) 25 µg of Proloid
(C) 10 µg of Cytomel
(D) 25 µg of Levothroid
(E) 100 mg of Thyrar

65mg thyrar
25mg Cytomel
65mg proloid

10g. Which of the following may be used to treat hyperthyroidism?

I. propylthiouracil

II. methimazole
III. sodium iodide ^{131}I

(A) I only
(B) III only
(C) I and II only
(D) II and III only
(E) I, II, and III

10h. The use of Synthroid by this patient is likely to

(A) increase the dosage requirement for warfarin
(B) prevent the oral absorption of warfarin
(C) decrease the dosage requirement for warfarin
(D) increase the likelihood of renal damage
(E) increase the likelihood of hepatic damage

10i. In a radiation emergency, which of the following would be appropriate to administer?

(A) propylthiouracil
(B) potassium iodide
(C) liotrix
(D) thyroglobulin
(E) Cytomel

10j. Thyroid hormone synthesis is controlled by

(A) TSH from the anterior pituitary
(B) Vasopressin from the posterior pituitary
(C) FSH from the anterior pituitary
(D) human chorionic gonadotropin
(E) LH from the anterior pituitary

10k. The use of Empirin/Codeine No. 3 by this patient is likely to

(A) increase the action of the Synthroid
(B) decrease the action of Synthroid
(C) increase the action of warfarin
(D) decrease the action of warfarin
(E) cause agranulocytosis

10l. Which of the following laboratory determinations may be used to monitor the patient's progress on warfarin?

(A) prothrombin time
(B) bilirubin
(C) amylase
(D) BUN
(E) creatine kinase

Levothyroxine – T4
Liothyronine – T3

Syn + Warfarin
↓ Warfarin

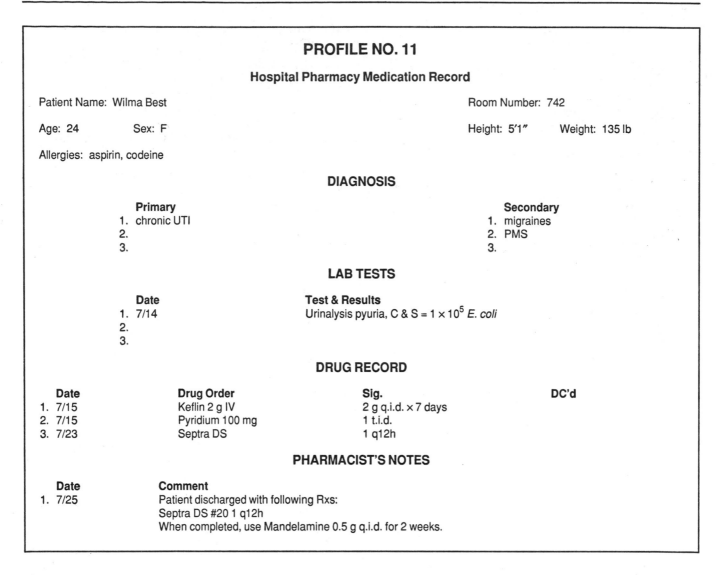

PROFILE NO. 11

Hospital Pharmacy Medication Record

Patient Name: Wilma Best   Room Number: 742

Age: 24   Sex: F   Height: 5'1"   Weight: 135 lb

Allergies: aspirin, codeine

DIAGNOSIS

Primary	Secondary
1. chronic UTI	1. migraines
2.	2. PMS
3.	3.

LAB TESTS

Date	Test & Results
1. 7/14	Urinalysis pyuria, C & S = 1×10^5 *E. coli*
2.	
3.	

DRUG RECORD

Date	Drug Order	Sig.	DC'd
1. 7/15	Keflin 2 g IV	2 g q.i.d. × 7 days	
2. 7/15	Pyridium 100 mg	1 t.i.d.	
3. 7/23	Septra DS	1 q12h	

PHARMACIST'S NOTES

Date	Comment
1. 7/25	Patient discharged with following Rxs:
	Septra DS #20 1 q12h
	When completed, use Mandelamine 0.5 g q.i.d. for 2 weeks.

DIRECTIONS (Questions 11a through 11m): Each of the numbered items or incomplete statements in this section is followed by answers or by completions of the statement. Select the ONE lettered answer or completion that is BEST in each case.

11a. The term "pyuria" indicates the presence of what substance in the urine?

(A) pyruvate
(B) pyridoxine
(C) pus
(D) red blood cells
(E) pyrogens

11b. *Escherichia coli* could also be described as

(A) pneumococci
(B) gram-negative bacilli
(C) gram-positive bacilli
(D) a systemic fungal organism
(E) a spirochete

11c. Keflin is an example of a

(A) penicillin
(B) 1st generation cephalosporin
(C) 2nd generation cephalosporin
(D) aminoglycoside
(E) 3rd generation cephalosporin

11d. Septra DS contains

(A) docusate sodium
(B) sulfisoxazole
(C) nalidixic acid
(D) trimethoprim
(E) methenamine

11e. An agent frequently administered with Mandelamine to facilitate its activity is

(A) sodium bicarbonate
(B) tyrosine
(C) mineral oil

(D) ascorbic acid *Keeping pH N5 no ppt in urine*
(E) sulfamethoxazole

11f. Patients using Septra DS or Mandelamine should be advised to
   I. drink a large amount of fluids ✓ *both*
   II. maintain an acid urine ✓ *mandelamine*
   III. avoid the use of folic acid-containing products *neither*

   (A) I only
   (B) III only
   (C) I and II only
   (D) II and III only
   (E) I, II, and III

11g. A patient wishes to test her urine to determine the presence of bacteriuria. Which of the following products would be suitable for this purpose?

   (A) Ictotest
   (B) Azostix
   (C) Microstix-3 — *test for presence of N which indicates bacteria urine*
   (D) Predict
   (E) Chemstrip K

11h. The Pyridium ordered for this patient can best be classified as a(n)

   (A) urinary antiseptic
   (B) aminoglycoside antimicrobial agent
   (C) buffer
   (D) antispasmodic
   (E) analgesic

11i. This patient should be advised that Pyridium may cause

   (A) temporary weight gain
   (B) abnormal hair growth
   (C) discoloration of the urine
   (D) dizziness
   (E) temporary infertility

11j. When used with Keflin, Pyridium should not be administered for longer than

   (A) 2 days
   (B) 5 days
   (C) 10 days
   (D) 14 days
   (E) 30 days

11k. Symptoms of PMS may include all of the following EXCEPT

   (A) backache
   (B) cramping
   (C) edema
   (D) irritability
   (E) weight loss

11l. Which of the following ingredients is(are) included in OTC PMS products?
   I. caffeine
   II. pamabrom — *Midol PMS Pamprin*
   III. HCTZ

   (A) I only
   (B) III only
   (C) I and II only
   (D) II and III only
   (E) I, II, and III

11m. If the UTI becomes chronic, the physician may wish to consider prescribing which of the following oral drugs?
   I. ciprofloxacin
   II. penicillin VK
   III. gentamicin

   (A) I only
   (B) III only
   (C) I and II only
   (D) II and III only
   (E) I, II, and III

PROFILE NO. 12

Hospital Pharmacy Medication Record

Patient Name: Marvin Lessard   Room Number: 241-2

Age: 64   Sex: M   Height: 5'11"   Weight: 188 lb

Allergies: none reported

DIAGNOSIS

Primary	Secondary
1. chronic myelocytic leukemia	1. oral candida
2.	2.
3.	3.

LAB TESTS

	Date	Test & Results		Date	Tests & Results
1.	6/4	WBC ($\times 10^3$) = 180; K = 4.5; Na = 138	4.	6/10	WBC ($\times 10^3$) = 6.5; K = 2.6; Na = 128
2.	6/6	WBC ($\times 10^3$) = 115; K = 3.8; Na = 136	5.	6/12	WBC ($\times 10^3$) = 0.9; K = 3.0; Na = 132
3.	6/8	WBC ($\times 10^3$) = 75; K = 3.1; Na = 134			

DRUG RECORD

	Date	Drug Order	Sig.	DC'd
1.	6/4	Colace 100 mg	1 or 2 daily	
2.	6/4	Dalmane 15 mg	1 hs 2	
3.	6/4	Daunorubicin	45 mg/m^2/day on days 1 to 3	
			2	
4.	6/4	Cytarabine	100 mg/m^2/day on days 1 to 7	
5.	6/4	Allopurinol	300 mg b.i.d. × 10 days	
6.	6/7	Mycostatin Liq.	q3h × 10 days	
7.	6/7	Mitrolan tabs	chew 1 q4h p.r.n.	

DIRECTIONS (Questions 12a through 12m) Each of the numbered items or incomplete statements in this section is followed by answers or by completions of the statement. Select the ONE lettered answer or completion that is BEST in each case.

12a. The patient's body surface area in square meters can best be determined with the use of a

(A) caliper
(B) tape measure
(C) picogram
(D) nomogram
(E) micrometer

12b. Daunorubicin is available in vials containing 20 mg of the drug. Assuming that the patient's body surface area was determined to be 1.85 m^2, how many vials of daunorubicin need to be supplied for each day's administration?

(A) 5
(B) 1

(C) 10
(D) 2
(E) 3

12c. Cytarabine can best be described as a(n)

(A) antibiotic
(B) mitotic inhibitor
(C) antimetabolite
(D) alkylating agent
(E) antiestrogen

12d. From the laboratory data provided, it appears that the patient is experiencing

(A) hypokalemia
(B) infection
(C) hyperkalemia
(D) myelosuppression
(E) hypernatremia

12e. Allopurinol is pharmacologically classified as a(n)

- (A) beta-adrenergic agonist
- (B) MAO inhibitor
- (C) xanthine oxidase inhibitor
- (D) antimetabolite
- (E) alkylating agent

12f. Patients using allopurinol should be advised to

- (A) drink adequate fluids
- (B) avoid dairy products
- (C) expect urine discoloration
- (D) avoid bruising
- (E) take at least 1 g of vitamin C daily

12g. In order to monitor the use of allopurinol, determinations should be made of

- (A) serum potassium
- (B) serum folate
- (C) urinary glucose
- (D) serum uric acid
- (E) urinary 5-HT

12h. An appropriate instruction for the use of Mycostatin liquid would be to

- (A) take with a large glass of water
- (B) swish and swallow
- (C) take on an empty stomach
- (D) mix it with fruit juice before administration
- (E) allow product to stand until it thickens

12i. If extravasation occurred with the administration of daunorubicin, which of the following would be recommended?

- (A) Inject subcutaneous epinephrine into the area.
- (B) Insert a catheter into the injection site.
- (C) Apply a corticosteroid cream to the injection site.
- (D) Inject sodium bicarbonate solution into the injection site.
- (E) Apply cold compresses to the injection site.

12j. A serious adverse effect associated with daunorubicin administration is

- (A) ocular degeneration
- (B) nephrotoxicity
- (C) cardiotoxicity
- (D) hypercalcemia
- (E) hyperkalemia

12k. While sleeping well at night, Mr Lessard appears to be unstable during the day and has fallen several times. The pharmacist should suggest that the Dalmane order be switched to

- (A) ethchlorvynol
- (B) glutethimide
- (C) phenobarbital
- (D) secobarbital
- (E) temazepam

SLUD

12l. Elderly patients consuming OTC sleep aid products containing either diphenhydramine or doxylamine may experience any of the following EXCEPT

- (A) constipation
- (B) blurred vision
- (C) dry mouth
- (D) confusion
- (E) urinary retention

12m. Mitrolan is prescribed for which of the following effects?

   I. antacid
   II. antidiarrheal
   III. treat constipation

- (A) I only
- (B) III only
- (C) I and II only
- (D) II and III only
- (E) I, II, and III

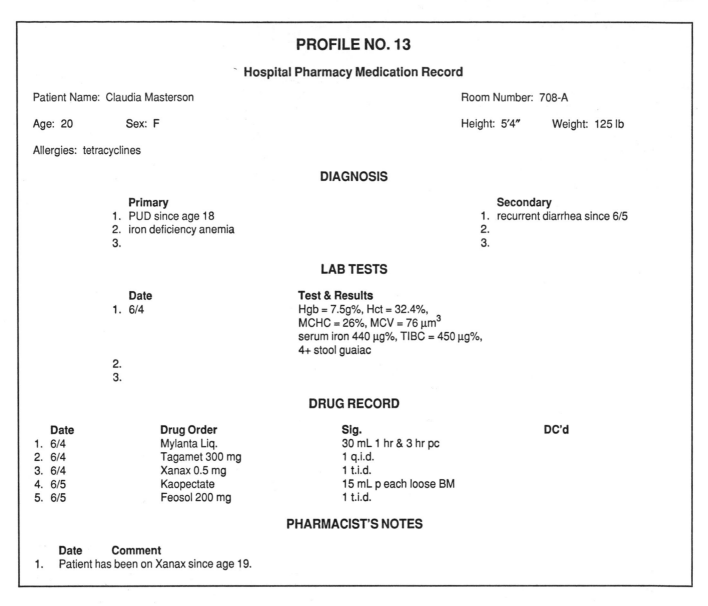

PROFILE NO. 13

Hospital Pharmacy Medication Record

Patient Name: Claudia Masterson

Room Number: 708-A

Age: 20   Sex: F

Height: 5'4"   Weight: 125 lb

Allergies: tetracyclines

DIAGNOSIS

Primary
1. PUD since age 18
2. iron deficiency anemia
3.

Secondary
1. recurrent diarrhea since 6/5
2.
3.

LAB TESTS

Date	Test & Results
1. 6/4	Hgb = 7.5g%, Hct = 32.4%, MCHC = 26%, MCV = 76 μm^3 serum iron 440 μg%, TIBC = 450 μg%, 4+ stool guaiac
2.	
3.	

DRUG RECORD

	Date	Drug Order	Sig.	DC'd
1.	6/4	Mylanta Liq.	30 mL 1 hr & 3 hr pc	
2.	6/4	Tagamet 300 mg	1 q.i.d.	
3.	6/4	Xanax 0.5 mg	1 t.i.d.	
4.	6/5	Kaopectate	15 mL p each loose BM	
5.	6/5	Feosol 200 mg	1 t.i.d.	

PHARMACIST'S NOTES

Date	Comment
1.	Patient has been on Xanax since age 19.

DIRECTIONS (Questions 13a through 13o): Each of the numbered items or incomplete statements in this section is followed by answers or by completions of the statement. Select the ONE lettered answer or completion that is BEST in each case.

13a. After 6 months of iron therapy, the patient's hemoglobin level should ideally be

(A) 4 to 6 g%
(B) 6 to 8 g%
(C) 8 to 10 g%
(D) 10 to 12 g%
(E) 12 to 14 g%

normal 14%

13b. 4+ stool guaiac is indicative of

(A) elevated serum guaiac levels
(B) hyperchlorhydria
(C) hepatic impairment
(D) renal impairment
(E) GI bleeding

13c. A likely cause of the patient's diarrhea is the use of

(A) Mylanta — MgOH
(B) Tagamet
(C) Feosol
(D) Xanax
(E) Kaopectate

13d. The use of Tagamet by this patient is likely to

(A) produce a hypersensitivity reaction
(B) increase Xanax activity
(C) decrease Xanax activity
(D) worsen the patient's anemia
(E) cause hyperchlorhydria

13e. A drug interaction is likely to occur with the concomitant use of
   I.   Tagamet and Mylanta
   II. Feosol and Mylanta ✓
   III. Tagamet and Xanax

   (A) I only
   (B) III only
   (C) I and II only
   (D) II and III only
   (E) I, II, and III

13f. Iron absorption may be increased by administering which of the following agents to this patient?

   (A) docusate sodium
   (B) ascorbic acid
   (C) benzalkonium chloride
   (D) pyridoxine hydrochloride
   (E) desferal mesylate

13g. Feosol contains

   (A) ferrous gluconate 11%
   (B) ferrous fumarate 33%
   (C) ferrous sulfate 20%
   (D) ferric chloride
   (E) ferric ammonium citate

13h. The active ingredient of Feosol is exsiccated. This means that the ingredient is

   (A) volatile
   (B) dried
   (C) in its hydrous form
   (D) able to absorb water when exposed to the atmosphere
   (E) chelated

13i. Examination of this patient's red blood cells is likely to reveal cells that are
   I.   microcytic ✓
   II. hypochromic ✓
   III. megaloblastic

   (A) I only
   (B) III only
   (C) I and II only
   (D) II and III only
   (E) I, II, and III

13j. A drug that may be more appropriate than Tagamet for use in this patient is

   (A) Zantac — doesn't interfere with P450
   (B) Imodium

   (C) Cephulac
   (D) Dialose Stool Softner
   (E) Doxinate Stool Softener

13k. Iron deficiency anemia patients often experience pica, which may present itself by

   (A) brittle fingernails
   (B) an abnormal craving for a single food
   (C) a pale color of the fingernails' moons
   (D) distorted vision
   (E) small discolorations under the skin

13l. Causes of megaloblastic anemia include a deficiency of
   I.   cyanocobalamin B12
   II. folic acid
   III. iron

   (A) I only
   (B) III only
   (C) I and II only
   (D) II and III only
   (E) I, II, and III

13m. Dietary sources rich in vitamin B_{12} include
   I.   apples
   II. broccoli
   III. liver

   animal products & shellfish

   (A) I only
   (B) III only
   (C) I and II only
   (D) II and III only
   (E) I, II, and III

13n. Which of the following statements concerning pernicious anemia is (are) true?
   I.   Condition caused by a deficiency in folic acid.
   II. Higher incidence occurs in women than in men.
   III. Occurrence appears to be both genetically and geographically biased.

   (A) I only
   (B) III only
   (C) I and II only
   (D) II and III only
   (E) I, II, and III

13o. Ferrous sulfate is available in all of the following dosage forms EXCEPT

   (A) elixir
   (B) oral drops
   (C) oral liquid
   (D) parenteral injection
   (E) tablets

PROFILE NO. 14

Community Pharmacy Medication Record

Patient Name: Joe Gaines   Address: 43 Pine St

Age: 38   Sex: M

Allergies: Chocolate

DIAGNOSIS

Primary	Secondary
1. mild hypertension	1. fits of depression
2. noninsulin-dependent diabetes	2.
3.	3.

DRUG RECORD

	Date	Rx No.	Prescriber	Drug	Refills
1.	6/4	132887	Long	HCTZ 25 mg #60 i qd	5
2.		132888	Long	Inderal 40 mg #120 1 b.i.d.	5
3.		132889	Long	Diabinese 250 mg #60 1 b.i.d.	5
4.		132890	Long	Slow-K 8 mEq #60 1 qd	5

PHARMACIST'S NOTES

	Date	Comment
1.		Joe enjoys his beer; be sure to warn about possible drug/alcohol interactions.
2.	6/12	Sold Joe some diet tablets (containing PPA). Check his progress next time in store.

DIRECTIONS (Questions 14a through 14n): Each of the numbered items or incomplete statements in this section is followed by answers or by completions of the statement. Select the ONE lettered answer or completion that is BEST in each case.

[14a-f] On June 15, Joe Gaines brings into the pharmacy a new prescription for penicillin VK 500 mg #40 with a Sig: one tablet q.i.d. until gone. He has been instructed by his physician to soak his swollen, infected thumb in alternate solutions of pHisoHex and epsom salts every two hours.

14a. The prescriber probably prescribed penicillin since he or she suspected an infection caused by

(A) *Chlamydia*
(B) *Staphylococcus epidermis*
(C) *Pseudomonas*
(D) *Streptococcus*
(E) fungus

14b. The above prescription could be filled by using any of the following EXCEPT

(A) Betapen
(B) Pentids
(C) Pen Vee
(D) Veetids
(E) V-Cillin

14c. pHisoHex is considered effective in treating infections caused by

I. fungus
II. gram-negative microorganisms
III. gram-positive microorganisms

(A) I only
(B) III only
(C) I and II only
(D) II and III only
(E) I, II, and III

14d. Which one of the following statements concerning pHisoHex is NOT true?

(A) active ingredient is hexachlorophene
(B) an occlusive dressing should be applied after the lotion is placed on the skin
(C) the lotion is a prescription item
(D) the product may darken upon exposure to sunlight
(E) the product is available in only one strength

14e. A more appropriate product for soaking would be one containing which one of the following chemicals?

(A) benzalkonium chloride
(B) chlorhexidine
(C) hydrogen peroxide

(D) iodine

(E) phenol

14f. Which one of the following pairings of active ingredient to product is INCORRECT?

  (A) chlorhexidine—Hibiclens

  (B) chlorhexidine—Peridex

  (C) iodine—Betadine

  (D) iodine—Cidex

  (E) benzalkonium chloride—Ionax

14g. Chemically, epsom salts is

  (A) aluminum sulfate

  (B) aluminum acetate

  (C) calcium sulfate

  (D) magnesium sulfate

  (E) a mixture of calcium and magnesium sulfates

14h. Mr Gaines requests a bottle of Percogesic. Which one of the following statements concerning Percogesic is true?

  (A) The active ingredient is acetaminophen only.

  (B) The active ingredients are acetaminophen and aspirin.

  (C) One of the active ingredients is phenyltoloxamine.

  (D) A prescription is required for dispensing.

  (E) One of the active ingredients is an antacid.

14i. Mr Gaines and his wife are planning a trip to an area of Central America that has poor sanitary facilities. Which one of the following products may both prevent and treat traveler's diarrhea?

  (A) Kaopectate *not prevent*

  (B) metronidazole

  (C) Mylanta

  (D) Paregoric

  (E) Pepto-Bismol

14j. Mr Gaines has returned from his trip with an infection of giardiasis. Which of the following drugs may successfully treat this condition?

  I. cefadroxil

  II. metronidazole

  III. quinacrine

  (A) I only

  (B) III only

  (C) I and II only

  (D) II and III only

  (E) I, II, and III

14k. A week after deer hunting, Mr Gaines exhibits symptoms of Lyme disease. Which of the following statements is(are) true of this condition?

  I. early signs are a skin rash and malaise

  II. late stages often result in chronic arthritis

  III. the disease is caused by a protozoa

  (A) I only

  (B) III only

  (C) I and II only   *Tick Deer*

  (D) II and III only

  (E) I, II, and III

14l. Successful treatment of Lyme disease includes

  I. doxycycline 100 mg b.i.d.

  II. ceftriaxone 2 g IV daily

  III. metronidazole 500 mg daily *NO*

  (A) I only

  (B) III only

  (C) I and II only

  (D) II and III only

  (E) I, II, and III

14m. Mr Gaines is placed upon 500 mg naproxen t.i.d. This drug may be prescribed as an

  I. anti-inflammatory

  II. analgesic

  III. antipyretic

  (A) I only

  (B) III only

  (C) I and II only

  (D) II and III only

  (E) I, II, and III

14n. Mr Gaines has read that aspirin will decrease the chance of heart attacks. How many 325 mg tablets should be suggested to him as a realistic dose?

  (A) 1 or less tablets daily

  (B) 1 or 2 tablets daily

  (C) 1 tablet twice a day

  (D) 1 tablet three times a day

  (E) 1 tablet four times a day

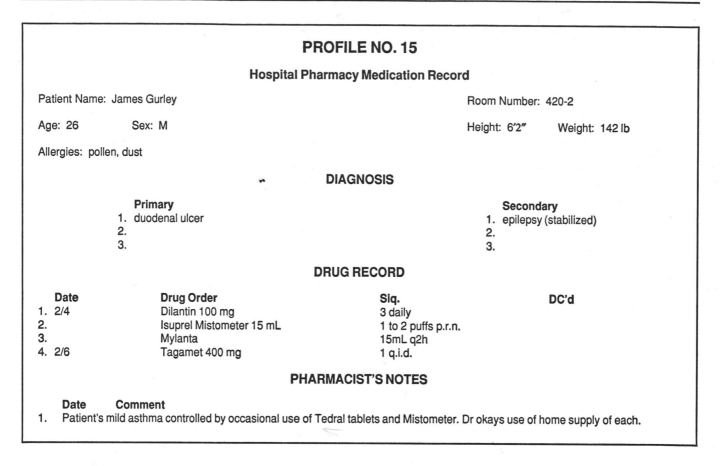

PROFILE NO. 15

Hospital Pharmacy Medication Record

Patient Name: James Gurley   Room Number: 420-2

Age: 26   Sex: M   Height: 6'2"   Weight: 142 lb

Allergies: pollen, dust

DIAGNOSIS

Primary
1. duodenal ulcer
2.
3.

Secondary
1. epilepsy (stabilized)
2.
3.

DRUG RECORD

	Date	Drug Order	Siq.	DC'd
1.	2/4	Dilantin 100 mg	3 daily	
2.		Isuprel Mistometer 15 mL	1 to 2 puffs p.r.n.	
3.		Mylanta	15mL q2h	
4.	2/6	Tagamet 400 mg	1 q.i.d.	

PHARMACIST'S NOTES

	Date	Comment
1.		Patient's mild asthma controlled by occasional use of Tedral tablets and Mistometer. Dr okays use of home supply of each.

DIRECTIONS (Questions 15a through 15p): Each of the numbered items or incomplete statements in this section is followed by answers or by completions of the statement. Select the ONE lettered answer or completion that is BEST in each case.

15a. The nursing staff reports that Mr Gurley is experiencing dizziness and has fallen down several times. It is advisable to

  (A) continue the drug regimen as the side effects are transient
  (B) increase the dose of Dilantin
  (C) decrease the dose of Tagamet
  (D) decrease the dose of Dilantin
  (E) take Tagamet with food to increase its absorption and decrease stomach irritation

15b. Mr Gurley's poor muscle coordination may be defined in medical terminology as

  (A) ataxia
  (B) atresia
  (C) dementia
  (D) hemiplegia
  (E) dysarthria

15c. Which one of the following drugs can be used in place of Tagamet?

  (A) diflunisal
  (B) famotidine
  (C) nylidrin
  (D) pentoxifylline
  (E) piroxicam

15d. Zollinger-Ellison syndrome is the result of adenomas in the

  (A) gallbladder
  (B) liver
  (C) stomach
  (D) pancreas
  (E) small intestine

↑gastric secretion

15e. Mr Gurley's physician calls the pharmacy for information concerning benzodiazepines that will not be affected by cimetidine. Which one of the following agents is most appropriate?

  (A) chlordiazepoxide
  (B) diazepam
  (C) flurazepam
  (D) alprazolam
  (E) oxazepam

[handwritten: 0.6–1.2 mEq/L]

15f. If the physician decides to maintain Mr Gurley on lithium therapy as an outpatient, which of the following guidelines should be followed?

    I. an oral dosing range of 900 to 1500 mg daily
    II. plasma lithium levels between 2 and 4 mEq/L *[handwritten: <1.2 mEq/L]*
    III. blood sampling 2 hours after dosing *[handwritten: 8hr]*

    (A) I only
    (B) III only
    (C) I and II only
    (D) II and III only
    (E) I, II, and III

15g. After 1 week of lithium therapy with a dosage regimen of 600 mg b.i.d., the patient is experiencing mild hand tremors and polyuria. The pharmacist should consult with the prescriber concerning the possibility of *[handwritten: occur on peaks of Li]*

    (A) giving the drug on a 300 mg q.i.d. schedule
    (B) increasing the dosage to 1500 mg daily
    (C) decreasing the dosage to 600 mg daily
    (D) giving the drug once a day in the morning
    (E) discontinuing the drug

15h. Lithium is probably being prescribed

    (A) to treat acute manic episodes
    (B) as an anti-Parkinson drug
    (C) an a hypnotic agent
    (D) to treat status epilepticus
    (E) to treat schizophrenia

15i. Five days after discharge from the hospital, Mr Gurley brings an antibiotic prescription into the pharmacy. He asks for an explanation of "nosocomial infection." The pharmacist can best explain nosocomial as being

    (A) communicable
    (B) hospital related
    (C) drug related
    (D) unknown origin
    (E) noncommunicable

15j. Mr. Gurley requests an OTC product to relieve a dry, nonproductive cough that he has developed. Which one of the following ingredients is indicated for this condition?

    (A) codeine
    (B) dextromethorphan
    (C) diphenhydramine
    (D) guaifenesin
    (E) ipecac

15k. Which of the following cough products contains diphenhydramine?

    I. Benylin (Liquid)
    II. Benylid D (Elixir)
    III. Benylin Expectorant *[handwritten: guiafen & DM]*

    (A) I only
    (B) III only
    (C) I and II only
    (D) II and III only
    (E) I, II, and III

15l. OTC products suitable for removing cerumen from the ear include

    I. Debrox
    II. S.T. 37
    III. Anbesol

    (A) I only
    (B) III only
    (C) I and II only
    (D) II and III only
    (E) I, II, and III

15m. Mr Gurley has a new prescription for Prozac 20 mg, which has the generic name of

    (A) amoxapine
    (B) desipramine
    (C) fluoxetine
    (D) trazodone
    (E) phenelzine

15n. The antidepressant activity of Prozac is believed due to

    (A) binding to beta-adrenergic receptors
    (B) prevention of reuptake of serotonin
    (C) blockage of reuptake of norepinephrine
    (D) blockage of reuptake of dopamine
    (E) being a dopamine antagonist

15o. Which of the following are potential side effects of Prozac.

    I. anorexia
    II. insomnia
    III. increase in heart rate

    (A) I only
    (B) III only
    (C) I and II only
    (D) II and III only
    (E) I, II, and III

15p. Prozac is available in which of the following dosage forms?

    I. capsules
    II. oral liquid
    III. parenteral liquid

    (A) I only
    (B) III only
    (C) I and II only
    (D) II and III only
    (E) I, II, and III

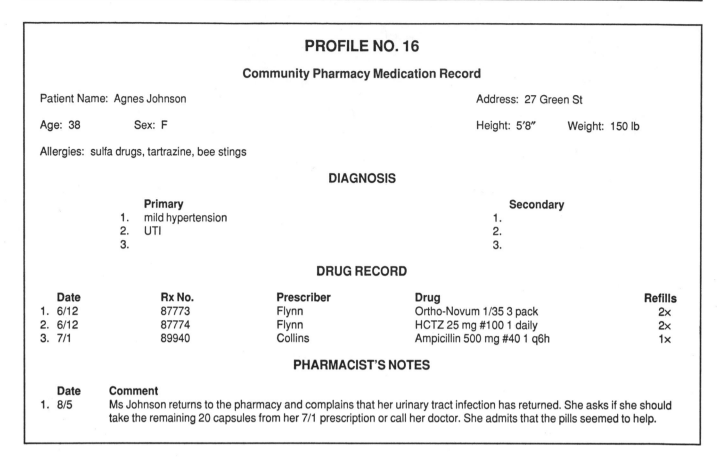

PROFILE NO. 16

Community Pharmacy Medication Record

Patient Name: Agnes Johnson

Address: 27 Green St

Age: 38   Sex: F

Height: 5'8"   Weight: 150 lb

Allergies: sulfa drugs, tartrazine, bee stings

DIAGNOSIS

Primary	Secondary
1. mild hypertension	1.
2. UTI	2.
3.	3.

DRUG RECORD

	Date	Rx No.	Prescriber	Drug	Refills
1.	6/12	87773	Flynn	Ortho-Novum 1/35 3 pack	2×
2.	6/12	87774	Flynn	HCTZ 25 mg #100 1 daily	2×
3.	7/1	89940	Collins	Ampicillin 500 mg #40 1 q6h	1×

PHARMACIST'S NOTES

	Date	Comment
1.	8/5	Ms Johnson returns to the pharmacy and complains that her urinary tract infection has returned. She asks if she should take the remaining 20 capsules from her 7/1 prescription or call her doctor. She admits that the pills seemed to help.

DIRECTIONS (Questions 16a through 16o): Each of the numbered items or incomplete statements in this section is followed by answers or by completions of the statement. Select the ONE lettered answer or completion that is BEST in each case.

16a. The pharmacist should advise her to

(A) finish the remaining capsules
(B) call the doctor for an increase in the ampicillin dose
(C) ask the doctor for another, more effective drug
(D) get a partial refill of ampicillin and use a total of 40 capsules
(E) use up the remaining 20 capsules but drink cranberry juice at the same time

16b. Which one of the following microorganisms accounts for the greatest percentage of urinary tract infections?

(A) *Escherichia coli*
(B) *Klebsiella aerogens*
(C) *Proteus mirabilis*
(D) *Pseudomonas aeruginosa*
(E) *Streptococcus fecalis*

16c. Dr Collins calls the pharmacy on Sept 2 starting that Ms Johnson has been noncompliant in completing regimens of therapy for her UTIs. Which of the following single-dose regimens is(are) appropriate?

I. Amoxil 500 mg 6 capsules
II. Septra DS 2 tabs
III. Furadantin 50 mg 1 capsule

(A) I only
(B) III only
(C) I and II only
(D) II and III only
(E) I, II, and III

16d. Phenazopyridine HCl is used in combination with antibacterials to treat urinary tract infections because it

(A) reduces the amount of antibacterial drug needed
(B) prolongs the duration of antibacterial activity
(C) speeds dissolution rate of sulfa drugs
(D) serves as an antiseptic and anesthetic
(E) maintains an acidic pH in the urine

16e. Ms. Johnson is concerned about the obesity of her 15-year-old daughter, Jenny, and requests a bottle of Diatrim. Which of the following is(are) present in this OTC product?

I. benzocaine
II. caffeine
III. phenylpropanolamine

(A) I only
(B) III only
(C) I and II only
(D) II and III only
(E) I, II, and III

16f. Obesity has been attributed to which of the following factors?

I. anxiety but not depression
II. derangement in the satiety center
III. genetic

(A) I only
(B) III only
(C) I and II only
(D) II and III only
(E) I, II, and III

16g. Jenny wants to go on a "crash diet" as described on TV. For her safety, the pharmacist should suggest weight losses of NOT more than _____ lb per week.

(A) 2
(B) 5
(C) 8
(D) 12
(E) 16

16h. Bulemia is characterized by all of the following behavior patterns EXCEPT

(A) consumption of large amounts of food at one sitting
(B) patient feels that he/she is too fat even when individual is underweight
(C) patient-induced vomiting
(D) compulsion for vigorous exercise to prevent overweight
(E) frequent use of laxatives

16i. Besides its use as an anorexigenic agent, phenylpropanolamine is included in pharmaceutical products as a(n)

(A) antihistamine
(B) antihypertensive agent
(C) local anesthetic
(D) nasal decongestant
(E) sleep aid

16j. Side effects of phenylpropanolamine may include any of the following EXCEPT

(A) constipation
(B) dry mouth
(C) hypertension
(D) mydriasis
(E) sedation

16k. Tartazine may be present in pharmaceuticals as a(n)

(A) antioxidant
(B) antimicrobial preservative
(C) antiseptic
(D) buffer
(E) coloring agent

16l. Ms Johnson presents the following prescription for Jenny to the pharmacist:

Rx		
Menthol		
Camphor	aa qs	1%
LCD		2%
Hydrophilic Ointment	qs	60 g
Sig: Apply to arms ut dict		

The amount of menthol required for this prescription is

(A) 0.3 g
(B) 0.5 g
(C) 0.6 g
(D) 1.0 g
(E) 1.2 g

16m. When preparing this ointment, the pharmacist may choose to

I. make a eutectic of the menthol and camphor
II. add isopropyl alcohol to dissolve the menthol and camphor
III. add polysorbate 80 (Tween 80) to solubilize the LCD

(A) I only
(B) III only
(C) I and II only
(D) II and III only
(E) I, II, and III

16n. The above prescription is most likely written for the treatment of

(A) dermatitis due to poison ivy
(B) insect bites
(C) acne
(D) localized abscesses
(E) psoriasis

16o. Patients using coal tar products should be cautioned that such products

I. may cause photosensitization
II. may have carcinogenic potential if placed on the rectal, genital, or groin area
III. should not be used as a shampoo

(A) I only
(B) III only
(C) I and II only
(D) II and III only
(E) I, II, and III

PROFILE NO. 17

Hospital Pharmacy Medication Record

Patient Name: Edward Coster   Room Number: 612-2

Age: 62   Sex: M   Height: 5'11"   Weight: 122 lb

Allergies: NK

DIAGNOSIS

Primary	Secondary
1. CA colon	1. hypertension
2.	2. lung rales
3.	3.

LAB TESTS

Date	Test & Results	Date	Test & Results
1. 10/6	WBC 8000	4. 10/6	BUN 10 mg/dL
2.	Hemoglobin 15 g/dL Hematocrit 40%	5.	Serum creatinine 1 mg/dL
3.	Glucose 100 mg/dL	6.	Albumin 4 g/dL
		7. 10/7	Electrolytes: Na = 138 mEq; K = 4 mEq; Cl = 120 mEq/L

DRUG RECORD

Date	Drug Order	Sig.	DC'd
1. 10/5	Digoxin 0.25 mg	1 qd p.o.	
2.	Propranolol 40 mg	1 b.i.d. p.o.	
3.	Colace 100 mg	p.r.n.	
4.	Dalmane 30 mg	1 hs p.r.n.	
5.	Lasix 40 mg	1 daily p.r.n. p.o.	
6. 10/7	usual preop per Dr Lachman		
7. 10/8	start TPN 1 L postop 1st day then 3 L daily; after 1st day start 500 mL Liposyn III 20% q.o.d.		

PHARMACIST'S NOTES

Date	Comment	
1. 10/8	Start following TPN as directed:	
	Amino acid sol. 8.5%	500 mL
	D50W	500
	Calcium chloride	8.6 mEq
	Potassium Cl	40
	NaCl	40
	MVI	1 vial
	Insulin	10 units
	Rate—50 mL 1st hr then 100 mL per hour	

DIRECTIONS (Questions 17a through 17o): Each of the numbered items or incomplete statements in this section is followed by answers or by completion of the statement. Select the ONE lettered answer or completion that is BEST in each case.

17a. Based upon the reported lab tests, Mr Coster is likely to have

    (A) a systemic infection   *normal 5000-10000*
    (B) an anemic condition
    (C) diabetes
    (D) renal impairment
    (E) none of the above

17b. Usually, antibiotic prophylaxis for surgical patients is started

    (A) 3 hours presurgery
    (B) 1 hour presurgery
    (C) during surgery
    (D) 1 hour postsurgery
    (E) 3 hours postsurgery

17c. Appropriate presurgical antibiotic prophylaxis for a patient undergoing intestinal surgery will be

    (A) gentamicin + tetracycline
    (B) erythromycin + neomycin
    (C) cephalosporin + neomycin

(D) penicillin + gentamicin
(E) amoxicillin + clavulanate potassium

17d. When selecting a commercial amino acid solution for the TPN order, the pharmacist would consider which of the following?
I. Aminosyn (Abbott)
II. FreAmine (Kendall McGaw)
III. NephrAmine (Kendall McGaw) — *for renal impairment*

all essential and none of the nonessential

(A) I only
(B) III only
(C) I and II only
(D) II and III only
(E) I, II, and III only

17e. Route(s) of administration for the TPN solution can include
I. central infusion
II. peripheral infusion
III. enteral

Glucose 10% or more not peripheral

(A) I only
(B) III only
(C) I and II only
(D) II and III only
(E) I, II, and III

17f. Before compounding the TPN formula, the prescriber should be consulted concerning the
I. high level of chlorides
II. level of dextrose
III. amount of multivitamins desired

(A) I only
(B) III only
(C) I and II only
(D) II and III only
(E) I, II, and III only

17g. The amount of nitrogen provided by each liter of the TPN formula will be approximately _____ g.

8.5% × 500 × 16% (N)

(A) 6.8
(B) 14
(C) 36
(D) 42.5
(E) 85

17h. The number of nonprotein calories present in each bottle will be approximately _____ kcal.

(A) 680
(B) 800
(C) 1200
(D) 1540
(E) 1800

17i. The best ratio of nonprotein calories to grams of nitrogen for TPN formulas is approximately

(A) 10:1
(B) 50:1

(C) 100:1
(D) 150:1
(E) 200:1

17j. The administration of Liposyn III is intended to prevent

(A) agranulocytosis
(B) decubitus ulcers
(C) EFAD
(D) BEE
(E) phlebitis

17k. The number of calories provided by each bottle of Liposyn III will be

500 × 20% = 100

(A) 100
(B) 500
(C) 1000
(D) 1200
(E) 1500

17l. After 4 days, the patient's surgical scar has not healed, and a bedsore has developed on the buttocks. Which one of the following ingredients may speed the healing process if added to the TPN?

(A) ascorbic acid
(B) folic acid
(C) iron
(D) selenium
(E) zinc

17m. Which one of the following is NOT appropriate as an aide in the healing of bedsores?

(A) DuoDerm
(B) egg crate cushions
(C) flotation cushions
(D) heat lamps
(E) water beds

17n. On the fifth day, the patient exhibits symptoms of Legionnaires' disease. Which of the following statements is(are) true concerning this disease?
I. causative agent is a fungus
II. transmission is by airborne inhalation
III. smokers are more susceptible than the general population

(A) I only
(B) III only
(C) I and II only
(D) II and III only
(E) I, II, and III

17o. The drug of choice in the treatment of Legionnaires' disease is

(A) cefaclor
(B) erythromycin *or Tetracycline*
(C) gentamicin
(D) penicillin VK
(E) acyclovir

PROFILE NO. 18

Hospital Pharmacy Medication Record

Patient Name: Frances Costello   Room No: 621

Age: 42   Sex: F   Height: 5'4"   Weight: 132 lb

Allergies: aspirin, penicillin?

DIAGNOSIS

Primary	Secondary
1. Hodgkin"s disease	1. Graves' disease
2.	2. essential hypertension (under control with diet)
3.	3. allergies

LAB TESTS

	Date	Test & Results		Date	Test & Results
1.	6/12	SMA-12	4.		
2.			5.		
3.			6.		

DRUG RECORD

	Date	Drug Order	Sig.	DC'd
1.	6/12	propylthiouracil	50 mg 2 b.i.d.	
2.		mechlorethamine	6 mg/m^2 on day 1	
3.		procarbazine	100 mg/m^2	
4.		prednisone	40 mg daily	
5.		vincristine	2 mg on day 1	
6.		Dalmane 30 mg	1 hs p.r.n.	
7.		Colace 100 mg	1 qd	
8.		APAP	2 tabs p.r.n. fever	

PHARMACIST'S NOTES

	Date	Comment
1.	6\12	Start MOPP therapy on 6/14 if blood work results are normal.

DIRECTIONS (Questions 18a through 18p): Each of the numbered items or incomplete statements in this section is followed by answers or by completions of the statement. Select the ONE lettered answer or completion that is BEST in each case.

18a. Which one of the following drugs is NOT a part of the chemotherapeutic regimen known as MOPP?

(A) mechlorethamine
(B) prednisone
(C) procarbazine
(D) propylthiouracil
(E) vincristine

18b. Which of the following drugs are given orally during MOPP treatment?
   I. mechlorethamine
  II. procarbazine
 III. prednisone

(A) I only
(B) III only
(C) I and II only
(D) II and III only
(E) I, II, and III

18c. Which one of the following forms of cancer is least responsive to chemotherapy?

(A) hepatocellular   (D) prostate
(B) Hodgkin's   (E) testicular
(C) ovarian

18d. The intern reports that Mrs Costello is experiencing extravasation of the mechlorethamine (Mustargen). Which of the following courses of treatment should be initiated?

(A) Apply warm compresses immediately
(B) Infiltrate sodium thiosulfate 1/6th N into area and apply cold compresses.
(C) Infiltrate sodium thiosulfate 1/6th N into area and apply warm compresses.
(D) Infuse heparin sodium 20,000 units into area.
(E) Withdraw infusion needle and apply compresses of sodium thiosulfate 10% W/V.

18e. How many grams of sodium thiosulfate USP (mol. wt. of the hydrated form is 248) are needed to prepare 100 mL of 1/6 Normal solution?

(A) 2.1   (D) 14.9
(B) 4.1   (E) 24.8
(C) 7.5

18f. The pharmacy only has the anhydrous form of the above chemical. How many grams are needed to prepare the above solution? (Hydrated sodium thiosulfate has five molecules of water present.)

(A) 2.6   (D) 5.6
(B) 3.8   (E) 0 (since anhydrous
(C) 4.4   form cannot be used)

18g. Three weeks after the start of MOPP therapy, the patient calls the oncology team to inform them that she is experiencing severe epistaxis. This condition is likely caused by

(A) blood pressure greater than 160/100
(B) blood pressure less than 100/60
(C) congestive heart failure
(D) low platelet counts
(E) a vasomotor disorder

18h. Adverse effects of chemotherapeutic agents, such as bone marrow depression, pass through three stages—onset, maximum depression, and recovery to normal. Which one of the following terms is used to indicate the time for maximum depression?

(A) climb   (D) nadir
(B) lag   (E) suppression time
(C) retention time

18i. Which one of the following drugs can be included in chemotherapy with little expectation of bone marrow depression?

(A) BCNU   (D) thiotepa
(B) mitomycin   (E) vincristine
(C) methotrexate

18j. Which of the following criteria is(are) used when selecting antineoplastic drugs for combination therapy?
   I. different mechanisms of cytotoxic activity
  II. different spectra of toxicity
 III. high therapeutic index *low index*

(A) I only   (D) II and III only
(B) III only   (E) I, II, and III
(C) I and II only

18k. The physician decides that the patient requires weekly parenteral cyanocobalamin (vitamin B_{12}) injections. Which of the following routes of administration are appropriate?
   I. subcutaneous
  II. intramuscular
 III. intravenous

(A) I only   (D) II and III only
(B) III only   (E) I, II, and III
(C) I and II only

18l. Mrs Costello has complained of back spasms that were not relieved with hot compresses. All of the following drugs may be prescribed as oral skeletal muscle relaxants EXCEPT

(A) carisoprodol (Soma)
(B) chlorzoxazone (Parafon Forte)
(C) baclofen (Lioresal)
(D) dantrolene (Dantrium)
(E) mefenamic acid (Ponstel) *NSAID*

18m. Mrs Costello's allergies have returned. Which of the following antihistamines may the pharmacist dispense without a prescription?
   I. brompheniramine
  II. chlorpheniramine
 III. clemastine

(A) I only
(B) III only
(C) I and II only
(D) II and III only
(E) I, II, and III

18n. Which of the following antihistamines is(are) not likely to cause drowsiness?
   I. astemizole
  II. terfenadine
 III. clemastine

(A) I only
(B) III only
(C) I and II only
(D) II and III only
(E) I, II, and III

18o. Which one of the following antihistamines has the slowest onset of action?

(A) astemizole *Hismanal*
(B) clemastine
(C) chlorpheniramine
(D) brompheniramine
(E) terfenadine

18p. Which of the following statements concerning Estraderm transdermal patches is (are) true?
   I. patch must be replaced once every week
  II. lower dosing is possible since drug administration avoids first-pass effect
 III. drug is as effective as Premarin in prophylaxis of osteoporosis and postmenopausal syndrome

(A) I only
(B) III only
(C) I and II only
(D) II and III only
(E) I, II, and III

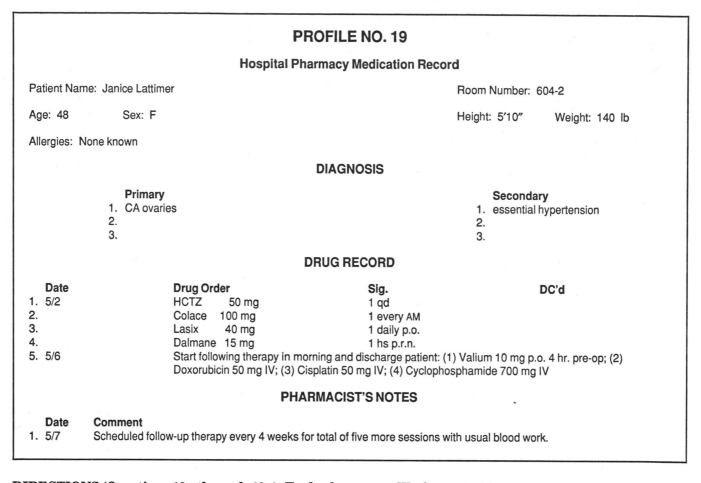

PROFILE NO. 19

Hospital Pharmacy Medication Record

Patient Name: Janice Lattimer   Room Number: 604-2

Age: 48   Sex: F   Height: 5′10″   Weight: 140 lb

Allergies: None known

DIAGNOSIS

Primary
1. CA ovaries
2.
3.

Secondary
1. essential hypertension
2.
3.

DRUG RECORD

	Date	Drug Order	Sig.	DC'd
1.	5/2	HCTZ 50 mg	1 qd	
2.		Colace 100 mg	1 every AM	
3.		Lasix 40 mg	1 daily p.o.	
4.		Dalmane 15 mg	1 hs p.r.n.	
5.	5/6	Start following therapy in morning and discharge patient: (1) Valium 10 mg p.o. 4 hr. pre-op; (2) Doxorubicin 50 mg IV; (3) Cisplatin 50 mg IV; (4) Cyclophosphamide 700 mg IV		

PHARMACIST'S NOTES

	Date	Comment
1.	5/7	Scheduled follow-up therapy every 4 weeks for total of five more sessions with usual blood work.

DIRECTIONS (Questions 19a through 19p): Each of the numbered items or incomplete statements in this section is followed by answers or by completions of the statement. Select the ONE lettered answer or completion that is BEST each case.

19a. Doxorubicin is available as

(A) Adriamycin
(B) CeeNu
(C) Cytosar-U
(D) DTIC
(E) Cytoxan

19b. Ms Lattimer should be warned of the possibility of alopecia when using which of the following drugs:
   I. cisplatin
  II. cyclophosphamide
 III. doxorubicin

(A) I only
(B) III only
(C) I and II only
(D) II and III only
(E) I, II, and III

19c. Significant side effects of doxorubicin include:
   I. cardiomyopathy
  II. leukopenia

 III. hepatotoxicity

(A) I only
(B) III only
(C) I and II only
(D) II and III only
(E) I, II, and III

19d. The dose of cyclophosphamide being administered is

(A) 5 mg/kg
(B) 11 mg/kg
(C) 24 mg/kg
(D) 700 mg/lb
(E) 700 mg/kg

19e. The pharmacist may wish to suggest the addition of metoclopramide to Ms Lattimer's therapy. This drug is used as a(an)

(A) antiemetic
(B) antihistamine
(C) local anesthetic
(D) antidepressant
(E) antivesicant

19f. All of the following cytotoxic agents exhibit vesicant properties except

(A) dactinomycin
(B) doxorubicin
(C) lomustine
(D) mithramycin
(E) mitomycin

19g. After two courses of therapy, Ms Lattimer's serum creatinine level is 3 mg/dL. The physician should be consulted to

(A) increase Lasix dose
(B) decrease cisplatin dose
(C) decrease cyclophosphamide dose
(D) decrease doxorubicin dose
(E) decrease dose of Valium

19h. A major toxic effect commonly observed in patients receiving cyclophosphamide (Cytoxan) therapy is

(A) anemia
(B) leukopenia
(C) hidrosis
(D) hepatotoxicity
(E) mental confusion

19i. Leucovorin (folinic acid) may be required after the administration of high doses of

(A) cisplatin
(B) doxorubicin
(C) cyclophosphamide
(D) methotrexate
(E) vincristine

19j. For which of the following drugs is the intrathecal route of administration acceptable?
I. thiotepa
II. methotrexate
III. vincristine

(A) I only
(B) III only
(C) I and II only
(D) II and III only
(E) I, II, and III

19k. Methotrexate is available in which of the following dosage forms?
I. oral solution
II. oral tablets
III. lyophilized powder for injection

(A) I only
(B) III only
(C) I and II only
(D) II and III only
(E) I, II, and III

19l. Janice brings a new prescription into your pharmacy for Vasotec. The generic name for this drug product is

(A) enalapril
(B) lisinopril
(C) labetalol
(D) captopril
(E) verapamil

19m. The mode of action of Vasotec for hypertension is as a

(A) alpha–adrenergic blocking agent
(B) alpha-beta–adrenergic blocking agent
(C) angiotensin-converting enzyme inhibitor
(D) calcium channel blocking agent
(E) centrally acting alpha agonist

19n. When dispensing the Vasotec prescription, the pharmacist should counsel the client that the drug may cause
I. dry coughing
II. precipitous fall in blood pressure during initial dosing
III. reflex tachycardia

(A) I only
(B) III only
(C) I and II only
(D) II and III only
(E) I, II, and III

19o. Which of the following antihypertensive agents is probably the safest to administer during pregnancy?

(A) captopril
(B) enalapril
(C) hydralazine
(D) hydrochlorothiazide
(E) nifedipine

19p. A second brand of Prinivil is

(A) Aldoril
(B) Isordil
(C) Triavil
(D) Vistaril
(E) Zestril

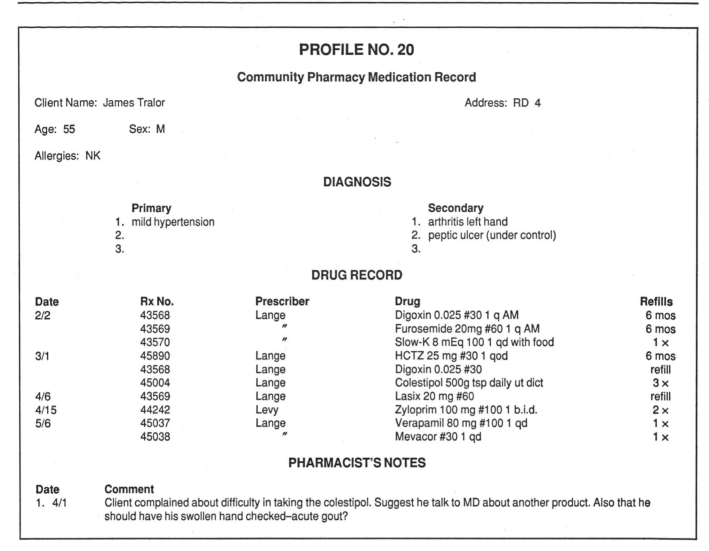

PROFILE NO. 20

Community Pharmacy Medication Record

Client Name: James Tralor

Address: RD 4

Age: 55   Sex: M

Allergies: NK

DIAGNOSIS

Primary
1. mild hypertension
2.
3.

Secondary
1. arthritis left hand
2. peptic ulcer (under control)
3.

DRUG RECORD

Date	Rx No.	Prescriber	Drug	Refills
2/2	43568	Lange	Digoxin 0.025 #30 1 q AM	6 mos
	43569	"	Furosemide 20mg #60 1 q AM	6 mos
	43570	"	Slow-K 8 mEq 100 1 qd with food	1 ×
3/1	45890	Lange	HCTZ 25 mg #30 1 qod	6 mos
	43568	Lange	Digoxin 0.025 #30	refill
	45004	Lange	Colestipol 500g tsp daily ut dict	3 ×
4/6	43569	Lange	Lasix 20 mg #60	refill
4/15	44242	Levy	Zyloprim 100 mg #100 1 b.i.d.	2 ×
5/6	45037	Lange	Verapamil 80 mg #100 1 qd	1 ×
	45038	"	Mevacor #30 1 qd	1 ×

PHARMACIST'S NOTES

Date	Comment
1. 4/1	Client complained about difficulty in taking the colestipol. Suggest he talk to MD about another product. Also that he should have his swollen hand checked–acute gout?

DIRECTIONS (Questions 20a through 20n): Each of the numbered items or incomplete statements in this section is followed by answers or by completions of the statement. Select the ONE lettered answer or completion that is BEST in each case.

20a. The pharmacist should consult Dr Lange concerning:
  I. Mr Tralor's compliance with HCTZ
  II. The desired strength of Mevacor
  III. A potential interaction between digoxin and Verapamil

  (A) I only
  (B) III only
  (C) I and II only
  (D) II and III only
  (E) I, II, and III

20b. Verapamil is available in which of the following dosage forms?
  I. extended release capsules
  II. extended release tablets
  III. parenteral solution

  (A) I only
  (B) III only
  (C) I and II only
  (D) II and III only
  (E) I, II, and III

20c. Verapamil is best classified as a(n)

  (A) adrenergic blocking agent
  (B) calcium entry blocker
  (C) ganglionic blocking agent
  (D) saluretic
  (E) vasopressor

20d. When given orally a high percentage of Verapamil undergoes the first-pass effect. This fact can be deduced by recognizing that
  I. the dose required for parenteral administration is much lower than oral dosing
  II. the apparent volume of distribution is high (420 L)
  III. the drug is approximately 90% protein bound in the blood

(A) I only
(B) III only
(C) I and II only
(D) II and III only
(E) I, II, and III

20e. The pharmacist will advise Mr Traler to consume the Mevacor

(A) before breakfast
(B) with breakfast
(C) after breakfast
(D) with any meal
(E) in the evening

20f. When selecting a generic brand of furosemide tablets, the pharmacist reviews the following relationships between brands A, B, C, and D:

Disintegration Times   A > B > C > D
Dissolution Times   C < B < A < D

Which brand should the pharmacist select as probably having the greatest bioavailability?

(A) A
(B) B
(C) C
(D) D
(E) either A or B

dissolution

20g. Niacin was likely prescribed

(A) as a vitamin supplement
(B) to prevent or treat peripheral neuritis
(C) prevent or treat beriberi
(D) improve the absorption of digoxin
(E) to reduce cholesterol levels

20h. Patients receiving niacin may experience
  I. constipation
  II. GI disorders
  III. flushing

(A) I only
(B) III only
(C) I and II only
(D) II and III only
(E) I, II, and III

20i. Niacin is available as an
  I. injection
  II. extended release capsule
  III. oral solution

(A) I only
(B) III only
(C) I and II only
(D) II and III only
(E) I, II, and III

20j. A desirable, realistic level of total cholesterol in the blood for an adult is

(A) < 100 mg/dL
(B) < 200 mg/dL
(C) < 250 mg/dL
(D) < 300 mg/dL
(E) < 500 mg/dL

20k. A significant increased risk of heart disease occurs when which of the following is(are) elevated?
  I. HDLP
  II. LDLP
  III. VLDLP

(A) I only
(B) III only
(C) I and II only
(D) II and III only
(E) I, II, and III

20l. The pharmacist should suggest all of the following dietary guides for reducing cholesterol EXCEPT

(A) increase intake of fruits and vegetables
(B) cook only with vegetable oils containing unsaturated fatty acids instead of saturated oils
(C) avoid red meats and chicken
(D) reduce intake of whole eggs to 2 or less per week
(E) increase intake of cereals and legumes

20m. Which one of the following antihyperlipidemic agents is considered the most potent?

(A) cholestyramine
(B) colestipol
(C) gemfibrozil
(D) lovastatin
(E) probucol

20n. Cholestyramine has the tendency to bind
  I. components of bile
  II. weakly acidic drugs
  III. weakly basic drugs

(A) I only
(B) III only
(C) I and II only
(D) II and III only
(E) I, II, and III

acidic drugs

PROFILE NO. 21

Community Pharmacy Medication Record

Client Name: Irma Jackson   Address: 12 Comfort Lane

Age: 77   Sex: F   Weight: 112 lb

Allergies: sensitive to aspirin, sulfas; limit chocolates

DIAGNOSIS

Primary
1. parkinsonism
2. glaucoma
3. CHF

Secondary
1. mild anemia
2. stroke (1 yr ago)
3.

PHARMACIST'S NOTES

	Date	Comment
1.		Do not use poison prevention closures.
2.		Irma is sometimes confused; explain all medicines to her. Whenever possible, suggest she take medications first thing in the AM with breakfast.
3.		OTCs-Mylanta 15 mL q AM and PM
		Tums-1 every night
		Vitamin C-500 mg q AM

DRUG RECORD

Date	Rx No.	Prescriber	Drug		Refills
8/4	82542	Puleo	Fe Sulfate	250 mg 60 1 q AM	2 ×
	82543	Puleo	Synthroid	50 µg 60 1 q AM	2 ×
	82544	"	Digoxin	0.25 mg 100 1 qd	1 ×
9/28	82543	Puleo	Ref. Synthroid	50 µg 60 1 qAM	1 ×
	89680	Puleo	Fe Sulfate	250 mg 100 2 qAM	2 ×
10/4	89890	Collins	Amantadine	8 oz 2 tsp b.i.d.	1 ×

DIRECTIONS (Questions 21a through 21m): Each of the numbered items or incomplete statements in this section is followed by answers or by completions of the statement. Select the ONE lettered answer or completion that is BEST in each case.

21a. Synthroid was prescribed to control

(A) hypothyroidism
(B) hyperthyroidism
(C) Graves' disease
(D) hyperparathyroidism
(E) hypoparathyroidism

21b. If Mrs Jackson misses a dose of Synthroid, she should be instructed to

(A) double the following morning's dose
(B) take 1 1/2 tablets the following morning
(C) increase her intake of iodized salt
(D) call her physician for advice
(E) continue with normal dosing the following morning

21c. When questioned about her recent weight loss, Mrs Jackson admitted that her breakfast and lunch consisted of two pieces of toast and herbal tea sweetened with Equal. The active ingredient in Equal is

(A) acesulfam
(B) aspartame
(C) fructose
(D) saccharin
(E) sucrose

21d. Factors contributing to Mrs Jackson's poor blood iron levels may be
 I. dietary intake
 II. antacid consumption
 III. daily consumption of vitamin C

(A) I only
(B) III only
(C) I and II only
(D) II and III only
(E) I, II, and III

21e. Amantadine may have been prescribed
   I. as a protectant against influenza B
   II. as a protectant against influenza A
   III. to treat the parkinsonism

(A) I only
(B) III only
(C) I and II only
(D) II and III only
(E) I, II, and III

21f. A tradename product of amantadine is

(A) Mellaril-S
(B) Propine
(C) Quinaglute
(D) Soma
(E) Symmetrel

21g. Mrs Jackson's daughter is worried that her mother is showing symptoms of Alzheimer's disease. What one of the following is the earliest symptom of this disease?

(A) incontinence
(B) inability to learn new skills
(C) loss of recent memory
(D) loss of remote memory
(E) wandering

21h. Drugs currently in use for Alzheimer's include
   I. papaverine
   II. ergoloid mesylates
   III. tacrine

(A) I only
(B) III only
(C) I and II only
(D) II and III only
(E) I, II, and III

21i. When dispensing the original prescriptions on 8/4, the pharmacist should have counseled the patient to take the digoxin

(A) first thing in the morning before food
(B) with breakfast
(C) after breakfast

(D) with lunch
(E) in the evening with the Mylanta

21j. The evening dose of Tums is probably intended to

(A) decrease gastric secretions
(B) decrease gastroesophageal reflux
(C) prevent osteoporosis
(D) provide magnesium ions
(E) serve as a mild laxative

21k. Pharmacokinetic changes in the elderly often include
   I. increase in plasma albumin levels
   II. increase in renal clearance
   III. increase in volume of distribution of lipophilic drugs

(A) I only
(B) III only
(C) I and II only
(D) II and III only
(E) I, II, and III

21l. How many mL of digoxin elixir are needed to replace the daily 0.25 mg dose of digoxin tablets based upon the following relationship in this patient?

	Strength	**"F value"**
digoxin tablet	0.25 mg	0.6
digoxin elixir	0.05 mg/mL	0.75

(A) 3
(B) 3.8
(C) 4
(D) 5
(E) 6.4

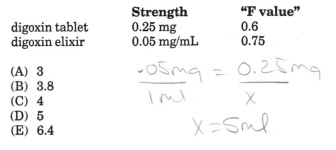

21m. An early sign of digoxin toxicity in Mrs Jackson is likely to be

(A) hazy vision
(B) hearing impairment
(C) tinnitus
(D) yellowish skin
(E) increase in appetite

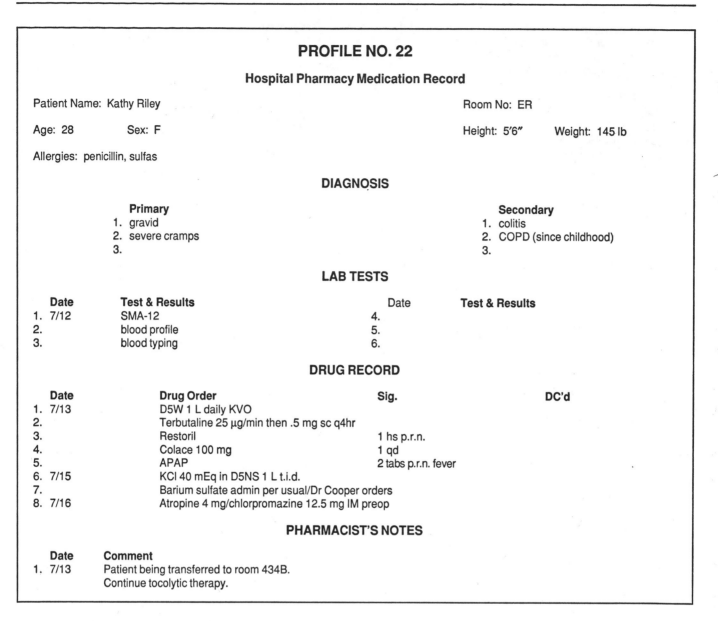

PROFILE NO. 22

Hospital Pharmacy Medication Record

Patient Name: Kathy Riley   Room No: ER

Age: 28   Sex: F   Height: 5'6"   Weight: 145 lb

Allergies: penicillin, sulfas

DIAGNOSIS

Primary	Secondary
1. gravid	1. colitis
2. severe cramps	2. COPD (since childhood)
3.	3.

LAB TESTS

Date	Test & Results	Date	Test & Results
1. 7/12	SMA-12	4.	
2.	blood profile	5.	
3.	blood typing	6.	

DRUG RECORD

Date	Drug Order	Sig.	DC'd
1. 7/13	D5W 1 L daily KVO		
2.	Terbutaline 25 µg/min then .5 mg sc q4hr		
3.	Restoril	1 hs p.r.n.	
4.	Colace 100 mg	1 qd	
5.	APAP	2 tabs p.r.n. fever	
6. 7/15	KCl 40 mEq in D5NS 1 L t.i.d.		
7.	Barium sulfate admin per usual/Dr Cooper orders		
8. 7/16	Atropine 4 mg/chlorpromazine 12.5 mg IM preop		

PHARMACIST'S NOTES

Date	Comment
1. 7/13	Patient being transferred to room 434B. Continue tocolytic therapy.

DIRECTIONS (Questions 22a through 22n): Each of the numbered items or incomplete statements in this section is followed by answers or by completions of the statement. Select the ONE lettered answer or completion that is BEST in each case.

22a. Terbutaline is being used as a tocolytic agent. The term tocolytic refers to a drug that   *premature labor*

(A) increases GI tract tone
(B) reduces GI tract motility
(C) reduces uterine contractility
(D) prevents emesis
(E) dilates bronchioles

22b. A tradename product of terbutaline is

(A) Alupent
(B) Brethine
(C) Pamelor

(D) Proventil
(E) Terazol

22c. The pharmacist places 2 mL of terbutaline injection (1 mg/mL) into 250 mL of D5W. How many drops per minute will be needed to deliver the terbutaline if the administration set delivers 15 drops to the mL?

(A) 6
(B) 11
(C) 23
(D) 46
(E) 120

22d. As compounded, for how many minutes will the above solution last on the patient?

(A) 40
(B) 80
(C) 100

(D) 160

(E) 480

22e. Barium sulfate is best described as a(n)

(A) antacid

(B) antidiarrheal

(C) diagnostic agent

(D) cleansing laxative

(E) protectant against colitis

22f. Which of the following concerning barium sulfate is (are) true?
I. practically insoluble in water
II. administered by the oral route
III. administered by the rectal route

(A) I only

(B) III only

(C) I and II only

(D) II and III only

(E) I, II, and III

22g. The purpose of the preop atropine is to

(A) relieve the patient's anxiety

(B) reduce secretions

(C) cause vasoconstriction of small blood vessels

(D) constrict the bronchioles

(E) lessen presurgical nervousness

22h. The pharmacist should question the atropine/chlorpromazine order because of
I. an acid/base reaction between the two ingredients
II. the combination is irrational
III. the high dose of atropine requested

(A) I only

(B) III only

(C) I and II only

(D) II and III only

(E) I, II, and III

0.4mg

22i. A second drug that has activity similar to that of atropine is

(A) glycopyrrolate (Robinul)

(B) haloperidol (Haldol)

(C) lorazapam (Ativan)

(D) ondansetron (Zofran)

(E) prochlorperazine (Compazine)

(22j–22n). Mrs Riley is discharged from the hospital on 7/21 with prescriptions for a Foley catheter, ostomy pouches, transderm dressings, Slo-Bid 100 mg t.i.d., Valium 2 mg 1 t.i.d. p.r.n., Metamucil plain 1 tbsp AM, and a multivitamin for pregnancy.

22j. For which of the following items is a prescription actually needed?
I. Foley catheter

II. ostomy pouches
III. transderm dressings

(A) I only

(B) III only

(C) I and II only

(D) II and III only

(E) I, II, and III

22k. Which of the following products is(are) intended for use during pregnancy and lactation?
I. Natalins Rx
II. Stuartnatal
III. Poly-Vi-Flor

(A) I only

(B) III only

(C) I and II only

(D) II and III only

(E) I, II, and III

22l. Ingredients in Metamucil include
I. docusate
II. sucrose
III. psyllium

(A) I only

(B) III only

(C) I and II only

(D) II and III only

(E) I, II, and III

22m. Mrs Riley should be counseled to consume the Metamucil by

(A) mixing the granules with 8 oz of water, stirring, and drinking immediately

(B) mixing the granules with one pint of water, stirring, and drinking immediately

(C) mixing the granules with 8 oz water, stirring, letting mixture sit for 20 minutes before drinking

(D) swallowing the granules, then drinking 8 oz of water

(E) allowing the granules to effervesce in 8 oz of water before consuming

22n. Products with therapeutic activity similar to that of Slo-Bid include
I. Klor-Con
II. Slow-K
III. Theo-Dur

(A) I only

(B) III only

(C) I and II only

(D) II and III only

(E) I, II, and III

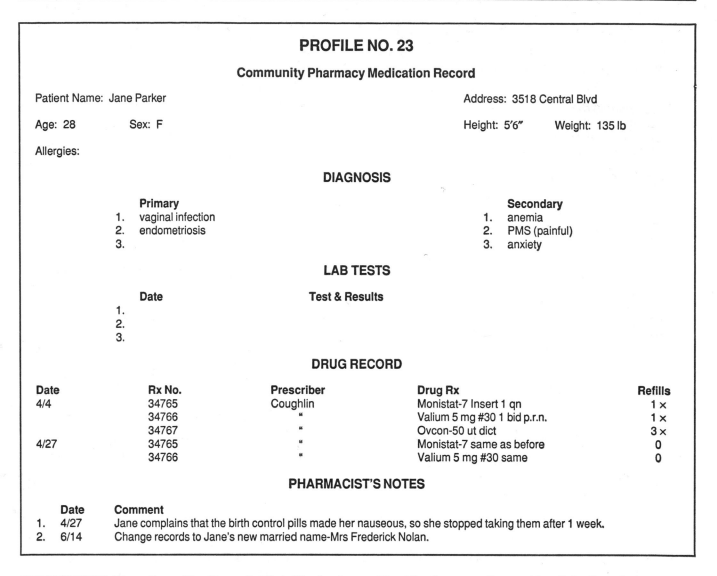

PROFILE NO. 23

Community Pharmacy Medication Record

Patient Name: Jane Parker

Address: 3518 Central Blvd

Age: 28   Sex: F

Height: 5'6"   Weight: 135 lb

Allergies:

DIAGNOSIS

Primary
1. vaginal infection
2. endometriosis
3.

Secondary
1. anemia
2. PMS (painful)
3. anxiety

LAB TESTS

	Date	Test & Results
1.		
2.		
3.		

DRUG RECORD

Date	Rx No.	Prescriber	Drug Rx	Refills
4/4	34765	Coughlin	Monistat-7 Insert 1 qn	1×
	34766	"	Valium 5 mg #30 1 bid p.r.n.	1×
	34767	"	Ovcon-50 ut dict	3×
4/27	34765	"	Monistat-7 same as before	0
	34766	"	Valium 5 mg #30 same	0

PHARMACIST'S NOTES

	Date	Comment
1.	4/27	Jane complains that the birth control pills made her nauseous, so she stopped taking them after 1 week.
2.	6/14	Change records to Jane's new married name-Mrs Frederick Nolan.

DIRECTIONS (Questions 23a through 23n): Each of the numbered items or incomplete statements in this section is followed by answers or by completions of the statement. Select the ONE lettered answer or completion that is BEST in each case.

23a. The Monistat prescription is probably being used to treat

(A) aspergillosis
(B) candidiasis
(C) gonorrhea
(D) genital herpes
(E) syphilis

23b. The most common causative microorganism of nongonococcal urethritis is

(A) *Candida cryptococcus*
(B) *Chlamydia trachomatis*
(C) *Klebsiella aerogenes*
(D) *Proteus mirabilis*
(E) *Treponema pallidum*

23c. The drug usually considered the first choice to treat all stages of syphilis is

(A) doxycycline
(B) erythromycin
(C) fluconazole
(D) penicillin
(E) ciprofloxacin

23d. The drug usually considered the first choice to treat chlamydia infections is

(A) doxycycline
(B) amoxicillin
(C) fluconazole
(D) penicillin
(E) ciprofloxacin

23e. Ms Parker asks what form of contraception is almost as effective as oral contraceptive tablets. The pharmacist should suggest

(A) condoms

(B) diaphragm
(C) IUD
(D) rhythm method
(E) spermicidal jellies

23f. Which of the following are acceptable lubricants for use with a condom or diaphragm?
  I. K-Y jelly
  II. spermicidal cream
  III. white vaseline

  (A) I only
  (B) III only
  (C) I and II only
  (D) II and III only
  (E) I, II, and III

23g. Which one of the following is inserted under the skin and offers up to 5 years of contraceptive protection?

  (A) Depo-Provera
  (B) nonoxynol-9
  (C) Norplant
  (D) ParaGard
  (E) Progestasert

23h. Ms Parker's endometriosis is best treated by the use of

  (A) Danocrine
  (B) Deltasone
  (C) Naprosyn
  (D) Sansert
  (E) Zantac

[23i–23n] Jane's husband confides in you that he is concerned by his wife's recent behavior. Fearing that she is going to become infected by bacteria, she wears a mask around the house, washes her hands every hour, and checks to make sure all windows are closed.

23i. The above behavior is characteristic of persons suffering from

  (A) generalized anxiety disorder (GAD)
  (B) obsessive-compulsive disorder (OCD)
  (C) panic disorder
  (D) posttraumatic stress disorder
  (E) social phobia

23j. A drug used in the treatment of OCD is

  (A) Anafranil
  (B) Ativan
  (C) Compazine
  (D) Haldol
  (E) Orudis

23k. Benzodiazepines are often used to treat anxiety disorders. Which one of the following is NOT a benzodiazepine?

  (A) alprazolam (Xanax)
  (B) chlordiazepoxide (Librium)
  (C) methylphenidate (Ritalin)
  (D) clorazepate (Tranxene)
  (E) lorazepam (Ativan)

23l. The mechanism of action of the benzodiazepines is believed to be

  (A) alpha$_1$ blockage
  (B) beta-adrenergic blockage
  (C) blockage of dopamine receptor sites
  (D) blockage of the reuptake of dopamine
  (E) potentiation of the inhibitory neurotransmitter GABA

23m. True statements concerning clozapine (Clozaril) include
  I. the drug is a dopamine-receptor antagonist
  II. there is a lower incidence of extrapyramidal effects than with chlorpromazine
  III. discontinue the drug if leukocyte levels fall below 3,000/mm^3.

  (A) I only
  (B) III only
  (C) I and II only
  (D) II and III only
  (E) I, II, and III

23n. Side effects occurring with clozapine include all of the following EXCEPT

  (A) drowsiness
  (B) hypersalivation
  (C) seizures
  (D) tachycardia
  (E) tardive dyskinesia

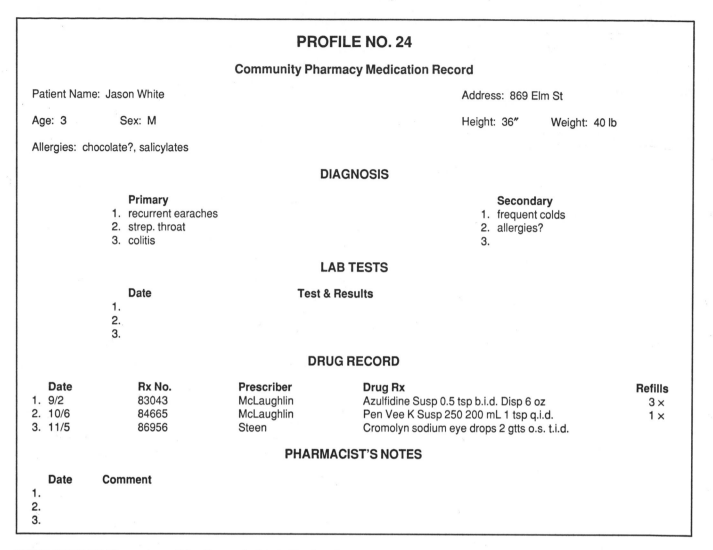

PROFILE NO. 24

Community Pharmacy Medication Record

Patient Name: Jason White

Address: 869 Elm St

Age: 3   Sex: M

Height: 36″   Weight: 40 lb

Allergies: chocolate?, salicylates

DIAGNOSIS

Primary
1. recurrent earaches
2. strep. throat
3. colitis

Secondary
1. frequent colds
2. allergies?
3.

LAB TESTS

Date	Test & Results
1.	
2.	
3.	

DRUG RECORD

	Date	Rx No.	Prescriber	Drug Rx	Refills
1.	9/2	83043	McLaughlin	Azulfidine Susp 0.5 tsp b.i.d. Disp 6 oz	3 ×
2.	10/6	84665	McLaughlin	Pen Vee K Susp 250 200 mL 1 tsp q.i.d.	1 ×
3.	11/5	86956	Steen	Cromolyn sodium eye drops 2 gtts o.s. t.i.d.	

PHARMACIST'S NOTES

	Date	Comment
1.		
2.		
3.		

DIRECTIONS (Questions 24a through 24n): Each of the numbered items or incomplete statements in this section is followed by answers or by completions of the statement. Select the ONE lettered answer or completion that is BEST in each case.

24a. Causative organisms of otitis media include
   I. *Heliobacter pylori*
   II. *Hemophilus influenzae*
   III. *Streptococcus pneumoniae*

   (A) I only
   (B) III only
   (C) I and II only
   (D) II and III only
   (E) I, II, and III

24b. Drugs of choice for otitis media include
   I. ampicillin
   II. amoxicillin
   III. cefaclor

   (A) I only
   (B) III only
   (C) I and II only
   (D) II and III only
   (E) I, II, and III

24c. When asked to suggest a drug to reduce Jason's fever and headache, the pharmacist could select products containing
   I. aspirin
   II. ibuprofen
   III. acetaminophen

   (A) I only
   (B) III only
   (C) I and II only
   (D) II and III only
   (E) I, II, and III

24d. Chemically, ibuprofen is a derivative of

   (A) fibric acid
   (B) phenylacetic acid
   (C) propionic acid
   (D) salicylic acid
   (E) xanthines

24e. When used to reduce fever, ibuprofen should not be used

(A) for more than 3 days
(B) for more than 10 days
(C) for less than 3 days
(D) for less than 10 days
(E) if the fever is greater than 104°F

24f. Aspirin dosage forms include all of the following EX-CEPT

(A) effervescent tablets
(B) elixir
(C) enteric coated tablets
(D) suppositories
(E) time-release tablets

[24g–24i] The eye drop prescription filled on 11/5 reads as follows:

Rx
Cromolyn sodium   2.5%   30 mL

Sig: gtt ii in o.s. t.i.d.
Make isotonic

24g. The pharmacist dilutes the commercially available 4% cromolyn solution with purified water. How many mg of sodium chloride are needed to render the solution isotonic, assuming that the 4% solution was isotonic?

(A) 100
(B) 170
(C) 330
(D) 540
(E) 900

24h. When preparing the above prescription using cromolyn capsules and purified water, the final solution must be passed through a _____ μ filter into a sterile dropper bottle.

(A) .22
(B) .45
(C) 1.0
(D) 5.0
(E) 10

24i. Opthalmic uses for the cromolyn solution include
I. to treat *Pseudomonas* infections
II. to relieve glaucoma
III. to treat conjunctivitis

(A) I only
(B) III only
(C) I and II only
(D) II and III only
(E) I, II, and III

24j. Mrs White's neighbor suggests that Jason be given daily doses of rose hips. The active ingredient in rose hips is

(A) ascorbic acid
(B) iron
(C) vitamin E
(D) ephedrine
(E) rose oil

24k. Which one of the following tricyclic antidepressants has been used successfully in treating bedwetting by children?

(A) amitriptyline (Elavil)
(B) doxepin (Sinequan)
(C) imipramine (Tofranil)
(D) nortriptyline (Pamelor)
(E) trimipramine (Surmontil)

24l. Which one of the following drugs would be appropriate as a sleep aid for Jason?

(A) flurazepam
(B) diphenhydramine
(C) dimenhydrinate
(D) estazolam
(E) triazolam

24m. Which one of the following drugs has the greatest potential for causing anterograde amnesia?

(A) flurazepam
(B) temazepam
(C) quazepam
(D) estazolam
(E) triazolam

24n. A therapeutic substitute for sulfasalazine is
(A) Bentyl
(B) Buspar
(C) Dipentum
(D) Imodium
(E) Lomotil

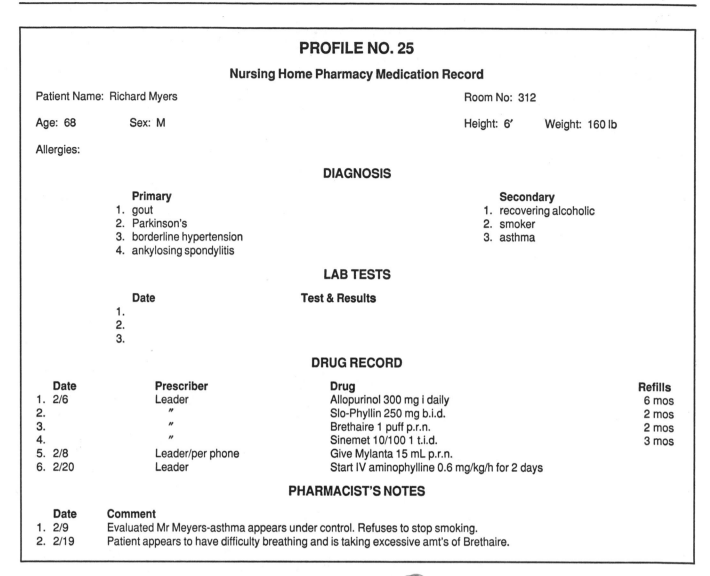

PROFILE NO. 25

Nursing Home Pharmacy Medication Record

Patient Name: Richard Myers

Room No: 312

Age: 68   Sex: M

Height: 6′   Weight: 160 lb

Allergies:

DIAGNOSIS

Primary
1. gout
2. Parkinson's
3. borderline hypertension
4. ankylosing spondylitis

Secondary
1. recovering alcoholic
2. smoker
3. asthma

LAB TESTS

	Date	Test & Results
1.		
2.		
3.		

DRUG RECORD

	Date	Prescriber	Drug	Refills
1.	2/6	Leader	Allopurinol 300 mg i daily	6 mos
2.		″	Slo-Phyllin 250 mg b.i.d.	2 mos
3.		″	Brethaire 1 puff p.r.n.	2 mos
4.		″	Sinemet 10/100 1 t.i.d.	3 mos
5.	2/8	Leader/per phone	Give Mylanta 15 mL p.r.n.	
6.	2/20	Leader	Start IV aminophylline 0.6 mg/kg/h for 2 days	

PHARMACIST'S NOTES

	Date	Comment
1.	2/9	Evaluated Mr Meyers-asthma appears under control. Refuses to stop smoking.
2.	2/19	Patient appears to have difficulty breathing and is taking excessive amt's of Brethaire.

DIRECTIONS (Questions 25a through 25o): Each of the numbered items or incomplete statements in this section is followed by answers or by completions of the statement. Select the ONE lettered answer or completion that is BEST in each case.

25a. Drugs of choice for treating acute attacks of gout include
   I.   allopurinol
   II. colchicine
   III. NSAIDs

   (A) I only
   (B) III only
   (C) I and II only
   (D) II and III only
   (E) I, II, and III

25b. Drugs of choice for controlling hyperuricemia include
   I.   allopurinol
   II. colchicine
   III. prednisone

   (A) I only
   (B) III only
   (C) I and II only
   (D) II and III only
   (E) I, II, and III

25c. Nursing should be advised that the allopurinol
   I.   should be consumed with a large amount of fluid
   II. may initially precipitate an attack of gout
   III. must be taken on an empty stomach to assure absorption

   (A) I only
   (B) III only
   (C) I and II only
   (D) II and III only
   (E) I, II, and III

25d. The new order for Mylanta may result in
   (A) increased absorption of Sinemet
   (B) decreased absorption of Sinemet
   (C) decreased absorption of Zyloprim

antacids ↑ levodopa

(D) increased absorption of magnesium ion
(E) calcium binding of the Sinemet

25e. Which of the following ingredients may be used in patients sensitive to aspirin?
   I. acetaminophen
   II. salicylamide
   III. ibuprofen

(A) I only
(B) III only
(C) I and II only
(D) II and III only
(E) I, II, and III

25f. Which one of the following is most likely to be prescribed to treat ankylosing spondylitis?

(A) fenoprofen
(B) flurbiprofen
(C) ketoprofen
(D) ibuprofen
(E) naproxen

25g. Mr Meyers is despondent because he is almost bald and asks about the drug that grows hair. The pharmacist should inform him that the drug is effective mainly in
   I. female patients
   II. patients younger than 40
   III. patients whose hair has thinned within the past 10 years

(A) I only
(B) III only
(C) I and II only
(D) II and III only
(E) I, II, and III

25h. Minoxidil is available in which of the following dosage forms?
   I. topical solution
   II. tablets
   III. topical ointment

(A) I only
(B) III only
(C) I and II only
(D) II and III only
(E). I, II, and III

25i. Based upon the order on 9/20, the pharmacist prepares an admixture of aminophylline 500 mg in 1 L D5W. What flow rate (gtt/min) should be set if the administration set delivers 15 drops to the mL?

(A) 2
(B) 10
(C) 15
(D) 22
(E) 46

25j. When prescribing the above dose, the prescriber took into consideration which of the following?

   I. Smoking decreases the half-life of theophylline.
   II. Aminophylline is more potent, mg to mg, than theophylline.
   III. The targeted theophylline serum level is 1 to 2 μg/mL.

(A) I only
(B) III only
(C) I and II only
(D) II and III only
(E) I, II, and III

25k. All of the following drugs will significantly increase the half-life of theophylline EXCEPT

(A) erythromycin
(B) cimetidine
(C) ciprofloxacin
(D) isoniazid
(E) ranitidine

25l. Theophylline's pharmacokinetics follow a two-compartment model when administered by IV bolus. Which of the following statements are true?
   I. The drug has faster initial distribution than elimination.
   II. When graphed, there will be two slopes.
   III. The half-lives of drugs following two-compartment modeling are longer than those following one-compartment modeling.

(A) I only
(B) III only
(C) I and II only
(D) II and III only
(E) I, II, and III

25m. Early symptoms of theophylline toxicity include nausea, anorexia, and

(A) bradycardia
(B) bleeding gums
(C) hypotension
(D) hypertension
(E) tachycardia

25n. Drugs that significantly increase the elimination of theophylline include all of the following EXCEPT

(A) carbamazepine
(B) isoproterenol
(C) phenytoin
(D) rifampin
(E) verapamil

25o. Drugs that have the tendency to impart an orange color to urine, sweat, and tears include

(A) carbamazepine
(B) isoniazid
(C) isoproterenol
(D) phenolphthalein
(E) rifampin

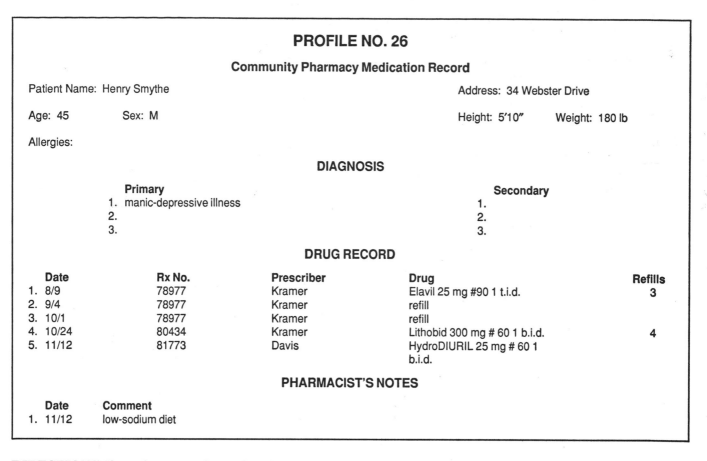

PROFILE NO. 26

Community Pharmacy Medication Record

Patient Name: Henry Smythe

Address: 34 Webster Drive

Age: 45   Sex: M

Height: 5'10"   Weight: 180 lb

Allergies:

DIAGNOSIS

Primary	Secondary
1. manic-depressive illness	1.
2.	2.
3.	3.

DRUG RECORD

	Date	Rx No.	Prescriber	Drug	Refills
1.	8/9	78977	Kramer	Elavil 25 mg #90 1 t.i.d.	3
2.	9/4	78977	Kramer	refill	
3.	10/1	78977	Kramer	refill	
4.	10/24	80434	Kramer	Lithobid 300 mg # 60 1 b.i.d.	4
5.	11/12	81773	Davis	HydroDIURIL 25 mg # 60 1 b.i.d.	

PHARMACIST'S NOTES

	Date	Comment
1.	11/12	low-sodium diet

DIRECTIONS (Questions 26a through 26j): Each of the numbered items or incomplete statements in this section is followed by answers or by completions of the statement. Select the ONE lettered answer or completion that is BEST in each case.

26a. Which of the following drugs is most similar in action to Elavil?

(A) Compazine
(B) Pamelor
(C) Nardil
(D) Loxitane
(E) Clozaril

26b. Which of the following is NOT a common adverse effect of Elavil?

(A) orthostatic hypotension
(B) sedation
(C) dry mouth
(D) urinary retention
(E) hirsutism

26c. Patients about to begin Elavil therapy should be advised that

(A) they must sign a consent form
(B) they will become more susceptible to infection
(C) it may take 1 to 4 weeks before any therapeutic action is evident

(D) they should not consume foods high in tyramine
(E) they should eat a high-protein diet while on the drug

26d. Patients using Elavil should not be using

(A) aspirin
(B) acetaminophen
(C) ibuprofen
(D) antimicrobial agents
(E) guanethidine

26e. Patients receiving Lithobid should be advised to

(A) avoid taking the drug at bedtime
(B) avoid taking the drug with milk
(C) drink 8 to 12 glasses of water/day while on the drug
(D) consume a low-sodium diet
(E) consume a low-potassium diet

26f. In using lithium products, toxicity commonly occurs when serum lithium levels exceed

(A) 1.5 mEq/L
(B) 1.5 mg/dL
(C) 1.5 mg/L
(D) 15 mg/L
(E) 300 µg/mL

26g. The addition of HydroDIURIL to this patient's regimen is likely to

(A) increase serum lithium levels
(B) decrease serum lithium levels
(C) decrease the absorption of lithium
(D) increase the absorption of lithium
(E) have no effect on lithium action

26h. In monitoring serum lithium levels, blood samples are usually drawn

(A) in the morning
(B) at bedtime
(C) just prior to taking a dose
(D) 1 to 3 hours after taking a dose
(E) at the midpoint between two doses

26i. HydroDIURIL can best be described as a(n)

(A) loop diuretic
(B) osmotic diuretic
(C) mercurial diuretic
(D) carbonic anhydrase inhibitor
(E) thiazide diuretic

26j. Lithobid is a

(A) slow-release capsule
(B) liquid-filled capsule
(C) slow-release tablet
(D) chewable tablet
(E) sublingual tablet

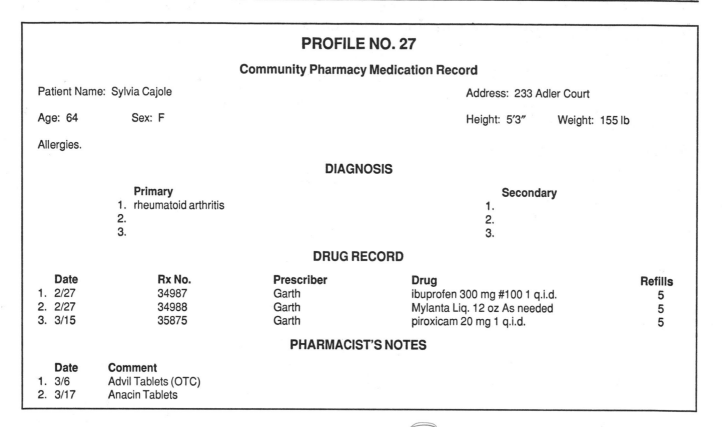

PROFILE NO. 27

Community Pharmacy Medication Record

Patient Name: Sylvia Cajole   Address: 233 Adler Court

Age: 64   Sex: F   Height: 5'3"   Weight: 155 lb

Allergies.

DIAGNOSIS

Primary	Secondary
1. rheumatoid arthritis	1.
2.	2.
3.	3.

DRUG RECORD

	Date	Rx No.	Prescriber	Drug	Refills
1.	2/27	34987	Garth	ibuprofen 300 mg #100 1 q.i.d.	5
2.	2/27	34988	Garth	Mylanta Liq. 12 oz As needed	5
3.	3/15	35875	Garth	piroxicam 20 mg 1 q.i.d.	5

PHARMACIST'S NOTES

	Date	Comment
1.	3/6	Advil Tablets (OTC)
2.	3/17	Anacin Tablets

DIRECTIONS (Questions 27a through 27j): Each of the numbered items or incomplete statements in this section is followed by answers or by completions of the statement. Select the ONE lettered answer or completion that is BEST in each case.

27a. In dispensing the prescription for ibuprofen, the pharmacist could have dispensed which of the following products?

(A) Rufen
(B) Orudis
(C) Ansaid
(D) Nalfon
(E) Lodine

27b. Ibuprofen is believed to act by

(A) antagonizing dopamine receptors
(B) stimulating dopamine receptors
(C) inhibiting xanthine oxidase
(D) increasing the production of prostaglandins
(E) decreasing the production of prostaglandins

27c. Which of the following statements is true?
  I. The active ingredient of Advil is ibuprofen.
  II. Ibuprofen should be administered three to four times daily
  III. Antacids should not be taken at the same time as ibuprofen.

(A) I only
(B) III only

(C) I and II only
(D) II and III only
(E) I, II, and III

27d. Mylanta Liquid contains

(A) calcium carbonate
(B) propylene glycol
(C) polyethylene glycol
(D) simethicone
(E) cation exchange resin

27e. When dispensing piroxicam, the pharmacist could dispense

(A) Nalfon
(B) Orudis
(C) Anaprox
(D) Torodol
(E) Feldene

27f. When the piroxicam prescription was filled the pharmacist should have advised the physician that

(A) it is not available in a 20-mg strength
(B) it should not be administered four times daily
(C) it should not be used for more than 10 days
(D) it is not to be used in patients with rheumatoid arthritis
(E) it is only used on a prn basis for acute pain

27g. Patients with rheumatoid arthritis who do not respond to NSAIDS may be given

(A) fluorouracil
(B) famotidine
(C) methysergide maleate
(D) allopurinol
(E) auranofin

27h. Misoprostol (Cytotec) can best be described as a(n)

I. synthetic prostaglandin analog
II. inhibitor of gastric acid secretion
III. H$_2$-receptor antagonist

(A) I only
(B) III only
(C) I and II only
(D) II and III only
(E) I, II, and III

27i. Misoprostol (Cytotec) is contraindicated for use in

(A) the elderly
(B) patients using aspirin
(C) patients with osteoarthritis
(D) pregnant women
(E) patients with hypertension

27j. Which of the following is an ingredient in Anacin?

I. caffeine
II. aspirin
III. acetaminophen

(A) I only
(B) III only
(C) I and II only
(D) II and III only
(E) I, II, and III

PROFILE NO. 28

Community Pharmacy Medication Record

Patient Name: Michael Teller

Address: 902 West 1st St

Age: 71   Sex: M

Height: 5'7"   Weight: 182 lb

Allergies:

DIAGNOSIS

Primary	Secondary
1. hypertension	1.
2. congestive heart disease	2.
3.	3.

DRUG RECORD

	Date	Rx No.	Prescriber	Drug	Refills
1.	6/23	90988	Wilson	Digoxin 0.25 #30 1 daily	3
2.	6/23	90989	Wilson	Lasix 40 mg #60 1 b.i.d.	3
3.	6/23	90990	Wilson	Klorvess 20 mEq #60 1 daily	3
4.	7/15	90988	Wilson	Refill	
5.	7/15	90989	Wilson	Refill	
6.	7/31	93889	Thomas	Amiloride 5 mg tab 1 daily in AM	3

PHARMACIST'S NOTES

	Date	Comment
1.	7/15	Baking soda to settle stomach

DIRECTION (Questions 28a through 28j): Each of the numbered items or incomplete statements in this section is followed by answers or by completions of the statement. Select the ONE lettered answer or completion that is BEST in each case.

28a. Digoxin can be described as an agent that produces a

 I. positive chronotropic effect
 II. positive inotropic effect
 III. vagomimetic effect

 (A) I only
 (B) III only
 (C) I and II only
 (D) II and III only
 (E) I, II, and III

28b. Patients with congestive heart disease who begin using digoxin are likely to experience

 (A) slowed heart rate
 (B) edema
 (C) decreased force of cardiac contraction
 (D) tardive dyskinesia
 (E) orthostatic hypotension

28c. Which of the following drugs is most closely related to digoxin?

 (A) hydralazine
 (B) mexiletine

 (C) flecainide
 (D) cyclandelate
 (E) deslanoside

28d. Which of the following would be suitable to use in a patient who needs a cardiac glycoside but has severe renal impairment?

 (A) digitoxin
 (B) disopyramide
 (C) digoxin
 (D) amiodarone
 (E) isradipine

28e. If this patient's medication were changed from digoxin tablets to Lanoxicaps, what would be an appropriate equivalent dose?

 (A) 2.5 mg
 (B) 25 µg
 (C) 200 µg
 (D) 0.25 mg
 (E) 0.125 mg

28f. Which of the following drugs would be appropriate to use in a patient who did not respond adequately to digitalis glycosides?

 (A) levarterenol
 (B) carteolol
 (C) amiodarone

(D) ramipril
(E) amrinone

28g. In dispensing Midamor the pharmacist should recommend to the prescriber that

(A) the dose of digoxin be increased by 50%
(B) the Klorvess be discontinued
(C) the dose of Klorvess be raised by 50%
(D) the dose of digoxin be decreased by 50%
(E) the dose of Klorvess be reduced by 50%

28h. Klorvess is available as a(n)
  I. effervescent granules
  II. effervescent tablet
  III. solution

(A) I only
(B) III only
(C) I and II only

(D) II and III only
(E) I, II, and III

28i. Bumex is most similar to

(A) Lasix
(B) HydroDIURIL
(C) Midamor
(D) Dyrenium
(E) Diamox

28j. The profile above reveals the possibility of
  I. patient noncompliance
  II. potential complexation
  III. a dosage error

(A) I only
(B) III only
(C) I and II only
(D) II and III only
(E) I, II, and III

PROFILE NO. 29

Community Pharmacy Medication Record

Patient Name: David Marchese   Address: 1904 Murray St

Age: 10   Sex: M   Height: 4'4"   Weight: 78 lb

Allergies: ragweed pollen

DIAGNOSIS

Primary	Secondary
1. bronchial asthma	1.
2. head lice	2.
3.	3.

DRUG RECORD

	Date	Rx No.	Prescriber	Drug	Refills
1.	7/9	38383	Charmin	Benadryl 25 mg caps #30 1 b.i.d.	1
2.	7/9	38384	Charmin	Kwell Shampoo 2 oz Apply ut dict	1
3.	7/15	39439	Charmin	Diprosone Cream 0.05% Apply as needed	

PHARMACIST'S NOTES

	Date	Comment
1.	7/9	hydrocortisone cream 0.5% (OTC)

DIRECTIONS (Questions 29a through 29j): Each of the numbered items or incomplete statements in this section is followed by answers or by completions of the statement. Select the ONE lettered answer or completion that is BEST in each case.

29a. Benadryl may have been prescribed for this patient as a(n)

   I. antipruritic
  II. sedative
 III. antihistamine

  (A) I only
  (B) III only
  (C) I and II only
  (D) II and III only
  (E) I, II, and III

29b. The active ingredient of Kwell Shampoo is

  (A) crotamiton
  (B) permethrin
  (C) piperonyl butoxide
  (D) undecylenic acid
  (E) lindane

29c. In counseling the parent of the patient receiving Kwell Shampoo, the pharmacist should stress the importance of avoiding

   I. contact with the eyes
  II. the use of metallic combs
 III. the use of vitamin A–containing foods

  (A) I only
  (B) III only
  (C) I and II only
  (D) II and III only
  (E) I, II, and III

29d. Another name for head lice is

  (A) *Sarcoptes scabiei*
  (B) *Pediculus pubis*
  (C) tinea capitis
  (D) *Pediculus capitis*
  (E) tinea versicolor

29e. Kwell Shampoo is usually administered

  (A) once daily for 3 days
  (B) once daily for 5 days
  (C) twice daily for 3 days
  (D) twice daily for 2 days
  (E) once in 7 days

29f. Diprosone Cream contains

  (A) hydrocortisone
  (B) betamethasone dipropionate
  (C) dexamethasone
  (D) triamcinolone acetonide
  (E) fluocinonide

29g. Diprosone Cream should not be used in patients with

   I. bacterial infection
  II. herpes simplex infection
 III. *Candida* infection

(A) I only
(B) III only
(C) I and II only
(D) II and III only
(E) I, II, and III

29h. Which of the following products for the treatment of head lice may be purchased over the counter (OTC)?

  I. Eurax
  II. Nix
  III. A-200 Pyrinate

(A) I only
(B) III only
(C) I and II only
(D) II and III only
(E) I, II, and III

29i. Patients with ragweed allergy should avoid lice remedies that contain

(A) EDTA
(B) organic solvents
(C) lindane
(D) pyrethrins
(E) pyrogens

29j. Scabies is a condition caused by a

(A) fungus
(B) virus
(C) flea
(D) protozoan
(E) mite

PROFILE NO. 30

Community Pharmacy Medication Record

Patient Name: Laura Machless   Address: 89 Noah Road

Age: 25   Sex: F   Height: 5'3"   Weight: 105 lb

Allergies:

DIAGNOSIS

Primary	Secondary
1. heroin abuse	1. PCP
2. AIDS-HIV	2.
3.	3.

DRUG RECORD

	Date	Rx No.	Prescriber	Drug	Refills
1.	5/16	39998	Malhous	Retrovir Caps 100 mg #100 2 q4h	2
2.	5/28	39999	Malhous	Pentam 300 × 10 Bring to office	

PHARMACIST'S NOTES

	Date	Comment
1.	6/1	Robitussin DM (OTC)

DIRECTIONS (Questions 30a through 30j): Each of the numbered items or incomplete statements in this section is followed by answers or by completions of the statement. Select the ONE lettered answer or completion that is BEST in each case.

(A) I only
(B) III only
(C) I and II only
(D) II and III only
(E) I, II, and III

30a. Which of the following agents would be appropriate to use in treating a patient with acute heroin overdose?

(A) naprosyn
(B) tolazamide
(C) cuprimine
(D) EDTA
(E) naloxone

30b. Another name for heroin is

(A) methylmorphine
(B) diacetylmorphine
(C) ethylmorphine
(D) nalorphine
(E) hesperidin

30c. "PCP" in the profile refers to

(A) phencyclidine
(B) pronounced cardiac pronation
(C) *Pneumocystis carinii* pneumonia
(D) *Pseudomonas Chlamydia* process
(E) postcardiac pressure

30d. Another name for Retrovir is
  I. AZT
  II. zidovudine
  III. ribavirin

30e. Patients receiving Retrovir must be monitored carefully for the development of

(A) pneumothorax
(B) malignant hypertension
(C) edema
(D) pulmonary fibrosis
(E) hematological suppression

30f. Retrovir capsules must be administered

(A) for not longer than 1 week
(B) around the clock
(C) for not longer than 1 month
(D) with milk or antacids
(E) on an empty stomach

30g. Patients on Retrovir should avoid the use of

(A) acetaminophen
(B) beta-adrenergic blockers
(C) penicillins
(D) iron products
(E) vitamin A

30h. Pentamidine (Pentam) is available in which of the following dosage forms?
  I. capsules
  II. aerosol
  III. injection

(A) I only
(B) III only
(C) I and II only
(D) II and III only
(E) I, II, and III

30i. Patients using Pentam must be monitored for the development of

(A) severe hypotension
(B) *Pseudomonas* infection
(C) kidney failure
(D) liver failure
(E) GI ulceration

30j. Which of the following are active ingredients in Robitussin DM?

  I. guaifenesin
 II. dextromethorphan HBr
III. codeine

(A) I only
(B) III only
(C) I and II only
(D) II and III only
(E) I, II, and III

Answers and Explanations

PROFILE NO. 1

1a. (D) The tinea fungus lives in dead, keratinous tissue. Athlete's foot is caused by tinea pedis. Candidal fungal infections generally involve warm, dark, and moist areas of the body such as the vagina, anus, and oral cavity. Thrush is a name for candidiasis involving the oral cavity. *(2:563)*

1b. (B) Tinea cruris is a fungal organism that survives only on dead, keratinized tissue. *(2:563)*

1c. (C) The active ingredient of Fulvicin P/G (griseofulvin) is ultramicrosized, ie, its particle size is dramatically reduced to improve its absorption.
(3:1798)

1d. (A) Polyethylene glycol is employed in the Fulvicin P/G formulation in order to help form the microcrystalline form of griseofulvin. *(3:1798)*

1e. (C) Patients who are using griseofulvin products need to be advised to avoid ultraviolet light since this drug may be a photosensitizing agent. Griseofulvin must be used consistently throughout the prescribed period in order to permit adequate levels of griseofulvin to accumulate in areas of the skin that are affected by the fungus. *(3:1796–8)*

1f. (B) Griseofulvin is derived from the same organism as penicillin. Patients who have a history of hypersensitivity reactions to penicillin, therefore, should use caution in the use of griseofulvin. *(3:1796)*

1g. (D) Grisactin Ultra also contains ultramicrosized griseofulvin as the active ingredient. Grifulvin V contains microsized griseofulvin, ie, griseofulvin particles that are larger in size than those in ultramicrosized products. *(3:1798)*

1h. (E) Tolnaftate (Tinactin) Cream is indicated for the topical treatment of tinea infections. It is available as an OTC product. *(3:2224)*

1i. (B) The use of potent topical corticosteroids on the skin reduces the defense mechanisms which the body has against fungi, bacteria, and viruses. This can result in worsening of the infection. *(3:2240)*

PROFILE NO. 2

2a. (D) Esidrix and Oretic are both brands of hydrochlorothiazide. Diuril is a brand of chlorothiazide. *(3:530–1)*

2b. (B) Slow-K is a formulation that contains potassium chloride crystals dispersed in a wax matrix. The wax matrix serves to provide a slow release for the potassium chloride and thereby reduces the irritant effect of the salt. *(3:47)*

2c. (A) The molecular weight of potassium chloride is 74. One milliequivalent of potassium chloride, therefore, contains 74 mg of potassium chloride. Eight milliequivalents of potassium chloride will contain 8 mEq × 74 mg/mEq = 592 mg of potassium chloride. *(3:47)*

2d. (D) Capoten (Captopril) is an angiotensin-converting enzyme (ACE) inhibitor that is indicated for the treatment of hypertension. *(3:779)*

2e. (C) Chlorthalidone (Hygroton) and HCTZ are thiazide diuretics. Bumetanide, furosemide, and ethacrynic acid are loop diuretics, while acetazolamide is a carbonic anhydrase inhibitor. *(3:534)*

2f. (B) Drixoral is a product that contains the antihistamine brompheniramine maleate and the decongestant pseudoephedrine. Because pseudoephedrine is a vasoconstrictor, its use in hypertensive patients is undesirable. *(3:889)*

2g. (C) Capoten decreases aldosterone production and, as a result, may increase serum potassium levels. The concomitant use of Capoten with potassium-sparing diuretics and/or potassium supplements may therefore result in hyperkalemia. *(3:774)*

2h. (A) Fosinopril sodium (Monopril) is also an angiotensin-converting enzyme (ACE) inhibitor. *(3:780)*

2i. (D) Dysgeusia is the impairment of taste. It may occur with the use of Capoten, but it tends to be reversible and self-limiting. *(3:777)*

2j. (C) Each Tylenol/Codeine No. 3 tablet contains 30 mg of codeine and 300 mg of acetaminophen. *(3:1059)*

2k. (C) Brompheniramine maleate is an H_1-receptor antagonist, which is in the alkylamine class of antihistaminic agents. *(3:911)*

PROFILE NO. 3

3a. (B) Micronor is a "minipill" oral contraceptive. Such products contain only progestin and are somewhat less effective than combination products that contain both an estrogen and progestin. Progestin-only products are taken daily rather than cyclically. *(3:361)*

3b. (B) Semicid is a contraceptive vaginal suppository that contains the spermicidal agent nonoxynol 9. *(2:2158)*

3c. (E) Grand mal seizures are currently more popularly referred to as tonic-clonic seizures. They are characterized by the initial presence of tonic muscle contractions, shortly followed by clonic contractions. *(11:845)*

3d. (D) Dilantin Kapseals contain phenytoin sodium extended. This product is suitable for single daily dosing or divided daily dosing. Products that contain phenytoin sodium, prompt, are suitable only for divided daily dosing. *(3:1371,1376)*

3e. (C) Gingival hyperplasia is characterized by an overgrowth of gum tissue within the oral cavity. This predisposes the patient to oral infection and loss of tooth integrity. Good oral hygiene is therefore absolutely essential for patients using phenytoin. *(11:858)*

3f. (A) Dilantin Kapseals are manufactured by Parke-Davis and contain phenytoin sodium, extended, as their active ingredient. *(3:1377)*

3g. (A) The therapeutic plasma concentration of phenytoin is 10 to 20 µg/mL. A phenytoin plasma concentration of 5 µg/mL several weeks after initiating therapy is indicative of inadequate dosing or noncompliance. *(3:1377)*

3h. (B) Phenytoin use may decrease the pharmacologic effect of the Micronor by increasing the hepatic metabolism of the progestin in Micronor. Since progestin-only products such as Micronor tend to be somewhat less effective in preventing pregnancy, this may result in an unwanted pregnancy. *(3:1373)*

3i. (C) The IM route for phenytoin sodium is generally avoided because the precipitation of phenytoin at the injection site may be painful and result in erratic absorption. Phenytoin is easily precipitated in the presence of an acidic substance in the IV admixture. The addition of phenytoin sodium to an IV infusion is therefore generally not recommended. *(3:1371)*

3j. (B) A morbilliform rash is one that resembles that of measles. *(3:1372)*

3k. (E) Nonoxynol 9 is a surfactant spermicide that is the active ingredient of Semicid. *(3:2158)*

3l. (B) Docusate sodium, the active ingredient of the stool softener Colace, is an anionic surfactant that promotes the penetration of water into the intestinal contents. This softens the contents and facilitates their evacuation. *(3:1573)*

3m. (A) Theragran-M is a therapeutic multivitamin product that also contains minerals. *(3:87)*

PROFILE NO. 4

4a. (B) Carbidopa serves as a dopadecarboxylase inhibitor that prevents the peripheral decarboxylation of levodopa and permits a greater proportion of the levodopa dose to enter the brain in its intact form. The use of carbidopa in combination with levodopa permits the use of lower levodopa doses than would be used without carbidopa. *(3:1468)*

4b. (E) Pyridoxine promotes the peripheral conversion of levodopa to dopamine, thereby decreasing the activity of the administered levodopa. *(3:1467)*

4c. (C) Darkening of the urine with the use of levodopa or Sinemet is normal and is a product of levodopa metabolism. It may be disregarded by the patient. *(3:1467)*

4d. (C) Benztropine mesylate (Cogentin) is an anticholinergic agent used in the treatment of Parkinson's disease. Such agents reduce the incidence and severity of akinesia, rigidity, and tremor in such patients. Anticholinergic drugs are used as adjuncts to levodopa in the treatment of Parkinson's disease. *(3:1463)*

4e. (E) The first four choices are anticholinergic agents used in treating Parkinson's disease. Tranylcypromine (Parnate) is a monoamine oxidase (MAO) inhibitor used in treating depression. *(3:1254)*

4f. (D) Amantadine (Symmetrel), in addition to being employed in the treatment of Parkinson's disease, is also used in the prevention and treatment of respiratory tract infections caused by influenza A virus. *(3:1862)*

4g. (A) Diplopia, or double vision, is sometimes experienced by patients receiving levodopa therapy. *(30:479)*

4h. (C) When a patient on levodopa is to be switched to Sinemet, at least 8 hours must be allowed to elapse from the last dose of levodopa to the first dose of Sinemet in order to decrease the likelihood of toxicity. Since the carbidopa in the Sinemet increases the proportion of intact levodopa that enters the brain, the dose of levodopa administered via Sinemet should be 75% to 80% less than that administered prior to the initiation of Sinemet therapy. *(3:1470)*

4i. **(C)** Levodopa is a precursor of dopamine, an agent that seems to be lacking in the brain of patients with Parkinson's disease. *(3:1465)*

4j. **(B)** Carbidopa is available by itself as Lodosyn. It should be employed in combination with levodopa to tailor-make a dosage combination for patients with Parkinson's disease. *(3:1468)*

4k. **(E)** Chlorpromazine is a phenothiazine antipsychotic agent that acts as a dopamine antagonist. With prolonged use, it can cause a variety of Parkinson-like effects. *(3:1257)*

PROFILE NO. 5

5a. **(E)** Pilocarpine acts to produce constriction of the pupil (miosis). This helps to increase the outflow of aqueous humor from the eye and lower intraocular pressure. *(3:2055)*

5b. **(E)** Carbachol, like pilocarpine, is a direct-acting miotic agent. Physostigmine and isoflurophate are also miotics; however, they work by inhibiting the enzyme acetylcholinesterase. *(3:2054)*

5c. **(B)** Intraocular pressure may vary considerably in the same individual, depending upon the time of day the measurement is taken as well as many other factors. A measurement of 14 mm Hg is well within the normal range of 10 to 20 mm Hg. *(11:810)*

5d. **(A)** The Ocusert Pilo-20 system is designed to release 20 μg of pilocarpine per hour for 1 week. This slow but steady drug administration permits better control of intraocular pressure and fewer adverse effects as compared to the use of pilocarpine eye drops. *(3:2057)*

5e. **(A)** The Ocusert Pilo-20 system must be replaced every 7 days. When first inserted, the pilocarpine is released from the system at about three times the rate indicated on the package. After about 6 hours, the rate of drug release diminishes to the labeled rate and remains within 20% of this rate for the rest of the 7 days. *(3:2057)*

5f. **(C)** Betaxolol (Betoptic), levobunolol (Betagan Liquifilm), and timolol (Timoptic) are beta-adrenergic blocking agents used ophthalmically in the treatment of glaucoma. They appear to act by decreasing the output of aqueous humor within the eye. Miochol contains acetylcholine, a direct-acting miotic agent. *(3:2051)*

5g. **(B)** Betaxolol (Betoptic) is a beta-adrenergic blocking agent that appears to be useful in the treatment of glaucoma because of its ability to reduce aqueous humor production within the eye. It is usually administered twice daily. *(3:2047)*

5h. **(C)** EDTA, or ethylenediamine tetraacetic acid, is a chelating agent that has the ability to remove trace quantities of metals that might promote the decomposition of the active drug. *(1:187)*

5i. **(B)** Visine contains tetrahydrozoline as its active ingredient. This agent is an imidazoline decongestant that tends to exhibit alpha-adrenergic agonist activity. Its use in the eye causes vasoconstriction and relief of "red eyes" and ophthalmic congestion. *(3:2069)*

5j. **(A)** The use of a beta-adrenergic blocking agent such as betaxolol (Betoptic) by a patient with a history of respiratory illness and breathing difficulty may be hazardous because beta blockers may cause bronchoconstriction. Even the relatively small amount of drug that enters the systemic circulation via an ophthalmic administration has been reported to cause breathing difficulty in susceptible patients. *(3:2050)*

5k. **(B)** Both Ecotrin Maximum Strength and Easprin are enteric-coated aspirin formulations. They each have an enteric coat on the surface of the tablet that dissolves only when the tablet reaches the more neutral-to-alkaline region of the small intestine. *(3:1096)*

PROFILE NO. 6

6a. **(D)** The active ingredient in Benzac is benzoyl peroxide, an agent that appears to act by providing antibacterial activity, especially against *Propionibacterium acnes*, the predominant organism in acne lesions. *(3:2172)*

6b. **(C)** Patients using tretinoin (Retin-A) products should be advised to avoid the use of the product near the eyes, mouth, angles of the nose, and mucous membranes since tretinoin may irritate these tissues. Patients using this product should also be advised to avoid excessive exposure to sunlight and sunlamps since the drug may increase the patient's susceptibility to burning. Although tretinoin is a vitamin A derivative, its topical use makes it unnecessary for patients to limit their intake of vitamin A–containing foods. *(3:2164)*

6c. **(B)** Butylated hydroxytoluene or BHT is an antioxidant that is commonly employed in food and topical products in order to reduce the likelihood of spoilage. *(1:1278)*

6d. **(C)** The use of clindamycin, the active ingredient of Cleocin T, has been associated with the development of diarrhea in some patients. If the diarrhea is severe and/or persistent, the patient's physician should be contacted since such a response may indicate the development of pseudomembranous enterocolitis, a serious and potentially life-threatening condition. *(3:1749)*

6e. **(B)** A product that contains 10 mg of drug per mL will contain 1000 mg or 1.0 g/100 mL. This is equivalent to a 1% (w/v) solution of the drug. *(3:2178)*

6f. (E) Accutane contains isotretinoin as its active ingredient. This is an isomer of retinoic acid, a metabolite of retinol (vitamin A). *(3:2169)*

6g. (E) Many adverse effects are associated with the use of Accutane. Cheilitis, an inflammation around the margins of the lips, is very common. Xerostomia (dry mouth) and conjunctivitis (inflammation of the conjunctival lining of the eye) are also common adverse effects associated with the use of this drug. *(3:2169)*

6h. (B) Because of the many adverse effects associated with the use of Accutane, a patient package insert must be dispensed by the pharmacist to any patient receiving this drug. *(3:2169)*

6i. (B) The use of Accutane in patients who are or may become pregnant is contraindicated because the use of this drug in pregnant patients has been shown to cause fetal abnormalities. Accutane has been given a pregnancy category X rating by the FDA because of this hazard. *(3:2169)*

6j. (A) Aluminum oxide is a water-insoluble material that is employed in the Brasivol formulation as an abrasive. When rubbed onto the affected area, the abrasive property is meant to help remove the comedone plugs and allow better drainage of the comedone. *(3:2181)*

6k. (E) Salicylic acid is a keratolytic agent; ie, it helps to remove keratin from the skin surface. This faciliates the opening of plugged comedones and decreases the likelihood of new comedone formation. *(2:624)*

6l. (E) Sebum is a lipid secretion of the sebaceous glands, which are associated with the hair follicle. Sebum acts as a protectant on the skin surface. When the esterified fatty acids of sebum are broken down to free fatty acids by microorganisms, the inflammatory lesion of acne may be formed. *(2:794)*

PROFILE NO. 7

7a. (C) Isoproterenol is a nonspecific beta-adrenergic agonist. It is capable of stimulating $beta_2$-receptors found in the respiratory tract to produce bronchodilation. It is also capable of stimulating $beta_1$-adrenergic receptors found in the heart, thereby producing cardiac stimulation. *(3:854)*

7b. (B) If the initial inhalation of Isuprel has not been successful in relieving an acute asthmatic attack, a second inhalation should be attempted 2 to 5 minutes after the first. It relief still does not occur, the patient should be advised to seek medical assistance. *(3:854)*

7c. (D) Theophylline is a methylxanthine, as is theobromine and caffeine. Methylxanthines tend to stimulate the central nervous system and the heart as well as increase diuresis. *(3:858)*

7d. (B) Theophylline, as well as most other methylxanthines, tends to cause stimulation of the central nervous system. *(3:858)*

7e. (A) Aminophylline, the ethylenediamine derivative of theophylline, is generally preferred for use in rectal suppository dosage forms since it is more water soluble than theophylline and will tend to be absorbed more readily through membranes. *(3:870)*

7f. (D) Intal solution contains cromolyn sodium, an agent that inhibits the degranulation of mast cells and thereby decreases the likelihood of an asthmatic attack. It is administered by inhalation. Intal is also available in a powder form that is administered by inhalation using a special device known as a Spinhaler. *(3:887)*

7g. (E) Cromolyn is the active ingredient in Intal. It is a drug that acts to decrease the degranulation of mast cells in the respiratory tract, thereby decreasing the likelihood of an asthmatic attack. *(3:887)*

7h. (D) The active ingredient in Vanceril is beclomethasone dipropionate, a corticosteroid. When administered by inhalation to asthmatic patients, Vanceril reduces the likelihood of future acute asthmatic attacks. Vanceril is not suitable for use during an acute attack. *(3:875)*

7i. (A) Patients who are to use Vanceril as well as a bronchodilator by inhalation such as Isuprel should be advised to use the bronchodilator several minutes before the corticosteroid is administered in order to facilitate penetration of the steroid into the bronchial tree. Vanceril is only to be used to prevent an acute asthmatic attack, not to abort an existing acute attack. Vanceril is only administered by inhalation. *(3:875)*

7j. (C) Cigarette and marijuana smoking tend to induce hepatic metabolism of theophylline, thereby decreasing its action in the body. Smokers may therefore require a 50% to 100% greater dose of theophylline than nonsmokers in order to control their disease. *(3:860)*

7k. (E) Tedral tablets contain theophylline, ephedrine, and phenobarbital. *(3:942)*

7l. (C) Terbutaline is a beta-adrenergic agonist, which is more specific in its action for $beta_2$-receptors in the respiratory tract than for $beta_1$-adrenergic receptors in the heart. Isoproterenol is relatively nonspecific in its effect. Terbutaline is therefore less likely to cause unwanted cardiac stimulation than isoproterenol. *(3:849)*

7m. (E) Beclovent and Vanceril are both inhalation products containing beclomethasone dipropionate. *(3:875)*

PROFILE NO. 8

8a. (A) Nitrostat is a nitroglycerin sublingual tablet that has been stabilized with polyethylene glycol in order to decrease the likelihood that volatilization of the nitroglycerin will take place. As a result, Nitrostat has a considerably longer shelf-life than non-stabilized nitroglycerin tablets. *(3:579)*

8b. (C) Nitrostat, as well as other oral nitroglycerin products, should be dispensed by the pharmacist in its original container since such containers are designed to minimize the loss of nitroglycerin during storage. *(3:579)*

8c. (A) Transdermal nitroglycerin patches should be applied onto a hairless site. Site rotation is important with each administration in order to decrease the likelihood of skin irritation. Transdermal patches should not be applied to distal portions of the extremities since these areas do not permit as reliable absorption of the nitroglycerin as other areas of the body. *(3:581)*

8d. (D) When discontinuing therapy with nitroglycerin transdermal systems, gradual reduction of both the dosage and frequency of application over a 4- to 6-week period is advisable in order to minimize the likelihood of sudden withdrawal reactions. *(3:581)*

8e. (C) Amyl nitrite is the only antianginal product administered by inhalation. It is available as a liquid packaged in small glass capsules covered by protectant cotton or gauze material. When required, the capsule is crushed and the vapors released are inhaled by the patient. A rapid response is generally evident. Dosage control is, however, a major drawback in the use of this drug. *(3:579)*

8f. (D) Dipyridamole (Persantine), in addition to being used in the treatment of angina, is also employed as an antiplatelet agent. It appears to act in this regard by inhibiting cyclic nucleotide phosphodiesterase activity. *(3:250)*

8g. (D) Nitroglycerin administered orally undergoes extensive first-pass hepatic deactivation, thereby limiting the usefulness of this route of administration. *(3:572)*

8h. (A) The use of alcohol in combination with nitroglycerin may produce a hypotensive response because of the vasodilating action of both of these drugs. The hypotensive response may be manifested as dizziness, fainting, and/or weakness. *(3:575)*

8i. (B) Nitroglycerin may be adsorbed onto the polyvinyl chloride (PVC) tubing used in most IV administration sets. This may result in loss of drug and inadequate dosing. Manufacturers of nitroglycerin for IV use supply non-PVC infusion tubing, which minimizes the adsorption of nitroglycerin. Such special tubing is generally recommended for use with nitroglycerin products. *(3:578)*

8j. (C) The dose of nitroglycerin topical ointment is measured in inches. It is applied to the skin with minimal rubbing, and the area to which it has been applied is covered with plastic wrap to facilitate drug absorption and to prevent staining of clothing. *(3:582)*

8k. (B) Nitrolingual Spray and sublingual forms of nitroglycerin provide the most rapid onset of action, ranging from 1 to 3 minutes. Transdermal patches have a 30- to 60-minute onset time. *(3:573)*

PROFILE NO. 9

9a. (D) Patients with type I diabetes mellitus are generally insulin dependent. Their disease generally begins early in life and is characterized by little or no insulin production by the pancreas. *(11:307)*

9b. (D) Humulin R insulin is human regular insulin that is prepared by recombinant DNA technology. As is the case with all regular insulin products, Humulin is a clear solution. *(3:467)*

9c. (A) The Humulin R insulin contains 100 units of activity per milliliter. Twenty-four units of insulin activity will therefore be contained in 0.24 mL of the product. *(3:471)*

9d. (E) Polydypsia refers to excessive thirst. This is frequently seen in type I diabetics because of the excessive urination (polyuria) that is associated with the body's attempt to eliminate excessive glucose in the blood. *(11:313)*

9e. (E) A fasting blood sugar of 100 mg/dL is well within the normal range of 70 to 110 mg/dL. *(11:311)*

9f. (B) Regular insulin is the only form of insulin available as a clear solution. The other forms are suspensions, which would be unsuitable for IV administration. *(3:467)*

9g. (A) When mixing two types of insulin, the clear regular insulin is always drawn into the syringe first in order to reduce the likelihood of contamination of the regular insulin with suspended particles of the second insulin. Insulin mixtures may be stored in a prefilled syringe for up to 1 week with refrigeration. *(3:470)*

9h. (A) Ascorbic acid found in multivitamin mixtures such as Optilets-M may interfere with Clinitest testing because the presence of a reducing substance such as ascorbic acid may be detected by the nonspecific test for reducing substances employed in the Clinitest. *(11:317)*

9i. (C) Clinitest employs the copper reduction mechanism for the detection of reducing substances. This is the same mechanism employed by the Benedict's test. The other tests listed all use the glucose oxidase mechanism for detecting glucose. Because they are more specific for detecting glucose, they are less susceptible to interference by other reducing substances that may be in the urine. *(11:317)*

9j. **(A)** Contac 12-Hour Caplets contain phenylpropanolamine, a sympathomimetic decongestant that is capable of inducing the conversion of glycogen to glucose in the body. This may increase glucose levels in the blood and increase the patient's insulin requirement. *(3:889)*

9k. **(B)** Lo-Dose syringes have a capacity of 0.5 mL. They are useful in situations where a low dose (< 50 units) of insulin must be administered. *(11:325)*

9l. **(A)** Glipizide (Glucotrol) is a second-generation sulfonylurea. Such agents are administered in lower doses than first-generation agents and tend to produce somewhat fewer adverse effects than first-generation agents. *(3:474)*

PROFILE NO. 10

10a. **(E)** Both warfarin and dicumarol are oral anticoagulants that interfere with vitamin K–dependent clotting factors. They are both derivatives of 4–hydroxycoumarin. *(3:260)*

10b. **(B)** The administration of chloral hydrate to a patient stabilized on warfarin is likely to result in increased warfarin activity because of the ability of a metabolite of chloral hydrate to displace warfarin from its protein binding sites. The other choices listed are agents that promote the hepatic metabolism of warfarin and would therefore decrease warfarin activity. *(3:262)*

10c. **(A)** Vitamin K is a specific antidote for warfarin toxicity. Treatment of hemorrhage caused by oral anticoagulant therapy generally consists of the administration of 10 to 20 mg of vitamin K_1 (phytonadione). *(3:264)*

10d. **(B)** Datril contains acetaminophen, an analgesic/antipyretic that does not appear to displace warfarin from plasma protein-binding sites. Ecotrin contains aspirin, and Advil contains ibuprofen. Both of these agents are capable of displacing warfarin from protein-binding sites and increasing warfarin activity. *(3:262)*

10e. **(D)** Synthroid contains levothyroxine, or T_4, as its active ingredient. *(3:498)*

10f. **(A)** 100 µg of Synthroid is approximately equivalent to 65 mg of Thyroid USP and Thyrar, 65 mg of Proloid, and 25 µg of Cytomel. *(3:488)*

10g. **(E)** Propylthiouracil and methimazole each inhibit the synthesis of thyroid hormones. Sodium iodide

$_{131}$I is a radioactive isotope that is concentrated in thyroid tissue and emits radiation that destroys thyroid tissue. Any of these agents may be used to treat hyperthyroidism. *(3:506)*

10h. **(C)** Synthroid and other thyroid hormone products appear to increase the catabolism of vitamin K–dependent clotting factors. This potentiates the action of warfarin and decreases the warfarin dosage requirement. *(3:491)*

10i. **(B)** In a radiation emergency, the administration of potassium iodide would saturate the thyroid with nonradioactive iodide, thereby making it less likely that radioactive iodides created in the emergency would accumulate in thyroid tissue. *(11:280)*

10j. **(A)** Thyroid hormone production in the body is controlled by the level of thyroid-stimulating hormone (TSH) produced by the anterior pituitary. *(11:267)*

10k. **(C)** Empirin/Codeine No. 3 contains aspirin. The aspirin may displace warfarin from protein-binding sites and may increase warfarin activity in the body. *(3:262)*

10l. **(A)** The prothrombin time (PT) is a screening test that measures clot formation via the extrinsic coagulation pathway. It can be used to gauge the success of warfarin therapy. *(11:223)*

PROFILE NO. 11

11a. **(C)** The term "pyuria" refers to pus in the urine. Such a condition is often associatied with a urinary tract infection (UTI). *(30:1302)*

11b. **(B)** *E coli* organisms are gram-negative bacilli commonly associated with the GI tract. They are commonly a causative organism in urinary tract infections as well as institutionally borne infections. *(4:1179; 6:1027)*

11c. **(B)** Cephalothin (Keflin) is classified as a first-generation cephalosporin. Such agents tend to have good activity against gram-positive bacteria and relatively modest activity against gram-negative microorganisms. *(6:1085)*

11d. **(D)** Septra and Bactrim products are combinations of sulfamethozazole and trimethoprim. The advantage of using such a combination as opposed to single-drug therapy is the ability of this combination to block two consecutive steps used by bacteria to produce tetrahydrofolic acid. Blocking two steps greatly diminishes the likelihood that bacterial resistance will develop. *(3:1880)*

11e. **(D)** Ascorbic acid and/or other urinary acidifiers such as mandelic and hippuric acids are used with Mandelamine in order to facilitate its action. In the presence of an acid urine, the methanamine component of Mandelamine is converted to formaldehyde, the active anti-infective agent. At neutral and alkaline pH levels, Mandelamine is of little therapeutic value.   *(6:1060)*

11f. (A) Patients using either Septra DS or Mandelamine should be advised to maintain adequate fluid intake in order to facilitate the urinary anti-infective action of the product as well as to prevent precipitation of poorly soluble drugs in the urinary tract. While urinary acidification is useful for patients using Mandelamine, it may cause precipitation of the sulfa component of Septra DS. There is no need for patients on either of these drug products to avoid the use of folic acid-containing foods.   *(3:1881,1919)*

11g. (C) Microstix-3 (formerly Microstix Nitrite Strips) are designed to test for nitrite in the urine. Elevated nitrite levels are indicative of the presence of bacteria in the urine, ie, bacteriuria.   *(3:2612)*

11h. (E) Phenazopyridine (Pyridium) is an azo dye employed as a urinary analgesic. It has no antiseptic activity. Phenazopyridine is often used to reduce pain in patients with urinary tract infections prior to the successful control of bacteria by antimicrobial agents.   *(6:1061)*

11i. (C) Phenazopyridine (Pyridium) is excreted unchanged into the urine. In doing so, it may cause a red-orange discoloration of the urine.   *(6:1061)*

11j. (A) When used with antimicrobial agents for the treatment of urinary tract infections, Pyridium should not be used for more than 2 days. This permits Pyridium's analgesic action to be employed during the early period of therapy when the infection is not yet under control. After 2 days, the infection should be under control and the continued use of Pyridium should not be required. In addition, the use of Pyridium beyond 2 days would mask pain that might be an indication of the failure of the antimicrobial therapy.   *(3:2558)*

11k. (E) Probably the most common psychological symptom of prementrual syndrome is tension characterized by irritability and depression. Weight gains of several pounds may be observed due to water retention. Several OTC products contain diuretics to combat this "bloating."   *(2:124)*

11l. (C) Caffeine in doses of 100 to 200 mg every 3 to 4 hours is a safe and effective diuretic but may cause sleeplessness. Pamabrom, a derivative of theophylline, is also effective in doses of 50 mg up to four times a day. Pamabrom is the active ingredient in Midol PMS and Pamprin.   *(2:126)*

11m. (A) Of the drugs listed, only ciprofloxacin (Cipro) is effective for treating urinary tract infections and for prostatitis. Usual dose ranges are 250 to 500 mg every 12 hours. The drug should not be used in pregnant women because it can cause permanent lesions in the weight-bearing joints.   *(6:1059)*

PROFILE NO. 12

12a. (D) A nomogram is a chart that permits the determination of a patient's body surface area (BSA) in square meters from the patient's known height and weight data. Nomograms are frequently employed in calculating doses for potent agents such as the antineoplastic drugs.   *(11:1339)*

12b. (A) The patient is to receive 45 mg of daunorubicin per square meter of body surface area per day. Since the patient's body surface area has been found to be 1.85 m^2, then $1.85 \text{ m}^2 \times 45 \text{ mg/m}^2 = 83.25$ mg of drug per administration. Since each vial contains 20 mg of drug, 5 vials will be required to supply the amount of drug needed.   *(10)*

12c. (C) Cytarabine (Arac) is a pyrimidine analog that is employed as an antimetabolite either alone or in combination with other antineoplastic drugs. Other pyrimidine antagonists include fluorouracil (5-FU) and the antiviral compound idoxuridine.   *(6:1900)*

12d. (D) Myelosuppression, or suppression of the bone marrow, commonly results in a sharp decrease in white blood cells as is seen on the patient's profile. This may be life-threatening because of the patient's increased susceptibility to infection.   *(15:278)*

12e. (C) Allopurinol is a xanthine oxidase inhibitor. Inhibition of xanthine oxidase enzyme results in a reduction in the formation of uric acid, a common metabolite formed in patients being treated with antineoplastic drugs. Allopurinol is, therefore, commonly employed in the prevention or management of hyperuricemia.   *(6:676)*

12f. (A) When allopurinol therapy is initiated, large quantities of uric acid are mobilized in the body and enter the urinary tract. Without adequate hydration, urates are likely to precipitate in the tract, causing pain and inflammation.   *(6:679)*

12g. (D) Since allopurinol is employed in managing uric acid levels in the body, the monitoring of serum urate levels will provide a means of determining the success of therapy.   *(6:679)*

12h. (B) When nystatin (Mycostatin) oral suspension is employed in the treatment of oral candidiasis infection, it is important that sufficient contact time be allowed between the drug and the mucosal surface of the oral cavity. This can be accomplished by having the patient swish the suspension in the mouth for several minutes prior to swallowing it.   *(4:1504)*

12i. (E) Extravasation is the leakage of injection fluid into tissue surrounding the injection site. When this occurs with the use of potent drugs such as daunorubicin, irritation and inflammation commonly occur. Once extravasation has occurred, the application of cold compresses to the injection site will relieve pain and minimize further dissemination of the drug into neighboring tissue.   *(3:2140)*

12j. (C) A serious adverse effect associated with the use of daunorubicin is cardiotoxicity. This is commonly manifested as congestive heart failure (CHF) and requires early diagnosis and aggressive treatment with sodium restriction, diuretics, and digoxin.
    (3:2419)

12k. (E) The active metabolite of Dalmane has a long half-life, and thereby accumulates over time. It also suppresses REM sleep even at low doses. The net result is impaired daytime functioning, especially in the elderly. Temazepam (Restoril) has a shorter half-life and is less likely to cause side effects.   *(11:969)*

12l. (E) The antihistamines may cause all of the listed anticholinergic effects except urinary retention. Urinary incontinence is a more likely effect.   *(2:229; 11:968)*

12m. (D) Mitrolan tablets contain calcium polycarbophil, which possesses both laxative and antidiarrheal properties. It quickly binds water in the GI tract, thus reducing fluidity by forming a bulk. *(2:325,350)*

PROFILE NO. 13

13a. (E) A normal hemoglobin level is considered to be 14 g% +/– 2 g%. When values drop below 10 g/dL, symptoms of iron deficiency anemia become evident. Six months of iron therapy is generally sufficient to raise hemoglobin levels to within a normal range. A better estimate of iron therapy effectiveness would be an increase in hemoglobin of 2 g/dL in the first 3- to 4-week period.   *(4:1528; 6:1289; 11:173)*

13b. (E) A stool guaiac test is employed to determine the presence of occult (hidden) blood. Such blood may be evident in a patient with a bleeding peptic ulcer or other conditions in which damage to the GI tract has been evident.   *(15:556)*

13c. (A) Mylanta Liquid contains magnesium hydroxide, aluminum hydroxide, and simethicone. The use of magnesium hydroxide-containing products is commonly associated with the development of diarrhea because the magnesium ion creates an osmotic effect in the GI tract.   *(3:1486)*

13d. (B) The use of cimetidine (Tagamet) is likely to increase Xanax activity because cimetidine reduces the hepatic metabolism of drugs such as alprazolam (Xanax) that are metabolized via the cytochrome P450 pathway.   *(3:1197,1201)*

13e. (E) The concomitant use of Tagamet and Mylanta may result in a decrease of Tagamet absorption. At least 1 hour should elapse between the administration of these two drug products. The use of antacids such as Mylanta with iron products is likely to result in a decrease in absorption of the iron since iron

tends to precipitate in an alkaline medium. The concomitant use of Tagamet and Xanax will likely increase the activity of the Xanax because cimetidine (Tagamet) has been shown to inhibit the metabolism of many of the benzodiazepines, including alprozolam (Xanax).   *(3:1522,1525)*

13f. (B) Iron absorption may be somewhat increased by the coadministration of approximately 200 mg of ascorbic acid per 30 mg of elemental iron administered. This appears to be the result of ascorbic acid's ability to maintain iron in the ferrous state, a form which is more absorbable than the ferric state.
    (3:200)

13g. (C) Feosol tablets contain exsiccated (dried) ferrous sulfate. The exsiccated form of ferrous sulfate contains approximately 30% elemental iron, considerably higher than that contained in hydrous ferrous sulfate, or ferrous gluconate.   *(3:202)*

13h. (B) The term "exsiccated" means dried; ie, water of hydration has been removed by a drying process. This process produces a more stable product with a higher content of elemental iron than hydrated forms of ferrous sulfate.   *(1:827)*

13i. (C) Patients who have iron deficiency anemia tend to have red blood cells that are microcytic; ie, smaller than normal, and hypochromic; ie, lacking in normal color. Megaloblastic cells are larger than normal cells. These are frequently seen in patients who have pernicious anemia.   *(11:174)*

13j. (A) Ranitidine (Zantac) is also an H_2-receptor antagonist that diminishes acid secretion in the stomach. An advantage of ranitidine over cimetidine is its relative lack of effect on hepatic metabolism of other drugs. Since this patient is using alprazolam (Xanax), a drug metabolized by hepatic enzymes, the use of ranitidine is more logical.   *(3:1525)*

13k. (B) Patients have a strong desire to eat unnatural foods such as chalk, clay, and ice, as well as specific individual foods.   *(11:173)*

13l. (C) A deficiency or impaired utilization of vitamin B_{12} and especially of folic acid may result in megaloblastic anemia. Other causes of the anemia include use of cytotoxins such as the antineoplastics or the immunosuppressive agents.   *(11:178)*

13m. (B) Foods from animal sources such as eggs, dairy products, and especially liver contain vitamine B_{12}. Another source is shellfish. Vegetables and fruit do not contain the vitamin.   *(11:179)*

13n. (D) Pernicious anemia is a progressive disease caused by a lack of the intrinsic factor resulting in malabsorption of vitamin B_{12}. The condition affects more adult women, especially black women, than men. Individuals living in temperate regions (North America or Northern Europe) are more susceptable than people living in the tropics. There also appears to be an increased rate in certain families, suggesting a genetic factor.   *(11:182)*

13o. **(D)** Because of potential local irritation, the only form of injectable iron is an iron dextran. Dosage forms of ferrous sulfate include tablets (Feosol), oral drops (Mol-Iron and Fer-In-Sol), oral liquid (Mol-Iron), and an elixir (Feosol).   *(11:176)*

PROFILE NO. 14

14a. **(D)** Most *Streptococcus* infections are sensitive to penicillin while *Staphylococcus* infections are not, with the exception of nonpenicillinase-producing *Staphylococcus* aureus. *Pseudomonas*, fungus, and *Chlamydia* are not sensitive to either penicillin G or V. The main advantage of penicillin V when compared to penicillin G is its greater absorption from the GI tract. When given in comparable doses, penicillin V will reach plasma concentration levels two to five times those of penicillin G.   *(6:1024)*

14b. **(D)** Pentids is Squibb's brand name for products containing penicillin G potassium.   *(6:968; 10)*

14c. **(B)** Routine use of pHisoHex has reduced the incidence and severity of pyogenic skin infections, especially those caused by gram-positive microorganisms, such as staphylococci. However, there is the possibility of superinfection of gram-negative microorganisms and *Candida*.   *(1:1166; 10)*

14d. **(B)** The hexachlorophene present in pHisoHex has the tendency to accumulate in the skin. An occlusive dressing may increase the amount absorbed and may result in systemic toxicity. Exposure to sunlight will cause a discoloration of the product but does not affect its activity.   *(6:969; 10)*

14e. **(B)** When compared to hexachlorophene, chlorhexidine is faster acting, results in greater decreases in microbial counts, and has a similar antibacterial spectrum.   *(4:1515)*

14f. **(D)** The active ingredient in Cidex is glutaraldehyde, used mainly as a disinfectant. Chlorhexidine is present in Hibiclens, which is used as a skin cleanser. Peridex also contains chlorhexidine. It is an oral rinse for the prevention of oral infections in immunocompromised patients.   *(4:1515)*

14g. **(D)** Magnesium sulfate has been used internally as a saline laxative. Topically, hot concentrated solutions are used as soaks or poultices in treating deep-seated infections.   *(1:786)*

14h. **(C)** Percogesic contains 325 mg acetaminophen and 30 mg phenyltoloxamine citrate per tablet. Phenyltoloxamine is classified as an antihistamine.   *(10)*

14i. **(E)** Pepto-Bismol contains bismuth subsalicylate, which appears to exert an antisecretory effect on intestinal mucosa and also binds both cytotoxins and enterotoxins. Doses of 60 mL or two tablets four times a day have been used prophylactically. If diarrhea occurs, doses of 30 mL every half hour for eight doses is used.   *(1:776; 2:331; 11:446)*

14j. **(D)** Giardiasis is a protozoal infection caused by *Giardia lamblia*. It mainly affects the intestinal tract, causing diarrhea, other GI disorders, and profound malaise. The drug of choice is metronidazole, which is better tolerated than the alternative quinacrine.   *(4:1583)*

14k. **(C)** The disease is caused by a spirochete carried by a tick. Serious cases can result in crippling arthritis.   *(4:1186)*

14l. **(C)** Doxycycline or tetracycline are first-line antibiotics in the treatment of Lyme disease. However, more serious cases are treated with intravenous ceftriaxone.   *(4:1186)*

14m. **(E)** Naproxen (Naprosyn) is a propionic acid derivative related to ibuprofen. It is useful for musculoskeletal and soft tissue inflammation, including arthritis and ankylosing spondylitis. Naproxen has also been used for acute gout, with an initial dose of 750 mg followed by 250 mg every 8 hours until the attack is under control. Side effects of the drug, such as GI heartburn, constipation, tinnitus, and nausea, may be expected. Anaprox is the sodium salt of naproxen.   *(9:28:08.04)*

14n. **(A)** Aspirin is an antiplatelet drug that blocks the production of thromboxane A_2. Several studies have shown that daily doses of 320 mg or less are effective in reducing the incidence of transient ischemic attacks and myocardial infarctions, especially in men. Doses above 320 mg are not advocated since side effects such as bleeding may occur.   *(6:1325)*

PROFILE NO. 15

15a. **(D)** The rate of metabolism for Dilantin has decreased probably because of Tagamet's ability to inhibit the hepatic oxidative enzyme system. The symptoms reported by the medical staff are consistent with high blood levels of phenytoin. The daily doses of phenytoin should be reduced. Another solution would be the replacement of Tagamet with another H_2-receptor antagonist.   *(1:1853)*

15b. **(A)** Ataxia is the inability to coordinate muscles controlling voluntary movement.   *(30:147)*

15c. **(B)** Famotidine is Merck's Pepcid. While the onset of action is similar to that of cimetidine and ranitidine, it is more potent and has a longer duration of activity. It is effective in the treatment of duodenal ulcers, acute gastric ulcers, and Zollinger-Ellison syndrome. A 20 mg tablet is available. The other two drugs are available as both tablets and injectable solutions. Cimetidine is also available as an oral solution. *(4:829)*

15d. **(D)** Zollinger-Ellison syndrome is a pathologic hypersecretory condition caused by adenomas of the gastrin-producing islet cells of the pancreas. Patients with this condition experience persistent ulcer pain and diarrhea. *(11:398)*

15e. **(E)** Since cimetidine is a competitive antagonist of the hepatic cytochrome P-450 oxidase system, there will be a delay in the metabolism of many benzodiazepines. Others such as lorazepam, oxazepam, and temazepam are not affected since they are metabolized by glucuronidation.
(1:1853; 11:396,914)

15f. **(A)** Daily doses of 900 to 1200 mg will maintain plasma lithium levels of 0.6 to 0.8 mEq/L. Toxic symptoms usually are manifested when plasma levels are greater than 1.5 mEq/L. Blood sampling is performed 10 to 12 hours after the last dose. Usually, it is convenient to draw the blood just before the morning dose. *(11:937)*

15g. **(A)** The reported symptoms are mild effects that probably relate to peaks in lithium levels. The first approach in correcting the problem is to spread the doses further apart. *(11:939)*

15h. **(A)** Lithium is usually considered to be the drug of choice in the treatment of acute manic episodes. Symptoms of this condition include delusions, irritability, hallucinations, polyuria, and polydipsia. Some of the first signs that signal manic episodes are euphoric moods with hyperactivity, excessive energy, and perceived need for little sleep. Lithium has been used in treating schizophrenia, but it is not the drug of choice. *(11:937)*

15i. **(B)** Nosocomial infections are those that have been acquired during hospital stays. *(19:45; 30:1063)*

15j. **(B)** Dextromethorphan (DM) is indicated for a dry nonproductive cough especially during the daytime when drowsiness is a serious side effect. An antihistamine, diphenhydramine will cause drowsiness and dryness. Guaifenesin is an expectorant without any antitussive activity. *(2:154)*

15k. **(C)** Both Benylin liquid and elixir contain diphenhydramine, while the expectorant contains guaifenesin and dextromethorphan. *(2:168–71)*

15l. **(A)** Debrox drops contain carbamide peroxide, which will soften ear wax, easing its removal. S.T. 37 is a mouthwash and topical anti-infectant with hexylresorcinol as the active ingredient. Anbesol is used in the treatment of cold sores. It contains both benzocaine and phenol. *(2:652,682,790)*

15m. **(C)** Fluoxetine is marketed under the tradename of Prozac by Lilly for the treatment of major depression. *(10)*

15n. **(B)** Prozac's antidepressive effects are believed to be due to the drug's ability to prevent the reuptake of serotonin. It appears to be more selective in its serotonin to norepinephrine reuptake inhibition than the tricyclic antidepressants. *(9:28:16.04; 11:932)*

15o. **(C)** Prozac's side effect of causing anorexia is being explored as a method for weight loss. Insomnia is expected to occur in a number of patients, but the drug appears to slightly decrease heart rate, not increase it. *(9:28:16.04; 11:932)*

15p. **(C)** Prozac is available as 20 mg capsules (Pulvules) and as an oral liquid (20 mg/5 mL), but no parenteral dosage form is marketed. *(9:28:16.04)*

PROFILE NO. 16

16a. **(D)** Conventional therapy of urinary tract infections with ampicillin requires treatment for 7 to 14 days. Apparently, Ms Johnson discontinued therapy after a few days, probably because the symptoms subsided. She should be encouraged to take a full dosage regimen to clear the infection. *(4:1182)*

16b. **(A)** *Escherichia coli* is the predominant causative agent of urinary tract infections. All of the other microorganisms have been implicated in UTIs. With the exception of *Streptococcus fecalis*, the cited microorganisms are gram-negative enteric bacteria.
(11:1110)

16c. **(A)** Large single doses of drugs have been successfully employed in treatment of UTIs in nonpregnant patients. Amoxicillin (Amoxil) 3 g has been recommended. Sulfamethoxazole and trimethoprim combinations (Septra or Bactrim) have been administered in daily doses of 1600 mg sulfamethoxazole plus 320 mg trimethoprim for 3 days. However, Ms Johnson is allergic to sulfa drugs. The suggested dose of Furadantin is too low for single-dose therapy.
(1:1174,1193,1215; 4:1181)

16d. **(D)** Phenazopyridine may provide relief of dysuria and urethral irritation because of its anesthetic properties. It should be used for only 1 to 2 days. Phenazopyridine is available as Pyridium tablets, 100 to 200 mg. It is also available in combination with sulfisoxazole (Azo Gantanol, Azo Gantrisin, and Thiosulfil Forte). *(1:1169)*

16e. **(D)** The sympathomimetic agent, phenylpropanolamine, has been found to be safe and effective for short-term weight control. The stimulant caffeine, acting as a thermogenic agent, may be effective in increasing physical activity with a corresponding expenditure of energy. *(2:233,568; 11:989)*

16f. **(D)** There is evidence that the hypothalamus contains a "satiety" center. Normal-weight individuals appear to have internal cues such as hunger sensation and response to caloric density of foods that reduce the overeating habit. The genetic factor is also important. Statistically, the incidence of obesity is greater in children when either or both of the parents were obese. Because obesity is often associated with neurotic traits, overeating is commonly considered to be a behavioral defect. Either anxiety or depression may cause a tendency for some individuals to overindulge in eating.   *(11:984)*

16g. **(A)** Unless there is an emergency, or the patient is under close medical supervision, a deliberate weight loss should be limited to not more than 1 kg (2.2 lb) per week. This limit may be exceeded during the first 2 weeks of dieting when much of the loss is obligatory water. This initial weight loss explains the short-lived success of "water pills."   *(11:986)*

16h. **(B)** Both bulimia and anorexia nervosa are eating disorders. The most common trait of the individual suffering from anorexia nervosa is the feeling of being overweight even when actually underweight. Usually, such individuals refuse to eat normal meals. Pharmacists should counsel clients, especially young females, who may be using enemas, appetite suppressants, or ipecac syrup for unrealistic weight control.   *(11:992)*

16i. **(D)** Several oral OTC products such as Trind, Triaminic, and Tussagesic contain phenylpropanolamine as the nasal decongestant.   *(2:192–94)*

16j. **(E)** Insomnia and restlessness are more likely to be experienced by patients consuming phenylpropanolamine.   *(2:568)*

16k. **(E)** Tartrazine (F.D. & C. Yellow #5) is included in both solid and liquid products. A percentage of the general population is sensitive to the dye and may respond with typical allergic responses.   *(20:397)*

16l. **(A)** The designation "aa qs" translates as "of each a sufficient quantity to make 1%." Therefore, 0.5% each of menthol and camphor is needed. (60 g × 0.5% = 0.3 g)

16m. **(A)** Incorporating the two solids, menthol and camphor, into an ointment is best accomplished if a liquid is first formed. Simple mixing of the two chemicals will result in an eutectic liquid, which would readily mix with the alcoholic coal tar solution (LCD). It is not advisable to use alcohols such as isopropyl alcohol as incorporating agents since the alcohol may slowly migrate to the ointment surface, carrying dissolved drugs with it. There is no need to add polysorbate 80 to the product since it is already present in the LCD as a dispersing agent.

16n. **(E)** Coal tar solution contains 20% coal tar in an alcoholic solvent. Coal tar especially in combination with UV radiation has been successful in the treatment of psoriasis. The combination is known as the Goeckerman regimen.   *(2:834)*

16o. **(C)** Coal tar is a photosensitizer. It increases a patient's tendency to sunburn for up to 24 hours after application. The patient medication record should also be reviewed for other photosensitizers such as the phenothiazines and tetracyclines. Coal tar is relatively safe when included in shampooing products partially because of the short contact period. There are several shampoos on the market, including Ionil T, Polytar, and Zetar.   *(2:834)*

PROFILE NO. 17

17a. **(E)** Upon reviewing the lab reports, the pharmacist concludes that none of the other conditions are present. The white blood count is within normal values (5000 to 10,000 cells/mm^3). The normal hemoglobin for males is 14 to 18 g/dL, and the hematocrit only slightly low (range of 40% to 54%). Diabetes is suspected when serum glucose levels are above 120 mg/dL. Both the BUN and serum creatinine values are normal.   *(1:496,498)*

17b. **(B)** Clinical data suggest that administration of an antibiotic 1 hour before surgery will significantly reduce the incidence of postsurgical infections. One drug choice is intravenous cefazolin 1 g.   *(11:1245)*

17c. **(B)** While an IV cephalosporin is indicated for most surgical procedures, erythromycin and neomycin, 1 g of each, is given orally for a total of three doses for colorectal surgery. The dosage regimen greatly reduces the incidence of infection.   *(11:1245)*

17d. **(D)** Both Aminosyn and FreAmine are standard formulas containing essential and nonessential amino acids. NephrAmine is a specially designed formula intended for use in renal-impaired patients. It contains a mixture of the essential amino acids, but none of the nonessential amino acids except histidine. NephrAmine is significantly more expensive than the other two products.   *(9:40:20)*

17e. **(A)** TPN solutions are intended for slow parenteral infusion by either central administration through the subclavian vein or by peripheral administration through smaller veins. However, the TPN formula listed for this patient is very hypertonic, which precludes peripheral routes since the small veins may be damaged. Glucose concentrations of 10% or more should not be infused peripherally.   *(19:30–32)*

17f. **(A)** The patient's chloride levels were 120 mEq/L, which is above the normal range of 98 to 109 mEq/L. While it is possible to monitor blood pH, the pharmacist should suggest that potassium and sodium acetates be used in place of the respective chlorides. The "1 vial" designation for MVI refers to the standard 10 mL product.   *(1:1483)*

17g. **(A)** 500 mL amino acid solution × 8.5% = 42.5 g of amino acids × 16% (average level of nitrogen present) = 6.8 g of nitrogen.   *(11:155; 22:316)*

17h. **(A)** 500 mL dextrose × 40% = 200 g of dextrose. 200 g dextrose × 3.4 cal/g = 680 kcal.

(11:157; 19:30–33; 22:317)

17i. **(D)** TPN formulas should provide sufficient nonprotein calories to convert the amino acids present to lean body mass. A ratio of nonprotein calories to each gram of nitrogen has been established. A value of 150:1 is ideal, with a range of 125 to 175:1 acceptable. When lower ratios are used, either other sources of calories must be employed (ie, body fats) or some of the amino acids will be used as calories.

(11:155; 22:317)

17j. **(C)** EFAD is a deficiency of essential fatty acids. Liposyn III is a parenteral fatty oil emulsion that will provide the linoleic acid needed in humans for cell membrane synthesis and stabilization. EFAD is characterized by scaly skin, alopecia, poor wound healing, and thrombocytopenia.   *(4:2051; 22:317)*

17k. **(C)** Parenteral fatty oil emulsions are available in both 10% and 20% mixtures. Each mL of 10% emulsions gives 1.1 kcal, while each mL of 20% emulsions contributes 2 kcal. Therefore, 500 mL of 20% emulsion × 2 kcal/mL = 1000 kcal. If one did not know the exact calories present, the value could be estimated knowing that every gram of oil has approximately 9 calories. Thus:

$$500 \text{ mL} \times 20\% = 100 \text{ g} \times 9 \text{ kcal} = 900 \text{ kcal}$$

(21:372)

17l. **(E)** Patients experiencing delayed healing of wounds or burns have responded to therapeutic doses of zinc.   *(1:1170; 11:785; 22:243)*

17m. **(D)** Heat lamps will dry out the wound, which will slow the healing process. There is little evidence that the heat will stimulate blood circulation, especially since the inflamed area is already congested with blood.   *(22:252)*

17n. **(D)** Legionnaires' disease occurs mainly in the summertime when the airborne gram-positive *Legionella pneumophilia* is present. Many victims are older males, especially smokers with chronic lung disease.

(11:1085)

17o. **(B)** Aggressive treatment with erythromycin is usually necessary. An alternate choice is the tetracyclines.   *(11:1085)*

PROFILE NO. 18

18a. **(D)** Long-term therapy for treatment of Graves' disease includes either propylthiouracil or methimazole. The disease involves a hyperfunctional goiter, with clinical symptoms similar to that of thyrotoxicosis.   *(1:681; 16:1703)*

18b. **(D)** A regimen of chemotherapy known as MOPP is used in the treatment of Hodgkin's disease. Procarbazine (Matulane) and prednisone are given by the oral route on each day of the 14-day schedule. Mechlorethamine (Mustargen) and vincristine (Oncovin) are given intravenously on the first and eighth days of therapy. Experience has shown that combining drugs that have different mechanisms of action increases remission rates and lowers the incidence and severity of side effects.   *(4:1891; 9:10:10)*

18c. **(A)** Hepatocellular, bronchogenic, and pancreatic carcinomas have shown poor responses to presently used chemotherapeutic drugs. Ovarian and prostatic carcinomas are moderately responsive, with palliation and probable prolongation of life. Prolonged survival and probably some cures are expected in patients with testicular cancer and Hodgkin's disease.

(4:1866)

18d. **(B)** Mechlorethamine is a potent vesicant. Serious localized damage may occur if the drug solution seeps into the area surrounding the infusion site. The thiosulfate ion will react with the nitrogen mustard. Cold compresses will relieve the burning sensation and slow the spread of mechlorethamine. Other solutions that have been infused are normal saline and sodium bicarbonate.   *(4:1878)*

18e. **(A)** A 1 molar solution of sodium thiosulfate will contain 248 g of chemical in 1 L of solution. A one-half normal strength will contain 248/2 = 124 g. A one-sixth strength solution will contain 124/6 = 2.1 g. *(1:98)*

18f. **(A)** Although the official form of sodium thiosulfate contains five waters of hydration, the correct amount of active ingredient can be obtained by using the anhydrous form. Simply subtract 90 (weight of water in the molecule) from 248 to obtain 158 (the weight of anhydrous sodium thiosulfate), then follow the procedure outlined in answer 18e.

18g. **(D)** Hemorrhaging, such as nosebleeds, may occur when blood platelet counts are subnormal. Drugs such as the nitroureas, mitomycin, thiotepa, and methotrexate depress platelets.   *(19:906)*

18h. **(D)** The dictionary defines nadir as the place or time of deepest depression. When discussing drug chemotherapy, the term usually refers to the length of time before maximum bone marrow depression occurs. Many oncologic drugs, especially the alkylating agents, cause a depression characterized by low leukocyte counts with increased susceptibility to infections. For example, the nadir for a given drug may be 7 to 10 days after the start of therapy, with bone marrow recovery in 14 to 18 days.   *(4:1868)*

18i. **(E)** Bone marrow suppression is often the dose-limiting factor for toxicity during chemotherapy. Vincristine appears to have little effect on bone marrow.

(1:1157)

18j. **(C)** Because neoplastic cells have properties similar to normal cells, it is virtually impossible to develop an antineoplastic agent that will not attack normal cells. Consequently, the antineoplastic drugs have very low therapeutic indexes, usually less than 1.0.

(1:1140)

18k. **(C)** Cyanocobalamin injection (Redisol, Rubramin PC) is a pink-colored solution available in strengths of 30, 100, and 1000 µg/mL. It is administered by either IM or subcutaneous injection, but not IV. The injection route offers better bioavailability than oral administration.   *(1:1022; 6:1299)*

18l. **(E)** The NSAID mefenamic acid is usually used in 250 mg capsules as an analgesic to relieve mild or moderate pain after dental extractions or for dysmenorrhea. It should not be used for longer than 1 week because of side effects.   *(1:1117; 11:893)*

18m. **(E)** Brompheniramine maleate is available as Dimetane tablets (4 mg). Chlorpheniramine is available as Chlor-Trimeton 4 mg tablets and Teldrin 4 mg tablets or prolonged release 12 mg capsules. Clemastine fumarate is now available OTC as Tavist liquid (0.5 mg/5 mL) and tablets (1.34 and 2.68 mg).

(4:1699–1701)

18n. **(C)** Advantages of dosing with astemizole (Hismanal 10 mg tablets) or terfenadine (Seldane 60 mg tablets) are that drowsiness or sedation are extremely rare. Seldane is available as 60 mg tablets given twice daily. Increasing the dose of Seldane does not increase its activity. A significant advantage of the drug is that it does not potentiate the action of alcohol, diazepam, or CNS depressants. *(4:1700)*

18o. **(A)** Astemizole (Hismanal) has a half-life between 18 and 20 days. Because of its slow onset of action, a 30 mg dose the first day and a 20 mg dose the second day are often given before establishing the usual 10-mg daily maintenance dose. The drug should not be taken with food, which will slow its absorption.

(4:1700)

18p. **(D)** Estradern patches deliver 50 or 100 mg of estradiol, which is equivalent to 0.625 or 1.25 mg of Premarin in the prevention of postmenopausal symptoms and osteoporosis. Transdermal administration avoids early liver metabolism. The patches are replaced twice a week.   *(4:2107)*

PROFILE NO. 19

19a. **(A)** Adriamycin is marketed in vials containing either 10 or 50 mg of powder for reconstitution.

(1:1150; 4:1917)

19b. **(D)** Both doxorubicin and cyclophosphamide cause alopecia in a significant number of patients.

(4:1876,1918)

19c. **(E)** The nadir for the drug is approximately 10 to 15 days after administration. Recovery from the leuko-

penia occurs in about 20 days. Cardiomyopathy is a delayed, cumulative, dose-related adverse effect.

(4:1918)

19d. **(B)** The patient weights 140 lb or 140 lb × 1 kg/2.2 lb = 64 kg. Since 700 mg of cyclophosphamide is being given, 700 mg/64 kg = 11 mg/kg.   *(23:83)*

19e. **(A)** Almost all patients receiving cisplatin experience nausea and vomiting. Metoclopramide (Reglan) is administered in doses of 1 to 2 mg/kg approximately 30 minutes before cisplatin and every 2 hours after cisplatin injection to control emesis. Reglan is also used orally to increase upper GI tract motility. Oral administration 30 minutes before meals will prevent gastroesophageal reflux.   *(1:793; 4:419)*

19f. **(C)** Lomustine (CCNU) is a nitrosourea derivative classified as an alkylating agent. It is rapidly absorbed from the GI tract and marketed by Bristol-Myers as 10, 40, and 100 mg capsules. It is used in the treatment of brain tumors and Hodgkin's disease. All of the other listed drugs are administered by injection and have vesicant properties, especially doxorubicin. Medical personnel must handle these injection solutions carefully and avoid spillage or sprays. Infusion sites must be carefully monitored for signs of extravasation.   *(1:1153; 9:10:10; 22:302)*

19g. **(B)** The elevated creatinine value (normal = 1 mg/dL) indicates renal damage. Cisplatin can cause proximal renal tubular damage that is not completely reversible. It is advisable to either discontinue the cisplatin or reduce the dosage while carefully monitoring the patient for acute renal failure.

(4:1887)

19h. **(B)** Bone marrow depression is the usual dose-limiting factor of cyclophosphamide therapy. High doses frequently result in sterile hemorrhagic cystitis. Patients should be counseled to maintain a high level of fluid intake and void frequently.

(4:1875)

19i. **(D)** High serum levels of methotrexate will result in passive diffusion of the drug into normal cells. To avoid the resulting cytotoxic effects on normal cells, an injection of leucovorin is administered approximately 24 hours after the methotrexate injection. Leucovorin is also used in treating megaloblastic anemia. It is administered by intramuscular injection.   *(4:1898)*

19j. **(C)** Methotrexate is sometimes given intrathecally since the drug does not normally enter the cerebrospinal fluid except if given at high levels (>1 g/m^2). Thiotepa is poorly absorbed from the GI tract. Since it is not a vesicant, it can be administered intravenously, by bladder irrigation, and intrathecal injection.   *(4:1880, 1899)*

19k. **(D)** Vials of lyophilized powder are available as Folex (Adria). Both 2.5 mg tablets and a Solution for

Injection (2.5 mg/mL) in 2 mL vials are available from Lederle. *(4:1899)*

19l. (A) The antihypertensive enalapril maleate (Merck's Vasotec) is available as 5, 10, and 20 mg tablets, with usual maintenance dosing of 10 to 40 mg daily. *(5:541; 11:590)*

19m. (C) Vasotec is an angiotensin-converting enzyme (ACE) inhibitor. *(5:541; 11:590)*

19n. (C) Several of the ACE inhibitors cause the unusual side effect of an occasional dry, nonproductive cough. Patients should also be warned of incidences of hypotension, especially during the first few days of therapy. The drugs also appear to increase alertness and produce mood elevation. Vasotec does not cause reflex tachycardia. *(10; 11:590)*

19o. (C) Hydralazine (Apresoline) is an alternative for methyldopa (Aldomet) in the controlling of severe hypertension during pregnancy. Dosing of 10 to 25 mg twice or three times a day is used. *(1:837; 11:590, 1470)*

19p. (E) Lisinopril is available under the tradenames of Prinivil (Merck) and Zestril (Stuart). *(1:841; 10)*

PROFILE NO. 20

20a. (C) The 30-day supply of HCTZ appears to have been dispensed only once with tablets depleted by April 1. Either Mr Tralor has had the prescription filled elsewhere or is not complying with the once daily dosing. This may explain why Dr Lange has issued a new prescription for the stronger-acting Verapamil. Mevacor is available in several strengths (10, 20, and 40 mg tablets). There is no significant interaction between Verapamil and digoxin. However, Verapamil does increase digoxin levels by 50% to 70%. *(1:858,1854)*

20b. (E) Verelan is an extended release capsule containing either 120 or 240 mg of drug in pellets. Extended release tablets are marketed as Calan SR (180 mg) and Isoptin SR (120, 180, and 240 mg). Both dosage forms offer better patient compliance than the regular tablets and more consistent blood levels. The drug is also available as a parenteral solution (2.5 mg/mL). *(9:24:04)*

20c. (B) Verapamil is a calcium entry or calcium channel blocker used as an antihypertensive agent, antianginal, and antiarrhythmic. *(1:855,1854)*

20d. (A) When drugs such as Verapamil have significant differences between the oral and parenteral doses administered, there are several explanations. One is poor absorption from the GI tract. Another is that the drug undergoes significant first-pass effect, usually due to rapid metabolism by the liver. Since this

occurs before the drug reaches sites of activity, the oral dose must be relatively high as compared to the intravenous dose, which avoids the first-pass effect. Another drug example is propranolol, which has an IV dose of 4 mg compared to the oral dose of 40 to 80 mg. *(9:24:2404)*

20e. (E) Taking Mevacor with the evening meal appears to maximize the GI absorption of the drug. *(6:885; 9:24:06)*

20f. (C) A fast disintegration time for tablets indicates that the tablet has broken into smaller pieces, which allows the dissolution process to occur. The fastest disintegration occurred with brand D, followed by brand C. However brand C dissolved faster than brand D. Since dissolution is critical for drug absorption and is usually the rate-limiting step, brand C probably has the greatest bioavailability. *(1:1452)*

20g. (E) Niacin is one of the most economical drugs in attempting to reduce blood triglycerides and cholesterol. It causes the catabolism of low-density lipoproteins (LDL). Pyridoxine is used to treat peripheral neuritis. *(11:340)*

20h. (D) The vasodilation effect of niacin causes peripheral flushing that may last up to 1 hour after administration. The drug may also irritate the stomach, causing abdominal discomfort. The flushing and pruritus can be prevented by administration of 325 mg of aspirin 30 minutes before the niacin. *(1:1024; 11:340)*

20i. (E) The injection solution contains 50 or 100 mg of niacin, while the oral solution has 50 mg per teaspoonful dose. There are also extended release capsules (150 or 300 mg), which are claimed to reduce the annoying side effects of the drug. *(1:1024)*

20j. (B) Screening is usually based upon total cholesterol, with a targeted goal of less than 200 mg/dL (5.17 mmol/L in the nonfasting adult). People with higher cholesterol levels should have their LDL (low-density lipoprotein) value calculated by determining their triglyceride and HDL (high-density lipoprotein) while in the fasting state. *(31:164)*

20k. (D) High levels of LDL and VLDL (very low-density lipoproteins) indicate a high atherosclerotic risk. Patients with LDL values greater than 130 mg/dL should consider both dietary changes and possible drug therapy. On the other hand, HDL (high-density lipoproteins) appear to be a scavenger of cholesterol and protect arteries from deposition of cholesterol. Generally, a LDL/HDL ratio of less than 3.0 is ideal. *(1:856; 31:165)*

20l. (C) While patients should limit their intake of meats, up to 6-oz per day of lean red meat or chicken with the skin removed is permissible. All of the other choices are good dietary guidelines. *(11:338)*

20m. (D) When comparing the dosing regimen of the listed drugs, lovastatin (Mevacor) has the lowest dose—20 mg daily. Cholestyramine (Questran)—4 g t.i.d.; colestipol (Colestid)—15 g daily; gemfibrozil (Lopid)—300 mg b.i.d.; and probucol (Lorelco)—250 mg b.i.d.   *(11:340)*

20n. (C) Weak acidic compounds such as warfarin, digoxin, and penicillin will bind to cholestyramine and colestipol. Bile acids also bind. This is the mechanism by which the resins exert their activity.
                                                 (1:856; 11:339)

PROFILE NO. 21

21a. (A) Hypothyroidism (myxedema) is characterized by the slowing of body processes because of a deficiency of thyroid hormone. The classical treatment was thyroid tablets. Today, this drug has been replaced with L-thyroxine (T_4), L-thyronine (T_3), and liotrix (a mixture of T_4 and T_3). Synthroid is levothyroxine sodium (L-thyroxine). Graves' disease is a form of hyperthyroidism (thyrotoxicosis).   *(11:273)*

21b. (E) Omission of a single dose of Synthroid will not have significant effects upon the disease state.   *(10)*

21c. (B) Acesulfam, aspartame, and saccharin are artificial sweeteners that are 200, 180, and 400 times sweeter, respectively, than sucrose. The agents are used in many dietary foods and in some pharmaceuticals. The use of saccharin in place of one teaspoonful of sugar saves the consumer from 33 calories. Because of a weak relationship between saccharin and cancer in animals, a warning label is required in stores selling foods or beverages containing saccharin. Similar relationships between acesulfam and aspartame have not been established.   *(2:572)*

21d. (C) The tannins in teas may react with iron to form insoluble iron tannates. It is well established that many antacids combine with iron, thereby reducing the absorption of iron.   *(3:456; 11:172)*

21e. (D) Amantadine is a selective antiviral agent for prophylactic action (200 mg daily) against influenza A, but not B. It is also useful in reducing the signs and symptoms of Parkinson's disease in which it augments dopamine release. Amantadine can be used as the sole agent or with levodopa.   *(4:358,1656)*

21f. (E) Amantadine is available in both 100 mg capsules and syrup (50 mg/5 mL) under the tradename of Symmetrel.   *(10)*

21g. (C) While there is some patient to patient variation, one of the earliest signs of Alzheimer's disease is the forgetfulness of current events; for example, what one has eaten for lunch. Although gradual, this memory loss becomes progressively worse.   *(11:1480)*

21h. (D) Ergoloid mesylates (Hydergine), an ergot drug, has been used for several years in attempts to improve patients' memories and increase the feeling of well-being. Tacrine (Cognex) is a cholinesterase inhibitor that has reduced the clinical symptoms of Alzheimer's.   *(11:1485–86)*

21i. (D) Normally, the patient would be counseled to take digoxin in the morning to assure compliance. However, she is taking an antacid in the morning and at night that may interfere with digoxin absorption. Either suggest that the digoxin be taken at noon or in the morning, separated by 2 hours from the antacid.   *(3:271)*

21j. (C) Women, especially postmenopausal, should increase their intake of calcium to avoid osteoporosis. Tums is available as 500 mg of calcium carbonate per tablet or as 750-mg chewable tablets (Tums E-X). While calcium carbonate could be used in the prevention of gastroesophageal reflux, there are better products on the market and the dosing regimen would be after each meal as well as at bedtime.   *(3:257,291,457)*

21k. (B) The volume of distribution of lipophilic drugs may increase if the individual has a lower body weight, usually because of dehydration, but a corresponding increase in relative amount of adipose tissue. Renal clearance rates are often lower in the elderly because of impaired kidney function. The plasma albumin levels are sometimes lower than normal, thereby affecting the amount of protein binding.   *(11:1490–91)*

21l. (C) If both dosage forms had 100% bioavailability (F value of 1.0), the answer would be 5 mL.

$$\frac{0.05 \text{ mg}}{1 \text{ mL}} = \frac{0.25 \text{ mg}}{x \text{ mL}}$$
$$x = 5 \text{ mL of elixir}$$

However, not all of the drug is available as reflected in the "F" values of 0.6 for the tablet and 0.75 for the elixir. Therefore,

$$Q_1 \times C_1 = Q_2 \times C_2$$
$$(0.25 \text{ mg})(0.6) = (x)(0.75)$$
$$x = 0.2 \text{ mg of digoxin absorbed}$$

Since the elixir contains 0.05 mg per mL.

$$\frac{0.05 \text{ mg}}{1 \text{ mL}} = \frac{0.2 \text{ mg}}{x \text{ mL}}$$
$$x = 4 \text{ mL of elixir}$$
                                                      (23:229)

21m. (A) Many of the elderly exhibit digoxin toxicity by having a hazy vision rather than the more classical halo and color vision changes that occur in the younger population. Rather than having an increase in appetite, anorexia often occurs.   *(11:1495)*

PROFILE NO. 22

22a. **(C)** The term tocolytic refers to a drug that will reduce uterine contractility, thereby preventing premature birthing.   *(28:1605)*

22b. **(B)** Terbutaline is available under the trade names of Brethine (Geigy) and Bricanyl (Marion Merrell Dow). To prevent preterm labor, it is administered either SC or IV. However, its greatest market is as a bronchodilator.   *(1:885; 12:12)*

22c. **(D)** The medication order calls for 25 µg of drug per minute. The pharmacist added 2 mL (2 mg or 2,000 µg) to 250 mL of diluent.

$$\frac{2000 \text{ µg}}{250 \text{ mL}} = \frac{25 \text{ µg}}{x \text{ mL}}$$
$$x = 3.125 \text{ mL}$$

$$\frac{15 \text{ gtt}}{1 \text{ mL}} = \frac{x \text{ gtt}}{3.125 \text{ mL}}$$
$$x = 46.8 \text{ drops per minute}$$
(23:207)

22d. **(B)** The total amount of drug present is 2000 µg and it is being administered at a rate of 25 µg/m.

$$\frac{250 \text{ mL}}{x \text{ min.}} = \frac{3.125 \text{ mL}}{1 \text{ min.}}$$
$$x = 80 \text{ minutes}$$
(23:207)

22e. **(C)** Barium sulfate is used to render the intestinal tract opaque for x-rays. A dose of 60 to 250 g is administered as a suspension.   *(1:1272)*

22f. **(E)** Barium sulfate is practically insoluble in water, thus there is little danger of toxicity from systemic absorption of the chemical. It is administered either orally or rectally, depending upon the portion of the GI tract to be x-rayed.   *(1:1272)*

22g. **(B)** Atropine is classified as an antimuscarinic/antispasmodic agent used to inhibit salivation and other excessive secretions during surgery. It may also prevent cholinergic effects such as cardiac arrhythmias, hypotension, and bradycardia during surgery.   *(9:12:08.08)*

22h. **(B)** The usual adult dose of atropine is 0.4 mg SC, IM, or even IV. Atropine sulfate and chlorpromazine HCl (Thorazine) will be compatible in a syringe. The purpose of chlorpromazine is to relieve presurgical apprehension and control nausea and vomiting during surgery.   *(9:12:08.08; 21:90)*

22i. **(A)** Glycopyrrolate is administered 30 minutes prior to surgery for action similar to that of atropine. It is also available as oral tablets (1 and 2 mg) to suppress gastric secretions for the treatment of peptic ulcers.   *(1:911)*

22j. **(A)** Because of their sizing and use, urinary cathe-

ters bear a Federal warning concerning dispensing without a prescription. Ostomy pouches are available in several sizes and designs, but the consumer may purchase them, as well as bandages and dressings, without a prescription.   *(1:1886,1888)*

22k. **(C)** Both Natalins Rx and Stuartnatal are well-rounded vitamin supplements intended to prevent deficiencies such as low folic acid levels during pregnancy.   *(10; 11:187)*

22l. **(D)** Metamucil contains psyllium as the active ingredient. Sucrose imparts sweetness to the product. A pharmacist may wish to counsel diabetics away from this type of product to one that contains an artificial sweetener; for example, Orange Flavor Metamucil Instant Mix.   *(2:374)*

22m. **(A)** Bulking agents such as Metamucil should be dispersed in water or a flavored vehicle such as orange juice, quickly stirred, then drunk immediately. Otherwise, the powder will swell, forming a gel that would be difficult to swallow.   *(2:349)*

22n. **(B)** Both Slow-Bid and Theo-Dur contain anhydrous theophylline for the prevention of asthma. Slow-Bid consists of timed release capsules (50, 100, 200, and 300 mg) while Theo-Dur is available as sustained action tablets and sustained action capsules.   *(10)*

PROFILE NO. 23

23a. **(B)** The active ingredient in Monistat-7 is miconazole, an antifungal agent effective against numerous species, including *Candida albicans* and *Trichophyton mentagrophytes,* which infect the vagina and the foot, respectively. Monistat-7 consists of suppositories for vaginal insertion. Many products containing miconazole are now OTC as 2% creams, powders, and sprays.   *(1:1235; 2:780,983)*

23b. **(B)** With the successful treatment of gonorrhea with either penicillin or tetracyclines, other causes of sexually transmitted urethritis have emerged. Over 50% of cases of nongonorrheal urethritis are caused by the obligate intracellular parasite *Chlamydia.*   *(11:1187)*

23c. **(D)** Syphilis is usually transmitted by direct contact with an active lesion containing spirochetes. While there are several stages and types of syphilis, the drug of choice is still parenteral penicillin, such as 2.4 million units of benzathine penicillin G. For patients allergic to penicillin, tetracycline is used.   *(11:1193)*

23d. **(A)** Primary treatment will be doxycycline 100 mg twice a day for seven days. Alternatives include erythromycin or ofloxacin 400 mg b.i.d. Ciprofloxacin has been used but is not as successful as doxycycline.   *(11:1189)*

23e. **(C)** Oral contraceptives appear to be the best

method to avoid conception, followed by intrauterine devices (IUDs).   *(2:709; 4:1046)*

23f. (C) White vaseline or any petrolatum product is not acceptable as a lubricant for either condoms or diaphragms, since small openings will develop due to the solvent characteristics of petrolatum toward rubber.   *(4:1046)*

23g. (C) Skin implants such as Norplant offer long-term contraceptive protection. Six capsules are implanted subcutaneously into the upper arm. A constant rate release of 20 to 30 µg of levonorgestrel occurs daily. The implants appear to be even more effective than oral contraceptives.   *(2:709; 4:1067)*

23h. (A) The testicular hormone danazol (Winthrop's Danocrine) is given orally in 100 to 200 mg doses to treat endometriosis, a condition characterized by menstrual-like bleeding and localized inflammation and pain, usually within the pelvis. A second drug successful in the treatment of endometriosis is Nafarelin acetate (Synarel), which is available as an intranasal spray.   *(1:998; 4:1039; 9:68:08)*

23i. (B) Obsessive-compulsive disorder (OCD) is an anxiety disorder characterized by compulsions such as a fear of dirt or microorganisms, recurrent fear that a stove has not been shut off, constant checking to see if lights have been turned off, or having persistent thoughts that one might injure a loved one.   *(11:908)*

23j. (A) The antiobsessional drug clomipramine (Ciba's Anafranil), is a tricyclic antidepressant related to imipramine (Tofranil). Its mode of action in the treatment of obsessive-compulsive disorders is believed to be that it inhibits reuptake of serotonin. Dosing has to be carefully adjusted to avoid adverse effects, especially seizures.   *(4:238)*

23k. (C) Methylphenidate (Ritalin) is classified as a centrally acting sympathomimetic. It is used in the therapy of attention-deficit hyperactivity disorder.   *(11:977)*

23l. (E) The benzodiazepines exert their antianxiety effects by potentiation of the inhibitory neurotransmitter GABA.   *(11:911)*

23m. (E) Therapy with clozapine should be reserved for severely ill schizophrenic patients. While the drug has many valuable attributes, blood monitoring is necessary. One serious side effect is the development of agranulocytosis.   *(4:264; 11:951,1499)*

23n. (E) The incidence of extrapyramidal effects, including tardive dyskinesia, is minimal with clozapine, especially when compared with other psychiatric drugs.   *(4:264; 11:950,1499)*

PROFILE NO. 24

24a. (D) These two microorganisms are major causes of both ear infections and sinusitis.   *(11:804)*

24b. (D) Other appropriate antibiotics include erythromycin + sulfisoxazole and amoxicillin + potassium clavulanate (Augmentin).   *(11:804,1067)*

24c. (B) All three drugs possess antipyretic activity. However, Jason is sensitive to salicylates and neither aspirin nor ibuprofen (to which he may also be sensitive) should be dispensed.   *(2:63,70)*

24d. (C) Ibuprofen is 2 (p-isobutylphenyl) propionic acid.   *(1:1116)*

24e. (A) Fever may be the sign of a serious systemic infection. If the fever is masked by the use of an antipyretic, prompt treatment may be delayed.   *(2:104; 11:1402)*

24f. (B) The rapid hydrolysis of aspirin into salicylic acid in the presence of water has made the development of a liquid aspirin product difficult.   *(1:253; 2:77–89)*

24g. (A) Amount of cromolyn needed for Rx is 30 mL × 2.5% = 0.75 g. Amount of the available 4% solution to use:

$$\frac{4\,g}{100\,mL} = \frac{0.75\,g}{x\,mL}$$

$$x = 19\,mL \text{ (therefore, must}$$
make only the remaining 11 mL isotonic)

$$11\,mL \times 0.9\%\,NaCl = 0.099\,g \text{ or } 99\,mg$$
                    (1:1490)

24h. (A) Removal of bacteria and fungi from extemporaneously prepared solutions may be accomplished by passage through a 0.20- or 0.22-micron filter into a sterile container.   *(1:1474)*

24i. (B) Ophthalmic solutions containing cromolyn sodium have been effective in treatment of allergic conjunctivitis. Chronic allergic conjunctivitis patients should also avoid using OTC sympathomimetic decongestants, which may cause rebound vasodilation.   *(6:632; 11:798)*

24j. (A) Ascorbic acid (vitamin C) is found in many natural sources including citrus fruits, melons, green vegetables such as lettuce and cabbage, and in rose hips.   *(1:1012)*

24k. (C) Tofranil in doses of 25 mg one hour before bedtime reduces the incidence of childhood enuresis. If unsuccessful, the dose may be increased up to 75 mg.   *(1:1093)*

24l. (B) Diphenhydramine (Benadryl) is a well-known antihistamine exhibiting drowsiness as a major side effect. It is sometimes prescribed as a sleep aid and is available in several commercial OTC sleep aid products including Compoz, Nytol, and Sominex.   *(2:240)*

24m. (E) Triazolam is an ultrashort hypnotic with a half-life of 2 to 3 hours. It is the least likely of any of the benzodiazepines to produce a morning hangover.

However, it does produce short-term amnesia in some patients. *(11:969)*

24n. **(C)** Sulfasalazine (Azulfidine) is usually administered for ulcerative colitis in doses of 500 mg q.i.d. A second drug, olsalazine (Dipentum), may also be used. It is a topical anti-inflammatory agent that forms 5 amino-salicylic acid in the intestines.

(1:1179; 10)

PROFILE NO. 25

25a. **(D)** Gout is a chronic metabolic disease characterized by hyperuricemia. The uric acid is an end product of protein catabolism. Either uric acid production increases or impaired renal clearance slows removal. To relieve an acute attack, an anti-inflammatory drug (NSAID) or colchicine is administered. Colchicine is most effective if given within the first 12 to 36 hours of the acute attack. Allopurinol is reserved for patients who appear to be refractory to colchicine or the NSAIDs. *(11:508,511)*

25b. **(A)** Allopurinol (Zyloprim) is the most commonly used agent for long-term control of chronic gout and is the drug of choice for patients that are over-producers of uric acid. Not only does allopurinol inhibit xanthine oxidase, which converts xanthine to uric acid, but allopurinol's metabolite, oxypurinol, also inhibits xanthine oxidase. *(11:517)*

25c. **(C)** Sufficient liquid intake of at least 2 L daily is necessary to prevent formation of xanthine calculi. Acute attacks of gout may occur on initial therapy; therefore, colchicine therapy should be continued for a few days. Because of possible stomach irritation, it is best to take allopurinol with food. *(1:1110; 10)*

25d. **(A)** Antacids appear to increase the absorption of levodopa by as much as a threefold factor. Since levodopa dosing for Parkinson's is usually by titration, either the addition or discontinuation of concurrent antacids may change plasma levels of levodopa significantly. *(2:272)*

25e. **(C)** Acetaminophen products are usually suggested for patients sensitive to aspirin and other salicylates. Salicylamide products may also be used since they do not form salicylic acid in the body. However, relatively high doses are needed. There have been reports of patients sensitive to aspirin who may also be sensitive to ibuprofen. *(2:68–71; 6:650)*

25f. **(E)** Of all the related NSAIDs listed, naproxen (Naprosyn) has been shown effective in the alleviation of ankylosing spondylitis. *(6:667)*

25g. **(D)** Minoxidil was originally marketed as Loniten, an antihypertensive agent. However, one side effect was stimulation of hair growth. The drug was further developed for the treatment of alopecia. Its greatest success is with males under 40 years of age who have had baldness for less than 10 years.

(1:837; 6:1587)

25h. **(C)** Loniten is available as 2.5 and 10 mg tablets. A topical 2% solution is marketed as Rogaine. *(1:837)*

25i. **(D)** The prescribed dose was 0.6 mg/kg/h. Since the patient weighs 160 lb:

step 1. 160 lb × 1 kg/2.2 lb = 77 kg

step 2. 77 kg × 0.6 mg/kg = 46.2 mg/h

step 3. $\dfrac{500 \text{ mg}}{1000 \text{ mL}} = \dfrac{46.2 \text{ mg}}{x \text{ mL}}$

$x = 92.4 \text{ mL/hr}$

step 4. $\dfrac{15 \text{ gtt}}{1 \text{ mL}} = \dfrac{x \text{ gtt}}{1.5 \text{ mL}}$

$x = 22.5 \text{ gtt}$

25j. **(A)** The half-life of theophylline in smokers is 4 to 5 hours, as compared to 7 to 9 hours in nonsmokers. Infusion rates of 0.7 mg/kg/h are needed, as compared to 0.4 mg/kg/h in nonsmokers. Aminophylline is the ethylenediamine salt of theophylline, and therefore has only 85% of the potency. The desired serum levels of theophylline are between 10 and 20 µg/mL.

(1:867; 11:557)

25k. **(E)** Since ranitidine does not interact with hepatic cytochrome P-450, it has minimal effect on the pharmacokinetics of theophylline. All of the other choices inhibit the metabolism of theophylline, thereby increasing its half-life.

(1:1863; 11:396,1099,1502,1853)

25l. **(C)** If the rate of initial distribution is not greater than the rate of elimination, two slopes will not be evident when the plasma drug levels are plotted on graph paper. Half-lives of drugs are not directly related to whether or not a one- or two-compartment model is present. The half-life relates to the clearance of the drug.

25m. **(A)** A faster heartbeat is a fairly early sign of theophylline overdosing. It is actually more reliable than nausea and anorexia, which do not occur in all patients. *(1:868; 11:554)*

25n. **(E)** Verapamil prolongs the activity of theophylline, probably by interfering with its metabolism.

(11:557)

25o. **(E)** Rifampin (Rifadin or Rimactane) discolors urine, sweat, and tears. The drug's major use is in the treatment of tuberculosis, usually in combination with isoniazid or pyrazinamide. *(1:1218; 11:1099)*

PROFILE NO. 26

26a. **(B)** Both amitriptyline (Elavil) and nortriptyline (Pamelor) are tricyclic antidepressants. Compazine is a phenothiazine, Nardil is a monoamine oxidase inhibitor, and Clozaril and Loxitane are antipsychotic agents. *(3:1227)*

26b. (E) Hirsutism or abnormal growth of hair has not been reported as a significant adverse effect of Elavil. *(3:1221)*

26c. (C) Patients using Elavil should be advised that the drug may require up to 30 days of continuous dosing in order to achieve a full therapeutic effect. A sedative effect may be apparent long before the antidepressant effect is seen. *(3:1226)*

26d. (E) Tricyclic antidepressants such as Elavil may antagonize the antihypertensive action of guanethidine by inhibiting its uptake into adrenergic neurons. *(3:1223)*

26e. (C) Patients using Lithobid should be advised to consume 8 to 12 glasses of water daily. This will stabilize lithium levels in the blood and prevent lithium toxicity. *(3:1293)*

26f. (A) Adverse reactions to lithium rarely occur when serum lithium levels are below 1.5 mEq/L. Mild to moderate toxic reactions may occur at a level of 1.5 to 2.5 mEq/L, and severe toxicity is seen above these levels. *(3:1295)*

26g. (A) The addition of HydroDIURIL to this patient's regimen is likely to increase serum lithium levels because, when sodium is depleted from the body, the body will conserve lithium, thereby resulting in lithium accumulation. *(3:1293)*

26h. (C) Blood samples are drawn just prior to taking a dose, since lithium levels will be steady at that time and will represent the trough value for lithium. *(3:1297)*

26i. (E) Hydrochlorothiazide (HydroDIURIL) is an example of a thiazide diuretic. *(3:531)*

26j. (C) Lithobid is a slow-release tablet that requires only twice-daily dosing instead of three-times-daily dosing, which is generally required for normal release products. *(3:1297)*

PROFILE NO. 27

27a. (A) The other agents are nonsteroidal anti-inflammatory drugs (NSAIDS). *(3:1119)*

27b. (E) Nonsteroidal anti-inflammatory drugs (NSAIDS) have analgesic and antipyretic action, which is believed to be related to their ability to inhibit cyclooxygenase activity and prostaglandin synthesis. *(3:1109)*

27c. (C) Advil is a nonprescription brand of ibuprofen. Ibuprofen is usually administered three to four times daily, although more frequent administration may be required in some cases. Antacids may be taken with ibuprofen to increase its GI tolerance. *(3:1119)*

27d. (D) Mylanta is an antacid containing aluminium

hydroxide, aluminum hydroxide, and simethicone. Simethicone is included in the formulation to dispel gas, which may otherwise accumulate in the stomach. *(3:1541)*

27e. (E) Piroxicam is available as the brand Feldene. *(3:1121)*

27f. (B) Piroxicam (Feldene) is a relatively long-acting NSAID that requires only a single daily 20 mg dose for most patients. *(3:1121)*

27g. (E) Auranofin (Ridaura) is an oral gold product used to treat rheumatoid arthritis that cannot be effectively or safely managed by NSAIDS and other more conservative forms of therapy. *(3:1141)*

27h. (C) Misoprostol is a synthetic prostaglandin analog that has both antisecretory activity and mucosal protective properties. It is primarily employed in preventing NSAID-induced gastric ulcers. *(3:1532)*

27i. (D) Misoprostol is contraindicated for use during pregnancy and is classified as a pregnancy category X drug by the US Food and Drug Administration. *(3:1533)*

27j. (C) Anacin is an OTC analgesic produce containing 400 mg of aspirin and 32 mg of caffeine in each tablet. *(3:1105)*

PROFILE NO. 28

28a. (D) Digoxin is a cardiac glycoside that produces a negative chronotropic effect (slowed heart rate), a positive inotropic effect (greater force of contraction), and a vagomimetic effect on the heart. *(3:559)*

28b. (A) Most patients using digoxin will experience a slowed heart rate (negative chronotropic effect). *(3:559)*

28c. (E) Deslanoside (Cedilanid-D) is a cardiac glycoside that is only administered intravenously. *(3:559)*

28d. (A) Digitoxin is a cardiac glycoside suitable for use in patients with renal impairment because most digitoxin is cleared by the liver. The other cardiac glycosides currently available are cleared primarily by the kidneys. *(3:559)*

28e. (C) Lanoxicaps are liquid-filled capsules that contain a solution of digoxin in polyethylene glycol. Since the digoxin is already in solution, the Lanoxicap dosage form provides greater bioavailability of digoxin than is achieved from digoxin tablets. A dose of 0.25 mg (250 µg) of digoxin from a tablet dosage form is equivalent to 0.2 mg (200 µg) from the Lanoxicap dosage form. *(3:568)*

28f. (E) Amrinone (Inocor) is a drug that produces a positive inotropic effect. It is useful for short-term management of patients with congestive heart failure who have not responded adequately to cardiac glycosides, diuretics, or vasodilators.   *(3:569)*

28g. (B) If amiloride (Midamor) is substituted for Lasix in this patient's regimen, the patient should no longer receive the potassium supplement Klorvess since amiloride is a potassium-sparing diuretic and the administration of the combined agents will result in hyperkalemia.   *(3:545)*

28h. (D) Klorvess is a potassium supplement available in a variety of different dosage forms, including effervescent granules and tablets as well as a solution.   *(3:46–7)*

28i. (A) Bumetanide (Bumex) and furosemide (Lasix) are both loop diuretics. Midamor and Dyrenium are potassium-sparing diuretics, and Diamox is a carbonic anhydrase inhibitor.   *(3:541)*

28j. (A) The patient appears to be noncompliant since he received a month's supply of digoxin but did not get a refill until about 1 1/2 months later.

PROFILE NO. 29

29a. (E) Diphenhydramine (Benadryl) is an ethanolamine antihistamine with both sedative and antipruritic properties.   *(3:917)*

29b. (E) Lindane, or gamma benzene hexachloride, the active ingredient in Kwell, is an ectoparasiticide and ovicide used for the treatment of human lice and scabies.   *(3:2233)*

29c. (A) When Kwell Shampoo is used, it is essential that the product not come in contact with the eyes since it can cause significant irritation. Kwell should not be used on the face or on open cuts or excoriated areas of the body.   *(3:2233)*

29d. (D) The term "pediculus" refers to lice. *Pediculus capitis* refers to head lice, while *Pediculus pubis* refers to pubic lice. *Sarcoptes scabiei* is the organism that causes scabies. The term "tinea" refers to a type of fungal organism.   *(3:2233)*

29e. (E) Kwell Shampoo is generally administered once. After working it thoroughly into the hair, it remains in place for 4 minutes and is then worked into a lather with water. It is then rinsed well from the hair, and the hair is towel-dried and combed to ensure the removal of any remaining nit shells. Retreatment may occur after 7 days if there is still evidence of living lice at that time.   *(3:2234)*

29f. (B) Diprosone Cream contains 0.05% betamethasone dipropionate in a hydrophilic emollient base.   *(3:2241)*

29g. (E) Diprosone Cream or any other potent corticosteroid topical product should not be used on areas of the skin that are infected by bacteria, fungi, or a virus since the corticosteroid will inhibit the body's defense mechanisms and potentially cause spreading of the infection.   *(3:2240)*

29h. (D) Both Nix (permethrin) and A-200 Pyrinate (pyrethrins, piperonyl butoxide, and petroleum distillate) are available for OTC use. Eurax (crotamiton) is available only by prescription.   *(3:2236–7)*

29i. (D) Pyrethrin-containing products should be avoided by people with ragweed allergy since pyrethrins are plant derivatives that may precipitate a hypersensitivity reaction in such patients.   *(3:2237)*

29j. (E) Scabies is a skin condition caused by the mite *Sarcoptes scabiei*. The mite burrows into the skin and causes severe itching and excoriation of the affected area. Lindane and crotamiton are effective drugs for the treatment of scabies.   *(3:2236)*

PROFILE NO. 30

30a. (E) Naloxone is a pure narcotic antagonist which, when administered parenterally, will rapidly reverse the effects of opioid narcotic agents such as heroin. Since it has no agonist action of its own, there is no danger in administering this agent to an unconscious patient even if the source of drug toxicity is unknown.   *(3:2508–9)*

30b. (B) Heroin is diacetylmorphine. Codeine is methylmorphine, while dionin is ethylmorphine.   *(11:1019)*

30c. (C) *Pneumocystis carinii* pneumonia (PCP) is a condition commonly seen in AIDS patients. It is an opportunistic infection that emerges when the immune system of a patient is suppressed by disease or drugs.   *(11:1083)*

30d. (C) Zidovudine or azidothymidine (AZT) is an antiviral agent commonly used in the management of patients with HIV infection who have evidence of impaired immunity. The drug is available by the brand name Retrovir.   *(3:1856–9)*

30e. (E) Patients on Retrovir are at risk of developing granulocytopenia or anemia that may require discontinuation of the medication or blood transfusions. It is therefore important to closely monitor the patient's hematological status while on Retrovir therapy.   *(3:1859)*

30f. (B) Retrovir capsules are administered every 4 hours around the clock, even though it may interrupt normal sleep. This is necessary because of the rapid absorption and rapid clearance of the drug from the body.   *(3:1856)*

30g. (A) Acetaminophen use may competitively inhibit the glucuronidation of zidovudine (Retrovir). This may increase the likelihood of granulocytopenia developing with the use of Retrovir.   *(3:1857)*

30h. (D) Pentamidine isethionate (Pentam 300, Nebu-

Pent) is an agent that is useful in the treatment of *Pneumocystis carinii* pneumonia. It is available as an injectable product that may be administered intravenously or intramuscularly and as an aerosol solution administered by inhalation using a nebulizer.

(3:1892)

30i. (A) Patients receiving pentamidine must be monitored for a variety of serious adverse effects, includ-

ing sudden, severe hypotension that may occur after a single parenteral dose. Other adverse effects include hypoglycemia, bronchospasm, and cough.

(3:1891)

30j. (C) Robitussin DM is an OTC product used for the treatment of cough. It contains guaifenesin, an expectorant, and dextromethorphan HBr, a cough suppressant.

(3:998)

CHAPTER 8

Practice Test

You have come a long way to get here. You have completed hundreds of test items and have studied thirty medication profiles and records. This practice test should confirm what you may already feel, ie confidence that your time and effort have been well spent. You should set aside about 2 hours of uninterrupted time to take this test. You should be able to answer 80 or more Practice Test questions without guessing, since most test the same competencies that you mastered in previous chapters.

Of course, the Practice Test is also a learning and self-assessment experience. Correct answers will build your confidence in the knowledge base that you have developed. Incorrect answers will enable you to focus on specific areas that may require more time for you to master. Good luck!

Questions

DIRECTIONS (Questions 1 through 100): Each of the numbered items or incomplete statements in this section is followed by answers or by completions of the statement. Select the ONE lettered answer or completion that is BEST in each case.

1. One course of fluorouracil therapy is 6 mg/kg twice a day for 4 days. How many mg will be given daily to a 140-lb patient?

   (A) 48
   (B) 380
   (C) 760
   (D) 1500
   (E) 3040

2. According to the National Bureau of Standards (NBS), the initial calibration mark on a 250-mL graduate should be

   (A) 10 mL
   (B) 25 mL
   (C) 50 mL
   (D) 75 mL
   (E) 100 mL

3. The most common type of drug transport in humans is

   (A) active transport
   (B) passive transport
   (C) facilitated transport
   (D) Newtonian transport
   (E) pinocytosis

4. The drug of choice for the treatment of estrogen–receptor–positive breast cancer is considered to be

   (A) mercaptopurine
   (B) methotrexate
   (C) procarbazine
   (D) prednisone
   (E) tamoxifen

5. Which of the following is NOT a common adverse effect associated with the use of tricyclic antidepressants?

   (A) hirsutism
   (B) sedation
   (C) orthostatic hypotension
   (D) dry mouth
   (E) urinary retention

6. An elixir contains 100 μg of drug per teaspoon dose. How many mg are present in each mL?

   (A) 0.02
   (B) 0.025
   (C) 0.1
   (D) 2.0
   (E) 20

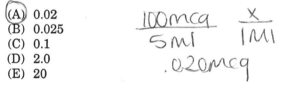

7. The most common ingredient in sodium-free salt substitute products such as Nu-Salt is

   (A) potassium chloride
   (B) calcium chloride
   (C) ammonium chloride
   (D) aluminum chloride
   (E) potassium nitrate

8. Generic product A has a greater AUC than generic product B, containing the same quantity of drug per dose. One can conclude that

   (A) product A is more bioavailable than B
   (B) product B is more bioavailable than A
   (C) product A has a shorter half-life than B
   (D) product B has a shorter half-life than A
   (E) product A is more readily excreted in the urine than B

9. Which one of the following drugs will NOT cause miosis of the pupil when instilled in the eye?

   (A) echothiophate
   (B) carbachol

(C) physostigmine
(D) pilocarpine
(E) timolol

10. Misoprostol (Cytotec) can best be described as a(n)

(A) ulcer-adherent complex
(B) anticholinergic
(C) H_2-receptor antagonist
(D) synthetic prostaglandin analog
(E) abortifacient

11. A hospital pharmacist adds 100 mL of Alcohol USP (95% V/V ethanol) to 1 L of cough syrup that contains 8% V/V ethanol. What is the new percentage of ethanol present in the mixture?

(A) 10
(B) 12
(C) 14
(D) 16
(E) 18

12. Which of the following needles is most suited for the administration of insulin products?

(A) 16G 5/8″
(B) 21G 1/2″
(C) 21G 5/8″
(D) 25G 5/8″
(E) 25G 1″

13. Assuming first-order kinetics, the characteristic that readily allows the calculation of time to reach plasma steady-state is the drug's

(A) AUC
(B) F value
(C) absorption constant
(D) elimination constant
(E) half-life

14. Midamor is most similar in action to

(A) Bumex
(B) HydroDIURIL
(C) Diamox
(D) Dyrenium
(E) Lasix

15. A patient with an abnormally elevated number of erythrocytes is said to have

(A) macrocytic anemia
(B) microcytic anemia
(C) purpura
(D) aplastic anemia
(E) polycythemia

16. A dietician adds 5 g of potassium chloride to 500 mL of an enteral formula. How many milliequivalents of potassium are present? (K = 39; Cl = 35.5; KCl = 74.5)

(A) 33.546.9
(B) 45
(C) 67
(D) 128
(E) 134

17. The agent most likely to precipitate when added to D5W or NS is

(A) folic acid (Folvite)
(B) ethacrynic acid (Edecrin)
(C) tobramycin sulfate (Nebcin)
(D) diazepam (Valium)
(E) ascorbic acid

18. Sodium bicarbonate is likely to increase the rate of urinary elimination of
   I. cocaine HCl
   II. penicillin G potassium
   III. phenobarbital sodium

(A) I only
(B) III only
(C) I and II only
(D) II and III only
(E) I, II, and III

19. Which one of the following cephalosporins has the greatest activity against gram-negative microorganisms?

(A) cefaclor (Ceclor)
(B) cefazolin (Ancef, Kefzol)
(C) cefonicid (Monocid)
(D) ceftizoxime (Cefizox)
(E) cephalexin (Keflex)

20. Peripheral veins are SELDOM used for the administration of

(A) TPN solutions
(B) cephalosporins
(C) vitamin infusions
(D) heparin
(E) electrolyte infusions

21. How many mL of glycerin would be needed to prepare 1 lb of an ointment containing 8.5% (W/W) glycerin? The density of glycerin is 1.25 g/mL.

(A) 10.6
(B) 18.5
(C) 30.9
(D) 32.6
(E) 48.2

Questions 22 through 25

Questions 22 through 25 are based on the following order received from a hospital outpatient clinic:

For: Happy Hospital Ophthalmology Clinic
Rx

Atropine sulfate	0.25%
Boric acid	1.0%
Pur. Water qs	60 mL

Please make isotonic and sterilize.
Label as "Atropine sulfate 0.25% ophthalmic solution"

22. Boric acid is present in the formula as a(n)
    I. antimicrobial preservative
    II. buffering agent
    III. chelating agent

    (A) I only
    (B) III only
    (C) I and II only
    (D) II and III only
    (E) I, II, and III

23. How many milligrams of sodium chloride are required to adjust the tonicity of the formula? (The following "E" values are available: atropine sulfate = 0.20; boric acid = 0.50.)

    (A) 210
    (B) 330
    (C) 425
    (D) 540
    (E) 900

24. The most practical method for sterilizing this ophthalmic solution is

    (A) autoclaving for 15 minutes
    (B) autoclaving for 30 minutes
    (C) membrane filtration through an 0.2-μ filter
    (D) membrane filtration through a 5-μ filter
    (E) the use of ethylene oxide gas

25. Kwell Lotion is indicated for the treatment of conditions caused by
    I. *Sarcoptes scabiei*
    II. *Pediculus capitis*
    III. tinea versicolor

    (A) I only
    (B) III only
    (C) I and II only
    (D) II and III only
    (E) I, II, and III

26. An administration set delivers 50 drops to the mL. How many drops per minute are needed to obtain 12 units of heparin per minute if the IV admixture contains 10,000 units of heparin per 500 mL of normal saline?

    (A) 30
    (B) 60
    (C) 20
    (D) 600
    (E) 40

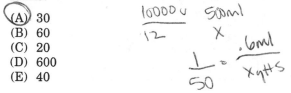

27. Which of the following would be likely to render benzalkonium chloride solution inactive?

    (A) acetic acid
    (B) *Pseudomonas aeruginosa*
    (C) ethanol
    (D) sodium stearate
    (E) sodium chloride

28. Fick's law is related to

    (A) complexation
    (B) viscosity
    (C) diffusion
    (D) adsorption
    (E) buffers

29. The naturally occurring enkephalins, endorphins, and dynorphins are chemically classified as

    (A) alkaloids
    (B) peptides
    (C) phospholipids
    (D) polysaccharides
    (E) prostaglandins

30. A drug approved by the FDA for the treatment of enuresis is

    (A) furosemide (Lasix)
    (B) nitrofurantoin (Macrodantin)
    (C) imipramine (Tofranil)
    (D) nadolol (Corgard)
    (E) hydroxyurea (Hydrea)

31. How many milliliters of a 1:150 stock solution of atropine sulfate would be needed to prepare the following prescription?

Rx

Atropine sulfate	0.5%	Normal
saline	qs.	30.0 mL

    (A) 45.0
    (B) 15.0
    (C) 66.7
    (D) 22.5
    (E) 17.8

32. The Henderson-Hasselbalch equation can be used to determine the pH of a
   I.   mixture of lactic acid and sodium lactate
   II. 0.15 mol/L hydrochloric acid
   III. 2% morphine sulfate solution

   (A) I only
   (B) III only
   (C) I and II only
   (D) II and III only
   (E) I, II, and III

33. A high F value for a drug indicates that the drug is

   (A) very bioavailable
   (B) very soluble in water
   (C) chemically unstable
   (D) susceptible to hepatic first pass metabolism
   (E) renally eliminated

34. The product Sinemet 25/100 contains

   (A) carbidopa 25 mg + levodopa 100 mg
   (B) carbidopa 100 mg + levodopa 25 mg
   (C) HCTZ 25 mg + propranolol 100 mg
   (D) HCTZ 25 mg + triamterene 100 mg
   (E) HCTZ 100 mg + triamterene 25 mg

35. A drug commonly employed in the treatment of acute morphine overdose is

   (A) naloxone
   (B) propranolol
   (C) chlordiazepoxide
   (D) metolazone
   (E) disulfiram

36. How many grams of hydrocortisone powder must be added to 2 lb of 1% W/W hydrocortisone cream to obtain a 4% W/W cream?

   (A) 20
   (B) 23
   (C) 27
   (D) 28
   (E) 38

Questions 37 through 39

Answer questions 37 through 39 based upon the following prescription:

Rx		
Phenylephrine HCl		0.5%
Menthol		
Thymol		aa 2.0%
Methyl salicylate		0.5%
Mineral oil	qs	30 mL

Sig: gtt ii both sides t.i.d.

37. Which of the following ingredients will NOT dissolve in the prescribed solvent?
   I.   menthol
   II. methyl salicylate
   III. phenylephrine HCl

   (A) I only
   (B) III only
   (C) I and II only
   (D) II and III only
   (E) I, II, and III

38. This prescription is intended for use in the

   (A) eyes
   (B) nose
   (C) ears
   (D) lungs
   (E) buccal cavity

39. In compounding this prescription, which of the following would be useful to employ?

   (A) eutexia
   (B) levigation
   (C) fusion
   (D) trituration by intervention
   (E) emulsification

40. An order for a TPN formula requests 500 mL of D30W. How many mL of D50W may be used if D30W is not available?

   (A) 200
   (B) 300
   (C) 400
   (D) 500
   (E) 600

41. The decay constant of a radioisotope is 0.69/h. The half-life of the radioisotope is

   (A) 100 h
   (B) 1 h
   (C) 10 h
   (D) 14 h
   (E) 69 h

42. Which of the following is true of active transport systems?
   I.   They do not consume energy.
   II. They never become saturated.
   III. They do not reach equilibrium.

   (A) I only
   (B) III only
   (C) I and II only
   (D) II and III only
   (E) I, II, and III

43. Which of the following agents are useful in the treatment of patients who are HIV positive and show signs of immunological deficiency?
    I. pentamidine isethionate
    II. zidovudine
    III. acyclovir

    (A) I only
    (B) III only
    (C) I and II only
    (D) II and III only
    (E) I, II, and III

44. Patients with PKU disease should avoid foods containing

    (A) arginine
    (B) sodium
    (C) tyramine
    (D) vitamin A
    (E) aspartame

45. A pharmacist has 80 mL of a 1.5% benzalkonium chloride solution. What will be the final ratio strength if he or she dilutes this solution to 1500 mL with purified water?

    (A) 1:1250
    (B) 1:120
    (C) 1:100
    (D) 1:1875
    (E) 1:2250

46. Which of the following are mixtures containing both aluminum hydroxide and magnesium hydroxide?
    I. ALternaGEL
    II. Riopan
    III. Mylanta II

    (A) I only
    (B) III only
    (C) I and II only
    (D) II and III only
    (E) I, II, and III

47. The peak of the serum concentration vs time curve approximates the time when

    (A) the maximum pharmacologic effect occurs
    (B) all of the drug has been absorbed from the GI tract
    (C) absorption and elimination of the drug has equalized
    (D) saturation of metabolizing enzymes has occurred
    (E) renal elimination of the drug begins

48. The pharmacist should advise a patient who has just received a prescription for prazosin 2 mg t.i.d. to take the initial dose

    (A) at noon
    (B) at bedtime

    (C) in the morning before breakfast
    (D) in the morning after breakfast
    (E) 1 hour before the evening meal

49. A disease characterized by inflammation of layers of the intestinal tract is

    (A) Bright's disease
    (B) Goeckerman's disease
    (C) Graves' disease
    (D) Crohn's disease
    (E) Cushing's disease

50. Which one of the following pharmaceutical adjuvants is most likely to cause asthma-like reactions in a certain number of patients?

    (A) benzalkonium chloride
    (B) benzyl alcohol
    (C) edetate
    (D) methylparaben
    (E) sodium bisulfite

51. A drug is said to have a biologic half-life of 2 hours. At the end of 8 hours, what percentage of the drug's original activity will remain?

    (A) 6.25
    (B) 12.5
    (C) 25
    (D) 50
    (E) 2.5

52. Moban is used as an

    (A) anticholinergic
    (B) immunosuppressant
    (C) antidepressant
    (D) antipsychotic
    (E) anti-inflammatory agent

Questions 53 through 56

Questions 53 through 56 refer to the following prescription:

For: David Harris	Age: 14
Rx	
Codeine phosphate	90 mg
Diphendydramine	900 mg
NAPAP	2500 mg
Ft. Cap. #12	
Sig: 1 q.i.d. p.r.n. pain	

Note: The pharmacist has 50 mg diphenhydramine capsules, each containing 130 mg of powdered contents as well as 1/4 grain codeine phosphate tablets, each weighing 90 mg. The NAPAP is available as a pure powder.

53. Which of the following statements concerning this prescription is (are) true?

   I. The amount of codeine being consumed per dose is an overdose.

   II. There is a chemical incompatibility between diphenhydramine and codeine phosphate.

   III. The patient should be cautioned about the possibility of drowsiness from the capsules.

   (A) I only
   (B) III only
   (C) I and II only
   (D) II and III only
   (E) I, II, and III

54. The final weight of each capsule will be approximately

   (A) 270 mg
   (B) 450 mg
   (C) 340 mg
   (D) 180 mg
   (E) 410 mg

55. Aminophylline Injection is likely to be compatible with which of the following parenteral solutions?

   I. Dopamine HCL
   II. Verapamil HCl
   III. Heparin

   (A) I only
   (B) III only
   (C) I and II only
   (D) II and III only
   (E) I, II, and III

56. To avoid coring of the rubber closure, the pharmacist should insert the needle at a _____ degree angle to the horizon.

   (A) 20
   (B) 45
   (C) 90
   (D) 120
   (E) 180

57. A tine test is employed in identifying patients who have been exposed to

   (A) acquired immunodeficiency syndrome
   (B) influenza
   (C) hepatitis virus
   (D) tuberculosis
   (E) herpes simplex

58. Nifedipine is classified as a(n)

   (A) narcotic antagonist
   (B) antihistamine
   (C) narcotic agonist
   (D) beta-adrenergic receptor blocker
   (E) calcium entry blocker

59. A patient is using hydrochlorothiazide (Hydro-DIURIL) and guanethidine (Ismelin) for the treatment of hypertension. This patient should not receive

   (A) potassium supplementation
   (B) tricyclic antidepressants
   (C) aluminum-containing antacids
   (D) folic acid supplementation
   (E) antihistamines

60. Which of the following is an example of an absorption base?

   (A) polyethylene glycol ointment
   (B) cold cream
   (C) Jelene
   (D) Eucerin w/o
   (E) white petrolatum

Questions 61 through 66

Answer questions 61 through 66 based upon the following prescription:

Rx	
Burow's solution	10 mL
Salicylic acid	4%
Phenol	1%
White petrolatum	qs 60 g

Sig: apply to affected area t.i.d.

61. The active ingredient in Burow's solution is

   (A) alum
   (B) acetic acid
   (C) aluminum chloride
   (D) calcium hydroxide
   (E) none of the above

62. When preparing this prescription the pharmacist may wish to include

   I. Aquaphor
   II. polysorbate 80
   III. alcohol

   (A) I only
   (B) III only
   (C) I and II only
   (D) II and III only
   (E) I, II, and III

63. The most appropriate way to incorporate salicylic acid into this product is by

   (A) levigation
   (B) fusion
   (C) dissolution in alcohol
   (D) trituration
   (E) attrition

64. The concentration (% W/W) of Burow's solution in the final preparation will be

    (A) 10
    (B) 16.7
    (C) 22.5
    (D) 20.0
    (E) 13.4

65. Which of the following may be employed as one of the ingredients of this prescription?

    (A) lactic acid
    (B) aspirin
    (C) thymol
    (D) salicylamide
    (E) carbolic acid

66. The function of salicylic acid in this product is as a(n)

    (A) preservative
    (B) local anesthetic
    (C) analgesic
    (D) keratolytic
    (E) abrasive

67. Which one of the following may be considered a viral disease?

    (A) pertussis
    (B) tuberculosis
    (C) hepatitis
    (D) cholera
    (E) typhoid fever

68. Retinoic acid is used therapeutically

    (A) by the oral route only
    (B) to accelerate the production of epithelial cells in the skin
    (C) to reverse the symptoms of psoriasis
    (D) to promote healing of actinic keratoses
    (E) to treat malignant melanoma

69. Which of the following drugs is indicated for the treatment of gout?
    I. colchicine
    II. probenecid (Benemid)
    III. sulfinpyrazone (Anturane)

    (A) I only
    (B) III only
    (C) I and II only
    (D) II and III only
    (E) I, II, and III

70. Oxidation will cause solutions of which of the following to turn pink?
    — I. epinephrine
    II. aminophylline
    III. vitamin B_{12}

    (A) I only
    (B) III only
    (C) I and II only
    (D) I and III only
    (E) I, II, and III

71. Which of the following is true of cholestyramine resin?

    (A) It is not absorbed from the GI tract.
    (B) It is a cationic exchange resin.
    (C) It increases the synthesis of cholesterol.
    (D) It is commercially available as a viscous syrup.
    (E) It will solubilize gallstones.

72. In addition to being used as an anticonvulsant, phenytoin (Dilantin) is also used in treating

    (A) tuberculosis
    (B) Parkinson's disease
    (C) systemic lupus erythematosus
    (D) cardiac arrhythmias
    (E) cataracts

73. The HLB system is used to classify

    (A) the danger of drugs in pregnant patients
    (B) droplet size of aerosols
    (C) pharmaceutical dyes
    (D) drug solubility
    (E) surfactants

74. Terfenadine (Seldane) can best be classified pharmacologically as an

    (A) antidepressant
    (B) H_1-receptor antagonist
    (C) antihypertensive agent
    (D) antipsychotic
    (E) H_2-receptor antagonist

75. A nurse informs you that a patient has polydipsia. This refers to

    (A) excessive urination
    (B) excessive craving for food
    (C) excessive thirst
    (D) diarrhea
    (E) double vision

76. Which one of the following body areas usually has the lowest (most acidic) pH?

    (A) blood
    (B) lacrimal fluid
    (C) oral cavity
    (D) skin
    (E) vagina

77. Monopril is most similar in action to

(A) Dyrenium
(B) Calan
(C) Minipress
(D) Lotrisone
(E) Capoten

78. A drug interaction is likely to occur when 6-mercaptopurine (Purinethol) is used with

(A) aspirin
(B) pyridoxine
(C) allopurinol (Zyloprim)
(D) streptokinase (Streptase)
(E) iron products

79. Phenolphthalein is employed in pharmaceutical products as a(n)

(A) buffer
(B) laxative
(C) chelating agent
(D) viscosity builder
(E) antifoaming agent

80. Acetylcysteine (Mucomyst) exerts its mucolytic effect by

(A) complexing with mucus protein
(B) altering the normal synthesis order of DNA
(C) altering the cellular synthesis of mucoproteins
(D) breaking chemical bonds of mucoproteins
(E) increasing the secretion of low viscosity mucus from the walls of the respiratory tract

81. A patient's chart reveals a hypersensitivity to penicillin. The patient should be suspected of exhibiting a similar reaction to

(A) cefixime (Suprax)
(B) erythromycin
(C) vancomycin (Vancocin)
(D) nystatin (Mycostatin)
(E) phenazopyridine (Pyridium)

82. An antacid that is most likely to induce gastric hypersecretion is

(A) calcium carbonate
(B) bismuth subgallate
(C) aluminum hydroxide
(D) magnesium hydroxide
(E) glycine

83. Which of the following is utilized in the treatment of viral infections?

(A) albuterol
(B) propranolol
(C) misoprostol
(D) amantadine
(E) bioflavonoid

84. A patient's blood test reveals an excessively high level of amylase. This may indicate a disease of the

(A) liver
(B) heart
(C) kidney
(D) lung
(E) pancreas

85. Basal thermometers and rectal thermometers are similar in that both
   I. have the same degree of accuracy
   II. can be used to determine ovulation
   III. can be used orally

(A) I only
(B) III only
(C) I and II only
(D) I and III only
(E) I, II, and III

86. Patients with estrogen-dependent neoplasms often benefit from the use of

(A) oral contraceptives
(B) methotrexate
(C) cyanocobalamin
(D) tamoxifen
(E) cisplatin

87. Another name for diacetylmorphine is

(A) codeine
(B) heroin
(C) dionin
(D) cocaine
(E) methadone

88. A patient receiving isocarboxazid (Parnate) should be advised to

(A) avoid foods high in potassium
(B) avoid foods high in tyramine
(C) avoid foods high in sodium
(D) avoid foods high in vitamin K
(E) consume a low-fat diet

89. Dextranomer (Debrisan) is employed pharmaceutically as a(n)

(A) topical corticosteroid
(B) plasma expander
(C) antipsoriatic agent
(D) abrasive cleanser for the skin
(E) absorbant for secreting wounds

90. The antidiarrheal Donnagel contains belladonna alkaloids and

(A) attapulgite
(B) bismuth subsalicylate
(C) docusate
(D) gelatin
(E) kaolin

91. A drug of choice for the treatment of typhoid fever is

    (A) nafcillin (Unipen)
    (B) vancomycin (Vancocin)
    (C) sulfasalazine (Azulfidine)
    (D) chloramphenicol (Chloromycetin)
    (E) ganciclovir (Cytovene)

92. Polyvinyl alcohol is commonly employed in pharmaceutical systems as a

    (A) viscosity builder
    (B) preservative
    (C) buffer
    (D) lubricant
    (E) solvent

93. Which of the following drugs exhibits H_2-receptor antagonist activity?
      I. Zantac
     II. Tagamet
    III. Pepcid

    (A) I only
    (B) III only
    (C) I and II only
    (D) II and III only
    (E) I, II, and III

94. The hub of a needle is

    (A) the portion that fits onto the syringe
    (B) the needle shaft
    (C) the portion of the needle that is ground for sharpness
    (D) the needle hole
    (E) the needle bevel

95. The use of which of the following drugs is associated with the development of a systemic lupus erythematosus (SLE)-like syndrome?

    (A) probenecid (Benemid)
    (B) phenobarbital
    (C) nitrofurantoin (Macrodantin)
    (D) diazepam (Valium)
    (E) hydralazine (Apresoline)

96. Which of the following drugs is least likely to interact with cholestyramine (Questran)?

    (A) phenobarbital
    (B) warfarin
    (C) codeine
    (D) chlorothiazide
    (E) penicillin

97. Folic acid supplementation should be provided to patients chronically using

    (A) phenytoin (Dilantin)
    (B) propranolol (Inderal)
    (C) levodopa (Larodopa)
    (D) sulindac (Clinoril)
    (E) tetracycline (Achromycin V)

98. Vasopressin is a hormone elaborated by the

    (A) anterior pituitary gland
    (B) posterior pituitary gland
    (C) adrenal gland
    (D) pancreas
    (E) kidney

99. An inverse relationship exists between the concentration of calcium in the blood and the blood concentration of

    (A) magnesium
    (B) thyroid hormone
    (C) testosterone
    (D) sodium
    (E) phosphorus

100. Drug metabolites are generally

    (A) more lipid soluble than their parent compound
    (B) referred to as "prodrugs"
    (C) eliminated more slowly from the body than their parent compound
    (D) more water soluble than their parent compound
    (E) incapable of producing pharmacologic effects

Answers

1. (C)	30. (C)
2. (C)	31. (D)
3. (B)	32. (E)
4. (E)	33. (A)
5. (A)	34. (A)
6. (A)	35. (A)
7. (A)	36. (D)
8. (A)	37. (B)
9. (E)	38. (B)
10. (D)	39. (A)
11. (D)	40. (B)
12. (D)	41. (B)
13. (E)	42. (B)
14. (D)	43. (C)
15. (E)	44. (E)
16. (C)	45. (A)
17. (D)	46. (A)
18. (D)	47. (C)
19. (D)	48. (B)
20. (A)	49. (D)
21. (C)	50. (E)
22. (C)	51. (A)
23. (A)	52. (D)
24. (C)	53. (B)
25. (C)	54. (B)
26. (A)	55. (B)
27. (D)	56. (E)
28. (C)	57. (D)
29. (B)	58. (E)

59. (B)	**81.** (A)
60. (D)	**82.** (A)
61. (E)	**83.** (D)
62. (A)	**84.** (E)
63. (A)	**85.** (D)
64. (B)	**86.** (D)
65. (E)	**87.** (B)
66. (D)	**88.** (B)
67. (C)	**89.** (E)
68. (B)	**90.** (C)
69. (E)	**91.** (D)
70. (E)	**92.** (A)
71. (A)	**93.** (E)
72. (D)	**94.** (A)
73. (E)	**95.** (E)
74. (B)	**96.** (C)
75. (C)	**97.** (A)
76. (B)	**98.** (B)
77. (E)	**99.** (E)
78. (C)	**100.** (D)
79. (B)	
80. (D)	

APPENDIX A

Frequently Dispensed Drugs

The practicing pharmacist should be familiar with commonly prescribed pharmaceutical products. If given the generic name, he or she should be able to match the following information with the drug:

1. brand or tradename
2. general pharmacological category or use
3. commonly available dosage forms
4. available strengths
5. names of other products with identical or similar ingredients

The table contains the following abbreviations:

COMPANIES		DRUGS	
B-W	Burroughs Wellcome	ASA	aspirin
M-J	Mead Johnson	APAP	acetaminophen
MSD	Merck Sharp & Dohme	HCTZ	hydrochlorthiazide
P-D	Parke-Davis	NSAID	nonsteroidal anti-inflammatory drug
R-PR	Rhone-Poulenc Rorer	PE	phenylephrine
SK-B	Smith Kline-Beecham	PPA	phenylpropanolamine
W-C	Warner Chilcott		
USV	United States Vitamin		

TABLE OF FREQUENTLY DISPENSED DRUGS

Generic Name	Tradename & Company	Category or Use	Dosage Forms and Strengths
Acetaminophen	Tylenol (McNeil)	analgesic	tablet; elixir
Acyclovir sodium	Zovirax (B-W)	treatment of herpes	injection vial (600 mg); cap 200 mg; ointment 5%; suspension
Albuterol repetabs; aerosol;	Proventil (Schering) Ventolin (Glaxo)	bronchodilator	tab (2 & 4 mg); syrup; inhalation nebulizer solution
Allopurinol	Zyloprim (B-W)	treatment of hyperuricemia (gout, etc)	tab (100 & 300 mg)
Alprazolam	Xanax (Upjohn)	treatment of anxiety	tab (0.25, 0.5, & 1 mg)
Amitriptyline HCl	Elavil (MSD)	antidepressant	tab (10, 25, 50, 75, 100 & 150 mg); injection
Amoxicillin	Amoxil (SK-B) Polymox (Apothecon) Trimox (Apothecon) Wymox (Wyeth)	broad-spectrum antibiotic	cap (250 & 500 mg); suspension
Amoxicillin + clavulanate K	Augmentin (SK-B)	broad-spectrum antibiotic	tab (250 & 500 mg); chewable tab (125 & 250 mg); suspensions
Ampicillin	Omnipen (Wyeth) Principen (Squibb) Polycillin (Bristol) Totacillin (Beecham)	same as above	capsules and suspensions (250 & 500 mg)
Aspirin with codeine	Empirin with codeine (B-W)	analgesic; antitussive	tabs–No. 1 (1/8 gr), No. 2 (1/4 gr), No. 3 (1/2 g), No. 4 (1 g)
Astemizole	Hismanal (Janssen)	antihistamine (H_1- receptor antagonist)	tab (10 mg)
Atenolol	Tenormin (ICI Pharma)	antihypertensive (beta-adrenergic blocking agent)	tab (50 & 100 mg)
Atenolol + chlorthalidone	Tenoretic (ICI Pharma)	same	tab 50 = 50 mg + 25 mg tab 100 = 100 mg + 25 mg
Beclomethasone dipropionate	Vanceril, Vancenase AQ (both Schering) Beconase AQ (Allen & Hanburys)	bronchodilator to treat rhinits	inhalation aerosol; aerosol nasal inhaler
Benztropine	Cogentin (MSD)	skeletal muscle relaxant (mainly for Parkinsonism)	tab (0.5, 1, & 2 mg) injection
Betaxolol HCl	Betoptic (Alcon)	treat open angle glaucoma	ophthalmic sol (0.5%)
Bismuth subgallate, resorcin comp, hydrocortisone	Anusol HC (P-D)	anorectal prep. (treatment of hemorrhoids)	suppositories, cream
Brompheniramine maleate	Dimetane (Robins)	antihistamine (OTC)	tab (4 mg); elixir; tab (8 & 12 mg)
Same + PE HCl + PPA HCl	Dimetapp (Robins)	antihistamine; nasal decongestant (OTC)	tab; elixir
Bumetanide Inj.	Bumex (Roche)	diuretic	tab (0.5, 1, & 2 mg)
Buspirone HCl	Buspar (M-J)	antianxiety	tab (5 & 10 mg)
Butalbital + ASA + caffeine	Fiorinal (Sandoz)	sedative; analgesic	tab; capsule

TABLE OF FREQUENTLY DISPENSED DRUGS

Generic Name	Tradename & Company	Category or Use	Dosage Forms and Strengths
Butalbital, ASA, caffeine, + codeine	Fiorinal with codeine (Sandoz)	same	same
Butalbital, APAP, caffeine	Fioricet (Sandoz)	same	tab
Carbamazepine	Tegretol (Geigy)	anticonvulsant	tab (200 mg); chewable tab (100mg)
Carbidopa + levodopa	Sinemet (MSD)	antiparkinson agent	tab 10/100 (10 mg + 100 mg); 25/250 (25 mg + 250 mg)
Cefaclor	Ceclor (Lilly)	antibiotic	cap (250 & 500 mg); suspension
Cefadroxil	Duricef (M-J)	antibiotic	tab (1 g); cap (500 mg); suspension (125, 250, & 500 mg)
Cefixime	Suprax (Lederle)	antibiotic	tab (200 & 400 mg); pwd for suspension
Cefuroxime	Ceftin (Allen & Hanburys) Kefurox (Lilly) Zinacef (Glaxo)	antibiotic	tab (125, 250, & 500 mg) pwd for injection same
Cephalexin	Keflex (Dista)	antibiotic	tab (250 & 500 mg); suspension
Cephalexin HCl monohydrate	Keftab (Dista)	antibiotic	tab (250 & 500 mg)
Chlorhexidine gluconate	Peridex (Procter & Gamble)	microbicide	0.12% oral rinse
Chlorpropamide	Diabinese (Pfizer)	oral hypoglycemic	tab (100 & 250 mg)
Chlorthalidone	Hygroton (Rorer)	antihypertensive	tab (25, 50, & 100 mg)
Cholestyramine	Questran (Bristol)	antihyperlipidemic	powder
Cimetidine	Tagamet (SK-B)	prevent and treat peptic ulcers	tab (200, 400, & 800 mg); liquid; injection
Ciprofloxacin	Cipro (Miles)	broad-spectrum antibiotic (a fluoroquinolone)	tab (250, 500 & 750 mg); injection solution
Clemastine	Tavist-1 (Sandoz)	antihistamine (OTC)	tab
Clemastine + PPA	Tavist-D (Sandoz)	treat allergic rhinitis (OTC)	tab
Clindamycin	Cleocin (Upjohn)	antibiotic	cap (75, 150, & 300 mg)
Clindamycin topical	Cleocin T (Upjohn)	treatment of acne	gel; solution; lotion (all 10 mg/mL)
Clofibrate	Atromid-S (Ayerst)	antilipidemia	cap (500 mg)
Clonidine HCl	Catapres (Boehringer)	antihypertensive	tab (0.1, 0.2, & 0.3 mg); transdermal patches
Clonazepam	Klonopin (Roche)	Treatment of petit mal seizures	tab (0.5, 1, & 2 mg)
Clotrimazole	Gyne-Lotrimin (Schering) Lotrimin (Schering) Lotrimin AF (Schering) Mycelex-G (Miles)	broad spectrum antifungal	vaginal cream (1%); vag. tab (100 mg) cream; lotion; & solution (all 1%) AF = antifungal; same conc. as above but OTC tab; cream

TABLE OF FREQUENTLY DISPENSED DRUGS

Generic Name	Tradename & Company	Category or Use	Dosage Forms and Strengths
Clotrimazole + betamethasone	Lotrisone (Schering)	antifungal and anti-inflammatory	cream
Cromolyn sodium	Intal (Fisons)	management of asthma & rhinitis	aerosol spray; solution for nebulizer
	Nasalcrom (Fisons)		nasal solution
Cyclo-benzaprine	Flexeril (MSD)	skeletal muscle relaxant	tab (10 mg)
Desipramine	Norpramin (Merrell Dow)	antidepressant (tricyclic) [inhibits uptake of serotonin & norepinephrine]	tab (10, 25, 50, 75, 100, & 150 mg)
Diazepam	Valium (Roche)	antianxiety	tab (2, 5, & 10 mg)
	Valrelease (Roche)		caps (15 mg)
Diclofenac	Voltaren (Geigy)	NSAID	tab
Diflunisal	Dolobid (MSD)	NSAID, analgesic, antipyretic	tab (250 & 500 mg)
Digoxin	Lanoxin (B-W)	cardiovascular agent	tab (0.125, 0.25, & 0.5 mg); pediatric elix.; injection
	Lanoxicaps		cap (50, 100, & 200 µg)
Diltiazem	Cardizem (Marion)	antianginal agent	tab (30, 60, 90, & 120 mg); SR caps (60, 90, & 120 mg) for hypertension
Diphenoxylate HCl + atropine	Lomotil (Searle)	antidiarrheal	tab (2.5 mg); liquid
Dipivefrin	Propine (Allergan)	antiglaucoma	0.1% solution
Dipyridamole	Persantine (Boehringer)	antianginal agent	tab (25, 50, & 75 mg)
Disopyramide	Norpace (Searle)	antiarrhythmic	cap (100 & 150 mg); CR (100 & 150 mg)
Doxepin	Sinequan (Roerig)	antianxiety	cap (10, 25, 50, 75, 100, & 150 mg)
Doxycycline	Vibramycin Vibra-Tab (Pfizer)	broad-spectrum antibiotic	cap (50 & 100 mg); tab (100 mg)
Enalapril	Vasotec (MSD)	antihypertensive	tab (2.5, 5, 10, & 20 mg)
Enalapril + HCTZ	Vaseretic (MSD)		
Ergoloid mesylates	Hydergine (Sandoz)	treat select symptoms in elderly (improve mood, reduce confusion)	sublingual tab (0.5 & 1 mg); tab (1 mg); liquid
Erythromycin	E-Mycin (Boots)	broad-spectrum antibiotic	tab (250 & 500 mg); suspensions
	Erythrocin (Abbott)		
	Ery-Tab (Abbott)		delayed release tab (250 & 500 mg)
	ERYC (P-D)		enteric coated pellets in delayed release cap (250 mg)
	PCE (Abbott)		tab with polymer-coated particles (500 mg)
Erythromycin ethylsuccinate	E.E.S. (Abbott)		powder for susp.; chewable tab (200 mg); tab (400 mg); liq (200 & 400)
same + acetyl sulfisoxazole	Pediazole (Ross)		granules for suspension (200 + 600 mg)

TABLE OF FREQUENTLY DISPENSED DRUGS

Generic Name	Tradename & Company	Category or Use	Dosage Forms and Strengths
Erythromycin Estolate	Ilosone (Dista)		cap (125 & 250 mg); suspension
Erythromycin Stearate	Erythrocin Stearate (Abbott)		film-coated tab (250 & 500 mg
Estradiol Transdermal	Estraderm (Ciba)	moderate symptoms of menopause	transdermal patches (4 and 8 mg)
Estradiol	Estrace (M-J)	same; treatment of atrophic vaginitis	tab (1 & 2 mg); vaginal cream
Estrogen combinations	Demulen (Searle) Ovral (Wyeth) Ovral-28 (Wyeth) Triphasil (Wyeth) Nordette (Wyeth) Tri-Levlen (Berlex)	oral contraceptives	tab
Estrogens, conjugated	Premarin (Wyeth-Ayerst)	replacement therapy in menopause and postmenopause	tab (0.3, 0.625, 1.25, & 2.5 mg)
Estropipate	Ogen (Abbott)	estrogen replacement	tab (0.625, 1.25, 2.5, & 5 mg)
Ethinyl estadiol + norethindrone (+ 75 mg ferrous fumarate)	Loestrin 21 & Fe (P-D)	monophasic oral contraceptive	tab
	Ovcon 35; 50 (M-J)		tab
Famotidine	Pepcid (MSD)	treatment of peptic ulcers	tab (20 & 40 mg); pwd for susp.; injection
Fenoprofen	Nalfon (Dista)	antirheumatic	cap (200 & 300 mg)
Fluocinonide	Lidex (Syntex)	antipruritic, anti-inflammatory	oint; cream; gel
Fluoxetine	Prozac (Dista)	antidepressant	pulvules (20 mg)
Flurazepam	Dalmane (Roche)	treat insomnia	cap (15 & 30 mg)
Flurbiprofen	Ansaid (Upjohn)	NSAID	tab (50 & 100 mg)
Fluoride + vit A, D, & C	Tri-Vi-Flor (M-J)	vitamin supplement; prevent dental caries	drops; chewable tab
same + vit E, B's, niacin, pantothenic & folic acids	Poly-Vi-Flor (M-J)	same	same
Furosemide	Lasix (Hoechst)	diuretic	tab (20, 40, & 80 mg); injection
Gamma benzene hexachloride (Lindane)	Kwell (Reed & Carnrick)	ectoparasiticide (kill head and pubic lice)	liquid shampoo
Gemfibrozil	Lopid (P-D)	antihyperlipidemic	cap (300 mg); tab (600 mg)
Gentamicin	Garamycin (Schering)	broad-spectrum antibiotic	oint; cream; ophth. sol & oint; injection
Glipizide	Glucotrol (Roerig)	antihyperglycemic	tab (5 & 10 mg)
Glyburide	Micronase (Upjohn) DiaBeta (Hoechst)	antidiabetic	tab (1.25, 2.5, & 5 mg)

TABLE OF FREQUENTLY DISPENSED DRUGS

Generic Name	Tradename & Company	Category or Use	Dosage Forms and Strengths
Guanfacine	Tenex (Robins)	antihypertensive	tab (1 mg)
Haloperidol	Haldol (McNeil)	antipsychotic	tab (1, 2, 5, & 10 mg); liquid; injection
Hydrochlorthiazide	Esidrix (Ciba) HydroDIURIL (MSD)	diuretic, antihypertensive	tab (25 & 50 mg)
HCTZ + reserpine	Hydropres (MSD)	same	same + reserpine 0.125 mg
Hydrocodone bitartrate + APAP	Vicodin (Knoll) Lortab (Russ)	narcotic analgesic; antitussive [C III]	tablets = 5 mg + 500 mg ES = 7.5 mg + 750 mg) tab = 2.5 mg + 500 mg liq. = 2.5 mg + 120 mg
Hydrocortisone + polymyxin & neomycin	Cortisporin (B-W)	antibacterial; anti-inflammatory	otic sol; topical oint.
Hydroxyzine HCl	Atarax (Roerig)	antianxiety agent	tab (10, 25, 50, & 100 mg); injection
Hydroxyzine pamoate	Vistaril (Pfizer)	same	cap (25, 50, & 100 mg)
Ibuprofen	Motrin (Upjohn) Rufen (Boots)	NSAID	tab (400, 600, & 800 mg)
Indapamide	Lozol (Rorer)	antihypertensive & diuretic	tablet (2.5 mg)
Indomethacin	Indocin (MSD)	anti-inflammatory	cap (25 & 50 mg); SR (75 mg); susp.; suppository
Iodinated glycerol	Tussi-Organidin (Wallace)	antitussive, mucolytic	liquid
Ipratropium Br	Atrovent (Boehringer)	bronchodilator	inhalation aerosol
Isosorbide dinitrate	Isordil (Wyeth) Sorbitrate (ICI Pharma)	treatment of angina pectoris	oral tab (5 & 10 mg); sublingual tab (2.5 & 5 mg); chewable tab (5 mg-Sorbitrate) Isordil Tembids 40 mg cap & tab; Titradose 5, 10, 20, 30, & 40 mg); chewable tab (10 mg)
Ketoconazole	Nizoral (Janssen)	antifungal	tab (200 mg); suspension (100 mg/5 mL); cream
Ketoprofen	Orudis (Wyeth-Ayerst)	NSAID	cap (25, 50, & 75 mg)
Labetalol	Normodyne (Schering)	antihypertensive	tab (100, 200, & 300 mg); injection
Levothyroxine	Synthroid (Boots)	management of thyroid	tablets (0.025 to 0.3 mg)
Lisinopril	Prinivil (MSD) Zestril (Stuart)	antihypertensive	tab (5, 10, 20, & 40 mg)
Lithium carbonate	Eskalith (SKF)	treat manic depression	cap (300 mg); controlled release (450 mg)
Loperamide	Imodium (Janssen)	antidiarrheal	capsule (2 mg)
Lorazepam	Ativan (Wyeth)	antianxiety agent [C IV]	tab (1, 2, & 5 mg); injection
Lovastatin	Mevacor (MSD)	antihyperlipidemic agent	tab (20 & 40 mg)

TABLE OF FREQUENTLY DISPENSED DRUGS

Generic Name	Tradename & Company	Category or Use	Dosage Forms and Strengths
Meclizine	Antivert (Roerig)	antiemetic	tablets (12.5 & 25 mg)
Medroxyprogesterone	Provera (Upjohn)	estrogen replacement	tab (2.5, 5, & 10 mg)
Metaproterenol	Alupent (Boehringer)	bronchodilator	tab (10 & 20 mg); syrup; inhalation aerosol
Methyldopa	Aldomet (MSD)	antihypertensive	tab (125, 250, & 500 mg)
Methyldopa + HCTZ	Aldoril 15 or 25 (MSD) Aldoril D30 or D50	same	tab (250 mg + either 15 or 25 mg HCTZ) tab (500 mg + either 30 or 50 mg HCTZ)
Methylphenidate	Ritalin (Ciba)	cortical stimulant	tab (5, 10, 20 mg); SR 20 mg
Methylprednisolone	Medrol (Upjohn)	anti-inflammatory	tab (2, 4, 8, 16, 24, & 32 mg); topical 0.25 & 1%; inj. (20, 40, & 80 mg)
Metoclopramide	Reglan (Robins)	antinauseant (esp. cancer chemotherapy); stimulate GI tract motility	tab (10 mg); syrup; injection (10 mg/2 mL)
Metoprolol	Lopressor (Geigy)	adrenergic blocking agent (antihypertensive)	tab (50 & 100 mg)
Metronidazole	Flagyl (Searle)	trichomonacide	oral tab (250mg); vaginal tab (500 mg); injection
Miconazole nitrate	Monistat 7 Monistat 3 (Ortho)	treatment of vulvovaginal candidasis	cream (2%); vaginal supp. (200mg) vaginal supp. (100mg)
Minocycline HCl	Minocin (Lederle)	broad-spectrum antibiotic	cap (50 & 100 mg); syrup
Minoxidil	Rogaine (Upjohn)	stimulate growth of hair	solution (20 mg/mL)
Mupirocin	Bactroban (SK-B)	treatment of impetigo	2% ointment
Nadolol	Corgard (Princeton)	antihypertensive, treatment of angina	tab (40, 80, 120, & 160 mg)
Naproxen	Naprosyn (Syntex)	antirheumatic	tab (250, 375, & 500 mg); suspension
Naproxen sodium	Anaprox (Syntex)	same	tab (275 mg); Anaprox DS tab (550 mg)
Neomycin, polymyxin B, & bacitracin	Neosporin (B-W)	antibiotic combination	topical oint; ophthal. oint.
Nicotine polacrilex	Nicorette (Lakeside)	smoker's aid	chewing pieces (2 mg)
Nifedipine	Procardia (Pfizer) Procardia XL	calcium channel blocker	capsule (10 mg); XL = extended release (30, 60, & 90 mg) extended release (once daily) 30, 60, & 90 mg
Nitrofurantoin macrocrystals	Macrodantin (Norwich Eaton)	urinary tract antibacterial	capsules (25, 50 & 100 mg)
Nitroglycerin	Nitroglycerin (Lilly) Nitro-Bid (Marion) Nitrostat (P-D) Transderm-Nitro (Summit) Nitro-Dur II (Key)	treatment of angina	sublingual tablets (0.15, 0.3, 0.4, & 0.6 mg) cap (2.5 mg); prolonged release (6.5 mg); oint (2%) regular and SR (2.5, 6.5, & 9 mg) patches oint (2%); inject; patches

TABLE OF FREQUENTLY DISPENSED DRUGS

Generic Name	Tradename & Company	Category or Use	Dosage Forms and Strengths
Nizatidine	Axid (Lilly)	treatment of duodenal ulcers	cap (150 & 300 mg)
Norfloxacin	Noroxin (MSD)	broad-spectrum antibacterial	tab (400 mg)
Norgestrel + ethinyl estradiol pilpak	Ovral Lo/Ovral (Wyeth)	oral contraceptive	tab (0.5 + 0.05 mg) tab (0.3 + 0.03 mg)
Norethindrone acetate	Norlestrin (P-D)	same	tab (1 & 2.5 mg)
same + ethinyl estradiol	Ortho-Novum (Ortho) Ortho-Novum 7/7/7 (Ortho)	same	tab (0.5 mg + 35 µg)
Norethindrone + mestranol	Norinyl 1/50 (Syntex) Tri-Norinyl (Syntex)	same	tab (1 mg + 0.05 mg)
Nortriptyline HCl	Pamelor (Sandoz)	antidepressant	cap (10, 25, 50, & 75 mg)
Nystatin	Mycostatin (Squibb)	antifungal	oral tab (500,000 units); vag tab (100,000 units)
Omeprazole	Prilosec (MSD)	short-term treat. of active duodenal ulcers	sustained release cap (20 mg)
Ondansetron	Zofran (Glaxo)	antiemetic	injection (2 mg/mL)
Oxazepam	Serax (Wyeth)	antianxiety; antispasmodic	capsules (10, 15, & 30 mg); tablets (15 mg)
Oxycodone HCl + O. terephthalate + ASA	Percodan (DuPont)	analgesic; antipyretic	tab
Oxycodone HCl + acetaminophen	Percocet-5 (DuPont) Tylox (McNeil)	same	tab
Papaverine HCl	Pavabid (Marion)	peripheral vasodilator	capsule (150 mg)
Penicillin V potassium (Potassium phenoxymethyl penicillin)	Beepen VK (SK-B) Betapen-VK (Apothecon) Ledercillin VK (Lederle) Pen-Vee K (Wyeth) V-Cillin K (Lilly) Veetids (Apothecon)	antibiotic for gram-positive microorganisms	tablets and susp. of various strengths (usually 125, 250, & 500 mg, which are equivalent to 200,000, 400,000 & 800,000 units)
Pentoxifylline	Trental (Hoechst)	treatment of intermittent claudication	tab (400 mg)
Perphenazine + amitriptyline	Triavil (MSD) Etrafon (Schering)	tranquilizer, antidepreseant	tabs (2 + 10; 2 + 25; 4 + 10; 4 + 25 mg)
Phenobarbital with hyoscyamine, atropine, and scopolamine	Donnatal (Robins)	anticholinergic, antispasmodic	tab; cap; elixir

TABLE OF FREQUENTLY DISPENSED DRUGS

Generic Name	Tradename & Company	Category or Use	Dosage Forms and Strengths
Phenylephrine HCl, PPA, & Guaifenesin	Entex (Norwich) Entex LA	decongestant; expectorant	tablets (LA formula does not have phenylephrine)
Phenylephrine + PPA, phentoloxamine, & chlorpheniramine	Naldecon (Bristol)	nasal decongestant	tab; syrup
Phenytoin	Dilantin (P-D)	anticonvulsant	cap (30 & 100 mg); susp.; infatabs (50 mg)
Piroxicam	Feldene (Pfizer)	NSAID	cap (10 & 20 mg)
Polymyxin B, neomycin, gramicidin, & hydrocortisone	Cortisporin (B-W)	broad-spectrum antibiotic	cream
Potassium bicarbonate & citrate	K-Lyte (Bristol)	potassium supplement	effervescent tab (25 mEq of potassium per tablet)
Potassium chloride	K-Tab (Abbott) Klotrix (M-J) Slow-K (Summit) Micro-K (Robins) Klor-Con (Upsher-Smith) K-Dur (Key)	same	tablets (4 to 10 mEq of potassium per tablet) wax matrix tab (8 mEq) pwd (20 & 25 mEq); tab (8 & 10 mEq) controlled release tab (10 & 20 mEq)
Prazepam	Centrax (P-D)	antianxiety	cap (5, 10, & 20 mg); tab (10 mg)
Prazosin	Minipress (Pfizer)	antihypertensive	cap (1, 2, & 5 mg)
Same + polythiazide	Minizide (Pfizer)		cap (same + 0.5 mg)
Prednisone	Deltasone (Upjohn)	glucorticoid	tabs (2.5, 5, 10, 20 & 50 mg)
Probucol	Lorelco (Merrell-Dow)	antihyperlipidemic agent	tabs (250 & 500 mg)
Procainamide HCl	Pronestyl (Princeton) Procan SR (P-D)	treat premature ventricular contractions	cap (250 & 500 mg); filmlok tab (250, 375, & 500 mg) sustained release (250, 500 & 750 mg)
Prochlorperazine	Compazine (SKF)	antianxiety; antiemetic	tab (5, 10, 25 mg); spansule (10, 15, 30, & 75 mg); suppositories (2.5, 5, & 25 mg)
Promethazine HCl	Phenergan (Wyeth)	antihistamine; antiemetic	tab (12.5 & 25 mg); supp. (25 & 50 mg)
Propranolol HCl	Inderal (Wyeth-Ayerst)	treat angina, arrhythmias, etc	tab (10, 20, 40, 60, & 80 mg); LA cap (80, 120, & 160 mg)
Propranolol + HCTZ	Inderide (Wyeth-Ayerst)	antihypertensive	tab (40 or 80 + 25 mg HCTZ); cap (80, 120, 160 + 50 mg)
Propoxyphene napsylate + acetaminophen	Darvocet-N (Lilly) Propacet (Lemmon)	analgesic	tab (50 & 100 mg with 325 or 650 mg APAP)
Ranitidine HCl	Zantac (Glaxo)	H_2 antagonist	tab (150 & 300 mg); syrup (150 mg/10 mL); injection (25 mg/mL)
Spironolactone	Aldactone (Searle)	antihypertensive; K-sparing diuretic	tab (25 mg)

TABLE OF FREQUENTLY DISPENSED DRUGS

Generic Name	Tradename & Company	Category or Use	Dosage Forms and Strengths
Same + HCTZ	Aldactazide (Searle)	same	tab (25 + 25 or 50 + 50 mg)
Sucralfate	Carafate (Marion)	treat peptic ulcers	tab (1 g)
Sulfonamide	Bleph-10 (Allergan)	ophthalmic antibacterial	ophthalmic solution (10%)
	Sulamyd (Schering)		ophth. sol. (10 & 30%)
Sulindac	Clinoril (MSD)	antiarthritic	tab (150 & 200 mg)
Tamoxifen	Nolvadex (ICI Pharma)	antiestrogen	tab (10 mg)
Temazepam	Restoril (Sandoz)	sedative/hypnotic	cap (15 & 30 mg)
Terazosin	Hytrin (Abbott)	antihypertensive	tabs (1, 2, 5, & 10 mg)
Terbutaline	Bricanyl (Marion Merrill Dow) Brethine (Geigy)	bronchodilator	tabs (2.5 & 5 mg)
Terconazole	Terazol (Ortho)	vaginal antifungal (candidiasis only)	Terazol 7 cream; Terazol 3 supp
Terfenadine	Seldane (Merrell)	treat seasonal rhinitis	tab (60 mg)
Tetracycline HCl	Achromycin V (Lederle) Robitet (Robins)	broad-spectrum antibiotic	cap (250 & 500 mg); suspension
Tetracycline Phosphate	Sumycin (Squibb)	broad-spectrum antibiotic	cap (250 & 500 mg); suspension
Theophylline	Elixophyllin (Forest)	treat bronchial asthma and reversible bronchospasms	elixir (80 mg/15 mL)
	Slo-Phyllin (R-P R)		cap (125 & 250 mg)
	Slo-bid (R-P R)	(contains anhydrous theo.)	cap (50, 100, 200, & 300 mg)
	Theo-Dur (Key)		sustained action tab (100, 200, 300, & 450 mg); sprinkle
Thioridazine HCl	Mellaril (Sandoz)	tranquilizer	tab (10, 25, 50, 100, 150, & 200 mg)
Thiothixene	Navane (Roerig)	antipsychotic	cap (1, 2, 5, 10, & 20 mg); liq. concentrate 5 mg/mL
Timolol maleate	Timoptic (MSD)	treat glaucoma	ophth sol (0.25 & 0.5%)
	Blocadren (MSD)	antihypertensive	tab (5, 10, & 20 mg)
Same + HCTZ	Timolide (MSD)	same	tab (10mg + 25mg HCTZ)
Trazodone HCl	Desyrel (M-J)	antidepressant	tab (50, 100, & 150 mg)
Tretinoin	Retin-A (Ortho)	treat acne vulgaris	cream; gel; liquid
Triamcinolone acetonide	Kenalog (Squibb)	anti-inflammatory	cream; oint; topical aerosol
	Azmacort (R-PR)	treatment of asthma	inhalation aerosol

TABLE OF FREQUENTLY DISPENSED DRUGS

Generic Name	Tradename & Company	Category or Use	Dosage Forms and Strengths
Triamterene + HCTZ	Dyazide (SKF)	antihypertensive; diuretic	cap (50 + 25 mg)
	Maxzide (Lederle)		tab (75 + 50 mg) Maxzide–25 (37.5 + 25 mg)
Triazolam	Halcion (Upjohn)	sedative/hypnotic	tab (0.25 & 0.5 mg)
Trimethobenzamide	Tigan (Beecham)	antiemetic	cap (100 & 200 mg) & supp.; injection
Trimethoprim + Sulfamethoxazole	Septra (B-W) Bactrim (Roche)	antibacterial (urinary tract infections)	tab (80 + 400 mg); DS = double strength (160 + 800 mg); infusion solution
Valproic acid	Depakote (Abbott)	anticonvulsant	tab (125, 250, & 500 mg)
	Depakene (Abbott)	same	liquid
Verapamil	Calan (Searle) Isoptin (Knoll)	treat angina (calcium channel blocker)	tab (40, 80, & 120 mg) SR = 240 mg; injection
Warfarin	Coumadin (DuPont)	anticoagulant	tab (2, 2.5, 5, 7.5, & 10 mg)

Trade Names and Generic Names

Trade Name	Generic Name
Achromycin V	Tetracycline
Adapin	Doxepin
Aldactone	Spironolactone
Aldactazide	Spironolactone + HCTZ
Aldomet	Methyldopa
Aldoril	Methyldopa + HCTZ
Alupent	Metaproterenol
Amicar	Aminocaproic acid
Amitriptyline	Elavil
Amoxil	Amoxicillin
Anaprox	Naproxen
Ansaid	Flurbiprofen
Antivert	Meclizine
Anusol HC	Bismuth subgallate, resorcin & hydrocortisone
Aspirin with codeine	Empirin with codeine
Atarax	Hydroxyzine
Ativan	Lorazepam
Atromid S	Clofibrate
Atrovent	Ipratropium
Augmentin	Amoxicillin + clavulanate K
Axid	Nizatidine
Azmacort	Triamcinolone acetonide
Bactroban	Mupirocin
Bactrim	Trimethoprim + sulfamethoxazole
Beconase	Beclomethasone diproprionate
Beepen VK	Potassium phenoxymethyl penicillin
Betapen-VK	Potassium phenoxymethyl penicillin
Betoptic	Betaxolol
Bleph-10	Sulfacetamide + prednisone
Blocadren	Timolol
Brethine	Terbutaline
Bricanyl	Terbutaline
Bumex	Bumetanide
Buspar	Buspirone
Calan	Verapamil
Capoten	Captopril
Carafate	Sucralfate
Cardizem	Diltiazem

Trade Name	Generic Name
Catapres	Clonidine
Ceclor	Cefaclor
Ceftin	Cefuroxime
Centrax	Prazepam
Cipro	Ciprofloxacin
Cleocin	Clindamycin
Clinoril	Sulindac
Compazine	Prochlorperazine
Cogentin	Benztropine
Corgard	Nadolol
Cortisporin	Polymyxin B; neomycin; bacitracin & hydrocortisone
Coumadin	Warfarin
Dalmane	Flurazepam
Darvocet N	Propoxyphene + acetaminophen
Deconamine	Chlopheniramine + pseudoephedrine
Deltasone	Prednisone
Demulen	Estrogens
Depakene	Valproic acid
Depakote	Valproic acid
Desyrel	Trazodone
DiaBeta	Glyburide
Diabinese	Chlorpropamide
Dilantin	Phenytoin
Dimetane	Brompheniramine maleate
Dimetapp	Brompheniramine, PE, & PPA
Dobutrex	Dobutamine
Dolobid	Diflunisal
Donnatal	Phenobarbital with hyoscyamine, atropine and scopolamine
Dopastat	Dopamine
Duricef	Cefadroxil
Dyazide	Triamterene + HCTZ
EES	Erythromycin ethylsuccinate
Elavil	Amitriptyline
Elixophyllin	Theophylline
E-Mycin	Erythromycin
Entex	Phenylephrine, PPA, & guaifenesin
Ery-Tab	Erythromycin
ERYC	Erythromycin

Trade Name	Generic Name	Trade Name	Generic Name
Erythrocin	Erythromycin	Lotrimin	Clotrimazole
Esidrex	Hydrochlorthiazide	Lotrisone	Clotrimazole + betamethasone
Eskalith	Lithium carbonate	Lorelco	Probucol
Estrace	Estradiol	Lozol	Indapamide
Estraderm	Estradiol	Lortab	Hydrocodone + APAP
Etrafon	Amitriptyline + perphenazine		
		Macrodantin	Nitrofurantoin
Feldene	Piroxicam	Maxzide	Triamterene + HCTZ
Fioricet	Butalbital, APAP, & caffeine	Medrol	Methylprednisolone
Fiorinal	Butalbital + ASA + caffeine	Mellaril	Thioridazine
Fiorinal with Codeine	Butalbital, ASA, caffeine, + codeine	Mevacor	Lovastatin
		Micro-K	Potassium chloride
Flagyl	Metronidazole	Micronase	Glyburide
Flexeril	Cyclobenzaprine	Minipress	Prazosin
		Minizide	Prazosin + polythiazide
Garamycin	Gentamicin	Minocin	Minocycline
Glucotrol	Glipizide	Monistat	Miconazole
Gyne-Lotrimin	Clotrimazole	Motrin	Ibuprofen
		Mycelex-G	Clotrimazole
Halcion	Triazolam	Mycostatin	Nystatin
Haldol	Haloperidol		
Hydergine	Ergoloid mesylates	Naldecon	Phenylephrine + PPA, phenyl-toloxamine, & chlorpheniramine
HydroDIURIL	Hydrochlorothiazide		
Hydropres	HCTZ + reserpine	Nalfon	Fenoprofen
Hygroton	Chlorthalidone	Naprosyn	Naproxen
Hytrin	Terazosin	Nasalcrom	Cromolyn
		Navane	Thiothixene
Ilosone	Erythromycin estolate	Neosporin	Neomycin, polymyxin B, & bacitracin
Imodium	Loperamide		
Inderal	Propranolol	Nicorette	Nicotine polacrilex
Inderide	Propanolol + HCTZ	Nitrobid	Nitroglycerin
Indocin	Indomethacin	Nitrostat	Nitroglycerin
Intal	Cromolyn	Nitro-Dur	Nitroglycerin
Intropin	Dopamine	Nizoral	Ketoconazole
Isoptin	Verapamil	Nolvadex	Tamoxifen
Isordil	Isosorbide dinitrate	Normodyne	Labetalol
		Norinyl	Norethindrone + mestranol
K-Dur	Potassium chloride	Norlestrin	Norethindrone acetate
K-Lyte	Potassium bicarbonate & citrate	Noroxin	Norfloxacin
K-Tab	Potassium chloride	Norpace	Disopyramide
Keflex	Cephalexin		
Keftab	Cephalexin HCl monohydrate	Ogen	Estropipate
Kefurox	Cefuroxime	Omnipen	Ampicillin
Kenalog	Triamcinolone acetonide	Ortho-Novum	Norethindrone + ethinyl estradiol
Klonopin	Clonazepam	Orudis	Ketoprofen
Klor-Con	Potassium chloride	Ovcon	Ethinyl estradiol + norethindrone
Klotrix	Potassium chloride	Ovral	Ethinyl estradiol + norgestrel
Kwell	Gamma benzene hexachloride		
		Pamelor	Nortriptyline
Lanoxin	Digoxin	Pavabid	Papaverine HCl
Lanoxicaps	Digoxin	PCE	Erythromycin
Lasix	Furosemide	Pediazole	Erythromycin ethylsuccinate + sulfisoxazole acetyl
Ledercillin VK	Potassium phenoxymethyl penicillin		
		Pepcid	Famotidine
Lidex	Fluocinonide	Percocet-5	Oxycodone HCl + acetaminophen
Lomotil	Diphenoxylate + atropine	Percodan	Oxycodone HCl + O. terephthalate + ASA
Lo-Ovral	Ethinyl estradiol + norgestrel		
Lopid	Gemfibrozil	Peridex	Chorhexidine gluconate
Lopressor	Metoprolol	Persantine	Dipyridamole

Pen-Vee K	Potassium phenoxymethyl penicillin	Tenormin	Atenolol
		Terazol	Terconazole
Phenergan	Promethazine	Theo-Dur	Theophylline
Polymox	Amoxicillin	Tigan	Trimethobenzamide
Poly-Vi-Flor	Fluoride + vitamins A, D, C, E, B's, & niacin, pantothenic & folic acids	Timoptic	Timolol
		Timolide	Timolol + HCTZ
		Totacillin	Ampicillin
Premarin	Conjugated estrogens	Transderm-Nitro	Nitroglycerin
Prilosec	Omeprazole	Tranxene	Chlorazepate
Principen	Ampicillin	Trental	Pentoxifylline
Prinivil	Lisinopril	Triavil	Perphenazine + amitryptyline
Polycillin	Ampicillin	Tri-Levlen	Estrogen combination
Procan SR	Procainamide	Trimox	Amoxicillin
Procardia	Nifedipine	Tri-Norinyl	Norethindrone + mestranol
Pronestyl	Procainamide	Triphasil	Ethinyl estradiol + levonorgestrel
Propine	Dipivefrin		
Proventil	Albuterol	Tri-Vi-Flor	Fluoride + vitamins A, D, & C
Provera	Medroxyprogesterone	Tussionex	Hydrocodone and clorpheniramine polistirexes
Prozac	Fluoxetine		
		Tussi-Organidin	Codeine + iodinated glycerol
Questran	Cholestyramine	Tylenol	Acetaminophen
		Tylox	Acetaminophen + oxycodone HCl
Reglan	Metoclopramide		
Restoril	Temazepam	Valium	Diazepam
Retin-A	Tretinoin	Valrelease	Diazepam
Ritalin	Methylphenidate	Vanceril	Beclomethasone dipropionate
Rogaine	Minoxidil	Vancenase	Beclomethasone dipropionate
Robitet	Tetracycline	Vasotec	Enalapril
Rufen	Ibuprofen	Vaseretic	Enalapril + HCTZ
		V-Cillin K	Potassium phenoxymethyl penicillin
Seldane	Terfenadine		
Septra	Trimethoprim + sulfamethoxazole	Veetids	Potassium phenoxymethyl penicillin
Serax	Oxazepam	Ventolin	Albuterol
Sincmet	Carbidopa + levodopa	Vibramycin	Doxycycline
Sinequan	Doxepin	Vicodin	APAP + hydrocodone
Slo-bid	Theophylline anhydrous	Vistaril	Hydroxyzine Pamoate
Slow-K	Potassium chloride	Voltaren	Diclofenac
Slo-Phyllin	Theophylline		
Sorbitrate	Isosorbide dinitrate	Wymox	Amoxicillin
Sulamyd	Sulfonamide		
Sumycin	Tetracycline	Xanax	Alprazolam
Suprax	Cefixime		
Synthroid	Levothyroxine	Zantac	Ranitidine
		Zinacef	Cefuroxime
Tagamet	Cimetidine	Zestril	Lisinopril
Tavist	Clemastine	Zofran	Ondansetron
Tegretol	Carbamazepine	Zovirax	Acyclovir
Tenex	Guanfacine	Zyloprim	Allopurinol
Tenoretic	Atenolol + chlorthalidone		